Crocus sativus L. Extract and Its Constituents: Chemistry, Pharmacology and Therapeutic Potential

Crocus sativus L. Extract and Its Constituents: Chemistry, Pharmacology and Therapeutic Potential

Editors

Nikolaos Pitsikas
Konstantinos Dimas

MDPI • Basel • Beijing • Wuhan • Barcelona • Belgrade • Manchester • Tokyo • Cluj • Tianjin

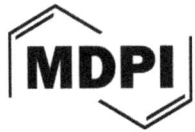

Editors
Nikolaos Pitsikas
Dept of Pharmacology,
Faculty of Medicine
University of Thessaly
Larissa
Greece

Konstantinos Dimas
Dept of Pharmacology,
Faculty of Medicine
University of Thessaly
Larissa
Greece

Editorial Office
MDPI
St. Alban-Anlage 66
4052 Basel, Switzerland

This is a reprint of articles from the Special Issue published online in the open access journal *Molecules* (ISSN 1420-3049) (available at: www.mdpi.com/journal/molecules/special_issues/crocus_sativus_extract).

For citation purposes, cite each article independently as indicated on the article page online and as indicated below:

LastName, A.A.; LastName, B.B.; LastName, C.C. Article Title. *Journal Name* **Year**, *Volume Number*, Page Range.

ISBN 978-3-0365-1806-0 (Hbk)
ISBN 978-3-0365-1805-3 (PDF)

© 2021 by the authors. Articles in this book are Open Access and distributed under the Creative Commons Attribution (CC BY) license, which allows users to download, copy and build upon published articles, as long as the author and publisher are properly credited, which ensures maximum dissemination and a wider impact of our publications.

The book as a whole is distributed by MDPI under the terms and conditions of the Creative Commons license CC BY-NC-ND.

Contents

About the Editors vii

Preface to "Crocus sativus L. Extract and Its Constituents: Chemistry, Pharmacology and Therapeutic Potential" ix

Nikolaos Pitsikas and Konstantinos Dimas
Crocus sativus L. Extract and Its Constituents: Chemistry, Pharmacology and Therapeutic Potential
Reprinted from: *Molecules* **2021**, *26*, 4226, doi:10.3390/molecules26144226 1

Nikolaos Pitsikas
Crocus sativus L. Extracts and Its Constituents Crocins and Safranal; Potential Candidates for Schizophrenia Treatment?
Reprinted from: *Molecules* **2021**, *26*, 1237, doi:10.3390/molecules26051237 5

Maria Anna Maggi, Silvia Bisti and Cristiana Picco
Saffron: Chemical Composition and Neuroprotective Activity
Reprinted from: *Molecules* **2020**, *25*, 5618, doi:10.3390/molecules25235618 17

Nikolaos Pitsikas and Petros A. Tarantilis
The $GABA_A$-Benzodiazepine Receptor Antagonist Flumazenil Abolishes the Anxiolytic Effects of the Active Constituents of *Crocus sativus* L. Crocins in Rats
Reprinted from: *Molecules* **2020**, *25*, 5647, doi:10.3390/molecules25235647 33

Nikolaos Pitsikas and Petros A. Tarantilis
Crocins, the Bioactive Components of *Crocus sativus* L., Counteract the Disrupting Effects of Anesthetic Ketamine on Memory in Rats
Reprinted from: *Molecules* **2021**, *26*, 528, doi:10.3390/molecules26030528 43

Laura Orio, Francisco Alen, Antonio Ballesta, Raquel Martin and Raquel Gomez de Heras
Antianhedonic and Antidepressant Effects of Affron®, a Standardized Saffron (*Crocus Sativus* L.) Extract
Reprinted from: *Molecules* **2020**, *25*, 3207, doi:10.3390/molecules25143207 57

Giulia Rossi, Martina Placidi, Chiara Castellini, Francesco Rea, Settimio D'Andrea, Gonzalo Luis Alonso, Giovanni Luca Gravina, Carla Tatone, Giovanna Di Emidio and Anna Maria D'Alessandro
Crocetin Mitigates Irradiation Injury in an In Vitro Model of the Pubertal Testis: Focus on Biological Effects and Molecular Mechanisms
Reprinted from: *Molecules* **2021**, *26*, 1676, doi:10.3390/molecules26061676 71

Suhrid Banskota, Hassan Brim, Yun Han Kwon, Gulshan Singh, Sidhartha R. Sinha, Huaqing Wang, Waliul I. Khan and Hassan Ashktorab
Saffron Pre-Treatment Promotes Reduction in Tissue Inflammatory Profiles and Alters Microbiome Composition in Experimental Colitis Mice
Reprinted from: *Molecules* **2021**, *26*, 3351, doi:10.3390/molecules26113351 85

Eleni Kakouri, Adamantia Agalou, Charalabos Kanakis, Dimitris Beis and Petros A. Tarantilis
Crocins from *Crocus sativus* L. in the Management of Hyperglycemia. In Vivo Evidence from Zebrafish
Reprinted from: *Molecules* **2020**, *25*, 5223, doi:10.3390/molecules25225223 95

Andromachi Lambrianidou, Fani Koutsougianni, Irida Papapostolou and Konstantinos Dimas
Recent Advances on the Anticancer Properties of Saffron (*Crocus sativus* L.) and Its Major Constituents
Reprinted from: *Molecules* **2020**, 26, 86, doi:10.3390/molecules26010086 . . . . **109**

Amr Amin, Aaminah Farrukh, Chandraprabha Murali, Akbar Soleimani, Françoise Praz, Grazia Graziani, Hassan Brim and Hassan Ashktorab
Saffron and Its Major Ingredients' Effect on Colon Cancer Cells with Mismatch Repair Deficiency and Microsatellite Instability
Reprinted from: *Molecules* **2021**, 26, 3855, doi:10.3390/molecules26133855 . . . . **125**

Evangelos Gikas, Nikolaos Stavros Koulakiotis and Anthony Tsarbopoulos
Phytochemical Differentiation of Saffron (*Crocus sativus* L.) by High Resolution Mass Spectrometry Metabolomic Studies
Reprinted from: *Molecules* **2021**, 26, 2180, doi:10.3390/molecules26082180 . . . . **143**

Aboli Girme, Sandeep Pawar, Chetana Ghule, Sushant Shengule, Ganesh Saste, Arun Kumar Balasubramaniam, Amol Deshmukh and Lal Hingorani
Bioanalytical Method Development and Validation Study of Neuroprotective Extract of Kashmiri Saffron Using Ultra-Fast Liquid Chromatography-Tandem Mass Spectrometry (UFLC-MS/MS): In Vivo Pharmacokinetics of Apocarotenoids and Carotenoids
Reprinted from: *Molecules* **2021**, 26, 1815, doi:10.3390/molecules26061815 . . . . **159**

About the Editors

Nikolaos Pitsikas

Nikolaos Pitsikas is a Professor in the Department of Pharmacology of the Faculty of Medicine of the University of Thessaly. He was a fellow at the Institute of Pharmacological Research "Mario Negri", and at the Department of Pharmacology of the Medical School of the University of Milan in Italy. He was also a fellow at the University of Utrecht, The Netherlands, and the University of Pennsylvania, USA. He has collaborated with various universities and research institutes, in Greece and abroad. He is the author/co-author of over 80 papers published in peer-reviewed journals, with over 2800 citations, and an h-index of 30, and 3 book chapters. He is a member of several scientific societies, and an editor and reviewer in international scientific journals. His research interests are focused on the field of behavioural pharmacology. He investigates the role of the NMDA, nitric oxide, 5-HT receptors, and the bioactive constituents of *Crocus sativus* L., in cognition, anxiety, and schizophrenia.

Konstantinos Dimas

Dr. Konstantinos Dimas is an Associate Professor in the Department of Pharmacology of the Faculty of Medicine of the University of Thessaly. He was the recipient of a fellowship from the International Organization for Research on Cancer (IARC, WHO) and has collaborated with various universities, research institutes (most recently the National Cancer Institute (NCI, NIH, USA)), and biotech companies. He is the author/co-author of over 100 papers published in peer-reviewed journals in pharmacology and cancer, with over 2600 citations and an h-index of 32, over 10 book chapters, and has five patents. He is a member of several scientific societies, and an editor and reviewer in international scientific journals. His research focuses on the study and development of new anticancer drugs, mainly from natural sources (e.g., plant derivatives), on the study of new S6 kinase inhibitors, and on sigma receptor ligands as potential targeting therapies for cancer and the development of animal models of cancer.

Preface to "*Crocus sativus* L. Extract and Its Constituents: Chemistry, Pharmacology and Therapeutic Potential"

Dear Colleagues,

the search for beneficial effects of plant extracts in therapy is a hot issue. *Crocus sativus* L. and its constituents are being studied intensively as potential candidates for the treatment of a wide range of diseases, including cancer, diabetes, cardiovascular diseases, neuropsychiatric disorders, and neurodegenerative diseases.

This book aims to assess new advances in the understanding of the therapeutic action of saffron and its constituents in targeting different pathologies. In this context, we strongly believe that it will be of great interest for pharmacologists and researchers not only working in the field of the therapeutic potential of *Crocus sativus* L. and its bioactive constituents, but for all these working in the field of natural products and their potential use as drugs.

As guest editors, we would like to express our gratitude to all the authors for their contributions to this book.

Nikolaos Pitsikas, Konstantinos Dimas
Editors

Editorial

Crocus sativus L. Extract and Its Constituents: Chemistry, Pharmacology and Therapeutic Potential

Nikolaos Pitsikas * and Konstantinos Dimas *

Department of Pharmacology, Faculty of Medicine, School of Health Sciences, University of Thessaly, Biopolis, Panepistimiou, 341500 Larissa, Greece
* Correspondence: npitsikas@uth.gr (N.P.); kdimas@uth.gr (K.D.)

Natural products or organic compounds isolated from natural sources as primary or secondary metabolites have inspired numerous drugs. It is not an overstatement that the majority of medicines in clinics, even in the 21st century, have been derived from natural resources despite the declining of industry research into natural products due to a variety of drawbacks [1].

Saffron crocus, considered to be the most valuable spice by weight [2], and its bioactive constituents, have been reported to have been studied for the treatment of a wide range of pathologies including neuropsychiatric and neurodegenerative disorders, cancer, diabetes, and even cardiovascular diseases.

In this special issue on the chemistry, pharmacology, and therapeutic potential of *Crocus sativus* L. extract and its constituents, two reviews report new data and advances in the fields of schizophrenia and cancer. In the first review, Pitsikas critically assesses advances in the research of these molecules for therapy for schizophrenia, a chronic, mentally devastating disease [3]. In the second review, Labrianidou and her colleagues provide an insight into the advances in research on the anticancer properties of saffron and its components, discussing preclinical data, clinical trials, and patents aiming to improve the pharmacological properties of saffron and its major ingredients [4].

This special issue of *Molecules* aims furthermore to assess new advances in the understanding of the therapeutic action of saffron and its constituents in targeting different pathologies. In this context, eight original research articles covering some recent advances in the therapeutic actions of saffron and its ingredients in different diseases are reported herein. Amin et al. present new data on the effects of saffron and its major ingredients, safranal and crocin, on colon cancer cells with mismatch repair (MMR) deficiency and microsatellite instability. In this study, saffron and its components are reported to show a significant anti-proliferative effect in cells with deficient MMR [5]. In another interesting work, Suhrid Banskota et al. present data which suggest that pre-treatment with saffron inhibits dextran sulfate sodium (DSS)-induced pro-inflammatory cytokine secretion; modulates gut microbiota composition; prevents the depletion of short-chain fatty acids (SCFA) such as isobutyric acid, acetic acid, and propionic acid; and reduces susceptibility to colitis, a result of special interest, as long-standing colitis is well-known to be associated with increased risk of colon cancer [6]. Four articles report novel findings on the effects of saffron and its ingredients on neuropsychiatric disorders. In the first of two articles, Pitsikas and Tarantilis report the beneficial effects of crocins on memory loss, induced by the widely used anesthetic ketamine, in rats [7]. In the second article, the same authors find that the anxiolytic properties of crocins are mediated by their agonistic action on the GABA$_A$-benzodiazepine receptor [8]. Orio et al. evidence the antidepressant effects of a standardized saffron extract, Affron®, suggesting that oral saffron may exert a beneficial action in anxious and depressive states [9]. The collection of the articles reporting new findings on neurological disorders is filled in nicely with a work by Maggi and colleagues, demonstrating the ability of saffron to cope with retinal neurodegeneration, and this beneficial action appears to be dependent on the presence of specific crocins and the contribution of other saffron components [10].

The interesting results of two studies performed by Rossi and colleagues [11] and Kakouri et al. [12] corroborate further for the therapeutic potential of saffron. Specifically, Rossi et al. demonstrate the efficacy of crocetin in alleviating irradiation injury in an in vitro model of the pubertal testis, suggesting the therapeutic potential of this bioactive constituent of saffron as a fertoprotective agent against ionizing radiation's deleterious effects in the pubertal period [11].

Additionally, Kakouri and her colleagues, in a nice, in vivo study conducted on the zebrafish, demonstrate that that the application of crocins reduces glucose levels in the zebrafish embryo and enhances insulin expression. They further show that following a single administration of crocins, the expression of phosphoenolpyruvate carboxykinase1 (pck1), a key gene involved in glucose metabolism, is increased, which is indicative of a putative role for crocins in glucose metabolism and insulin management [12].

The collection of this special issue is completed with two articles on two novel methods regarding the bioanalysis of saffron extracts. Gikas et al. report the use of high-resolution mass spectrometry metabolomics studies as novel tools to develop a fingerprint of the various saffron extracts which obviously, given the health-promoting effects of the extracts, can be of great importance for the selection of the appropriate saffron sample [13]. Finally, Girme et al. report the development and application of the pharmacokinetics of a new bioanalytical method based on a sensitive and ultra-fast liquid chromatography (UFLC)-tandem mass spectrometry method with high assay-based precision and accuracy on analytical quality control levels and excellent recoveries in plasma samples [14]. These latter results, as the authors state, suggest that this new procedure may be an appropriate bioanalytical method for preclinical/clinical trials on *Crocus sativus* extract's main ingredients.

In conclusion, in this special issue of *Molecules*, we are delighted to have received several works that we hope provide new and interesting information for the scientific community on the chemistry, pharmacology, and therapeutic potential of *Crocus sativus* L. extract and its constituents.

Acknowledgments: The guest editors would like to express their gratitude to all the authors for their contributions to this special issue.

Conflicts of Interest: The authors declare no conflict of interest.

References

1. Atanasov, A.G.; Zotchev, S.B.; Dirsch, V.M.; The International Natural Product Sciences Taskforce; Supuran, C.T. Natural products in drug discovery: Advances and opportunities. *Nat. Rev. Drug Discov.* **2021**, *20*, 200–216. [CrossRef] [PubMed]
2. Kafi, M.; Koocheki, A.; Rashed, M.H.; Nassiri, M. (Eds.) *Saffron (Crocus sativus) Production and Processing*, 1st ed.; Science Publishers: Washington, DC, USA, 2016; ISBN 978-1-57808-427-2.
3. Pitsikas, N. *Crocus sativus* L. Extracts and Its Constituents Crocins and Safranal; Potential Candidates for Schizophrenia Treatment? Nikolaos Pitsikas *Mol.* **2021**, *26*, 1237. [CrossRef]
4. Lambrianidou, A.; Koutsougianni, F.; Papapostolou, I.; Dimas, K. Recent Advances on the Anticancer Properties of Saffron (*Crocus sativus* L.) and Its Major Constituents. *Molecules* **2020**, *26*, 86. [CrossRef] [PubMed]
5. Amin, A.; Farrukh, A.; Murali, C.; Soleimani, A.; Praz, F.; Graziani, G.; Brim, H.; Ashktorab, H. Saffron and Its Major Ingredients' Effect on Colon Cancer Cells with Mismatch Repair Deficiency and Microsatellite Instability. *Molecules* **2021**, *26*, 3855. [CrossRef] [PubMed]
6. Banskota, S.; Brim, H.; Kwon, Y.H.; Singh, G.; Sinha, S.R.; Wang, H.; Khan, W.I.; Ashktorab, H. Saffron Pre-Treatment Pro-motes Reduction in Tissue Inflammatory Profiles and Alters Microbiome Composition in Experimental Colitis Mice. *Molecules* **2021**, *26*, 3351. [CrossRef] [PubMed]
7. Pitsikas, N.; Tarantilis, P. Crocins, the Bioactive Components of *Crocus sativus* L., Counteract the Disrupting Effects of Anesthetic Ketamine on Memory in Rats. *Molecules* **2021**, *26*, 528. [CrossRef] [PubMed]
8. Pitsikas, N.; Tarantilis, P.A. The GABA$_A$-Benzodiazepine Receptor Antagonist Flumazenil Abolishes the Anxiolytic Effects of the Active Constituents of *Crocus sativus* L. Crocins in Rats. *Molecules* **2020**, *25*, 5647. [CrossRef] [PubMed]
9. Orio, L.; Alen, F.; Ballesta, A.; Martin, R.; Gomez de Heras, R. Antianhedonic and Antidepressant Effects of Affron®, a Standardized Saffron (*Crocus sativus* L.) Extract. *Molecules* **2020**, *25*, 3207. [CrossRef] [PubMed]

10. Maggi, M.A.; Bisti, S.; Picco, C. Saffron: Chemical Composition and Neuroprotective Activity. *Molecules* **2020**, *25*, 5618. [CrossRef] [PubMed]
11. Rossi, G.; Placidi, M.; Castellini, C.; Rea, F.; D'Andrea, S.; Alonso, G.L.; Gravina, G.L.; Tatone, C.; Di Emidio, G.; D'Alessandro, A.M. Crocetin Mitigates Irradiation Injury in an In Vitro Model of the Pubertal Testis: Focus on Biological Effects and Molecular Mechanisms. *Molecules* **2021**, *26*, 1676. [CrossRef] [PubMed]
12. Kakouri, E.; Agalou, A.; Kanakis, C.; Beis, D.; Tarantilis, P.A. Crocins from *Crocus sativus* L. in the Management of Hyper-glycemia. In Vivo Evidence from Zebrafish. *Molecules* **2020**, *25*, 5223. [CrossRef] [PubMed]
13. Gikas, E.; Koulakiotis, N.S.; Tsarbopoulos, A. Phytochemical Differentiation of Saffron (*Crocus sativus* L.) by High Resolution Mass Spectrometry Metabolomic Studies. *Molecules* **2021**, *26*, 2180. [CrossRef] [PubMed]
14. Girme, A.; Pawar, S.; Ghule, C.; Shengule, S.; Saste, G.; Balasubramaniam, A.K.; Deshmukh, A.; Hingorani, L. Bioanalytical Method Development and Validation Study of Neuroprotective Extract of Kashmiri Saffron Using Ultra-Fast Liquid Chromatography-Tandem Mass Spectrometry (UFLC-MS/MS): In Vivo Pharmacokinetics of Apocarotenoids and Carotenoids. *Molecules* **2021**, *26*, 1815. [CrossRef]

Crocus sativus L. Extracts and Its Constituents Crocins and Safranal; Potential Candidates for Schizophrenia Treatment?

Nikolaos Pitsikas

Department of Pharmacology, School of Medicine, Faculty of Health Sciences, University of Thessaly, Biopolis, Panepistimiou 3, 415-00 Larissa, Greece; npitsikas@med.uth.gr; Tel.: +30-2410-685-535

Abstract: Schizophrenia is a chronic mental devastating disease. Current therapy suffers from various limitations including low efficacy and serious side effects. Thus, there is an urgent necessity to develop new antipsychotics with higher efficacy and safety. The dried stigma of the plant *Crocus sativus* L., (*CS*) commonly known as saffron, are used in traditional medicine for various purposes. It has been demonstrated that saffron and its bioactive components crocins and safranal exert a beneficial action in different pathologies of the central nervous system such as anxiety, depression, epilepsy and memory problems. Recently, their role as potential antipsychotic agents is under investigation. In the present review, I intended to critically assess advances in research of these molecules for the treatment of schizophrenia, comment on their advantages over currently used neuroleptics as well-remaining challenges. Up to our days, few preclinical studies have been conducted to this end. In spite of it, results are encouraging and strongly corroborate that additional research is mandatory aiming to definitively establish a role for saffron and its bioactive components for the treatment of schizophrenia.

Keywords: *Crocus sativus* L.; crocins; schizophrenia

1. Schizophrenia

Schizophrenia is a serious chronic mental disease that affects up to 1% of the world population. It is a complex heterogeneous psychiatric disorder that impairs social, occupational and individual functioning and causes an adjective decrease in the quality of life of patients. This disease usually is manifested in late adolescence or early adulthood. Schizophrenics display serious psychotic symptoms, which can be classified into three major categories: positive symptoms (e.g., hallucinations, delusions, disordered thinking, catatonic behavior), negative symptoms (e.g., social withdrawal, anhedonia, avolition, neglect of hygiene) and cognitive disturbances (e.g., in attention, executive functioning and memory) [1].

Schizophrenia's causes and pathophysiology are not yet elucidated. Nevertheless, it is widely acknowledged as a composite neurodevelopmental disease affected by genetic and environmental factors [2,3]. Specifically, it has been revealed that monozygotic siblings of schizophrenics have a 50–80% risk of developing the disease. Further, incomplete maturation of the brain and abnormal synaptic connections between different brain areas are also evidenced [4] Interestingly, an increasing number of reports propose the implication of oxidative stress in the pathophysiology of schizophrenia [5].

Additionally, several lines of evidence suggest that malfunctioning of different neurotransmitter systems, as are dopamine (DA), glutamate, cholinergic, serotonergic and the GABAergic systems is associated with the appearance of this disease [6]. In particular, positive symptoms of schizophrenia are associated with overactivation of dopaminergic neurotransmission in the striatum, while negative symptoms and cognitive impairments appear to be dependent on dopaminergic hypofunction in the prefrontal cortex [7].

Glutamate hypofunction seems also to be involved in the pathophysiology of schizophrenia. Abnormal glutamatergic transmission is related to secondary dopaminergic dysfunction in the striatum and prefrontal cortex. In this context, it has been shown that pharmacological blockade of NMDA receptor induces negative symptoms and cognitive deficits that were not alleviated by neuroleptics [7]. Moreover, the functionality of the GABAergic system, the major inhibitory neurotransmitter in the brain, is compromised in schizophrenia [8]. Since GABAergic firing modulates dopaminergic transmission in the prefrontal cortex, the malfunctioning of GABA interneurons seems to play a role in the appearance of some of the clinical symptoms of schizophrenia [9].

Clinical findings indicate that conventional antipsychotics (either those of the first generation, or atypical) display a certain efficacy in the alleviation of positive symptoms but are inefficacious in relieving negative symptoms and cognitive impairments of schizophrenia patients. These medications, however, are associated with important side effects which compromise their benefit. Specifically, motor side effects (Parkinsonism) are related with the administration of traditional neuroleptics (e.g., chlorpromazine, haloperidol). Conversely, the administration of atypical antipsychotics (e.g., clozapine, olanzapine, risperidone) does not produce Parkinsonism but causes weight gain. In addition, 30% of patients are resistant to the above-described treatments. Collectively, these results suggest that there is a pressing necessity to find novel compounds which could provide alleviation of negative symptoms and cognitive deficits typical features of schizophrenia patients [10,11].

Among the different alternative approaches for the therapy of schizophrenia, the involvement of the plant saffron and its bioactive components as potential anti-schizophrenia agents has lately been suggested. In the current analysis, I intend to assess with critical feeling the potential beneficial action of saffron and its components for the treatment of schizophrenia.

2. *Crocus sativus* L. (Saffron)

Crocus sativus L. (CS), is a perennial herb and a member of the Iridaceae family, of genus *Crocus*, the line of Liliaceae. This plant is cultivated in a number of countries such as Azerbaijan, China, France, Greece, Egypt, India, Iran, Israel, Italy, Mexico, Morocco, Spain and Turkey. The spice saffron is the end product of this plant. Saffron, in filaments, is the dried dark-red stigmas of CS flower. The weight of a single stigma is circa 2 mg and each flower has three stigmata; 150.000 flowers must be thoroughly selected separately to gain 1 kg of spice. Saffron has a characteristic color, taste and smell. From ancient to modern times the history of saffron is full of applications. It is widely utilized as a perfume, as a spice for flavoring and staining food and drink preparations. The most common way to consume saffron is still to mix it with food or to add it to any hot or warm drink [12,13].

Additionally, saffron is commonly utilized in traditional medicine, as a beneficial agent for the therapy of various pathologies of the cardiovascular, respiratory, gastrointestinal and nervous system For review see [14].

2.1. Chemistry of CS

The prevailing non-volatile components of the saffron are crocins, crocetin, safranal picrocrocin and flavonoids (quercetin and kaempferol) [12]. The coloring components of saffron are crocins ($C_{44}H_{64}O_{24}$), which are unusual water-soluble carotenoids (glycosyl esters of crocetin). The major component is a digentiobiosyl ester of crocetin ($C_{44}H_{64}O_{24}$, 8,8'-diapo-Ψ,Ψ'-carotenedioic acid bis (6-0-β-D-glucopyranosyl-β-D-glucopyranosyl) ester). Safranal ($C_{10}H_{14}O$, 2,6,6-trimethyl-1,3-cyclohexadiene-1- carboxaldehyde), which is responsible for the characteristic aroma of saffron is a monoterpene aldehyde. The principal bitter-tasting substance is picrocrocin a glycoside of safranal ($C_{16}H_{26}O_7$, 4-(β-D-glucopyranosyloxy)-2,6,6-trimethyl-1-cyclohexene-1- carboxaldehyde) [15–17].

In Figure 1 the molecular structures of CS and its constituent crocins, picrocrocin and safranal are illustrated.

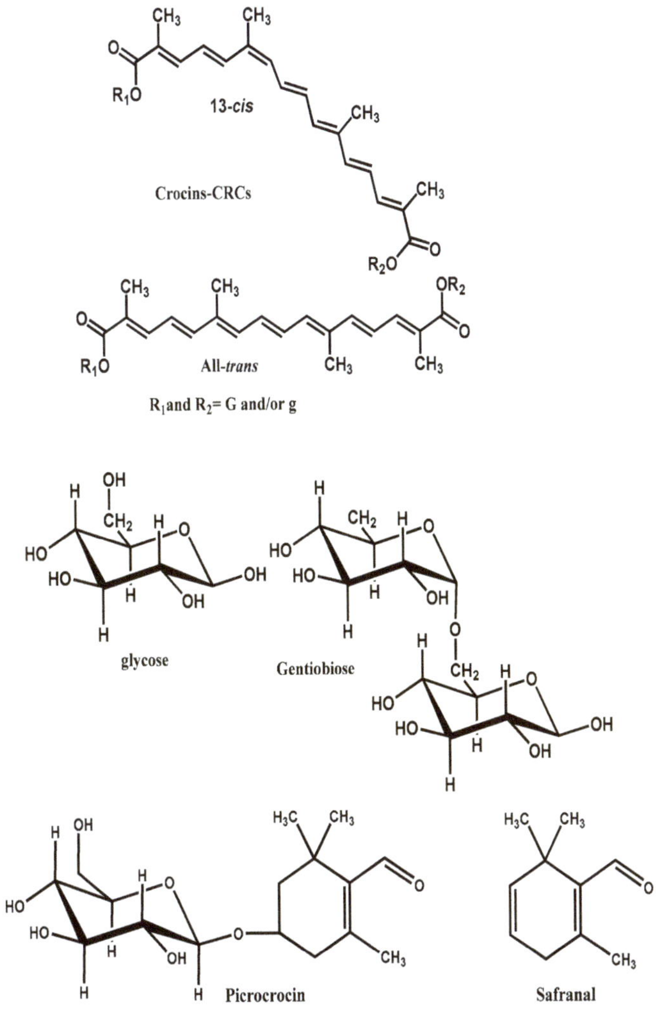

Figure 1. Chemical structures of saffron bioactive components. Crocins (CRCs): Glucosyl ester of Crocetin, R_1 = â-D-Geotiobiosyl, R_2 = â-D-Geotiobiosyl, R_1 = â-D-Gentiobiosyl, R_2 = â-D-glucosyl., R_1 = â-D-Gentiobiosyl, R_2 = H, R_1 = â-D-glucosyl, R_2 = â-D-glucosyl., R_1 = â-D-glucosyl, R_2 = H, Crocetin R_1 = H, R_2 = H., B. Picrocrocin., C. Safranal.

2.2. Pharmacology of CS and Its Bioactive Components

Based on a conspicuous number of preclinical and clinical data an exciting pharmacological profile of saffron and its bioactive ingredients is turning up.

2.2.1. Effects of CS and Its Constituents on Non-Neurological/Neuropsychiatric Pathologies

In a series of preclinical in vitro and in vivo studies the anti-cancer, anti-nociceptive and anti-inflammatory properties of saffron have been revealed. Additionally, it has been reported that *CS* and its bioactive ingredients reduced atherosclerosis and hepatotoxicity, diminish hyperlipidemia, display a protective action on myocardial injury and consistently reduce blood pressure [14,18,19].

As a whole, what emerges from these preclinical findings is that CS and its active components appear to express a beneficial action in preclinical models of different non-neurological/neuropsychiatric pathologies. Until now, however, there is a lack of clinical results validating the therapeutic efficiency of saffron observed in the above-mentioned preclinical pathological models. Thus, clinical studies should be designed and conducted in order to properly address this important issue.

2.2.2. Effects of CS and Its Constituents on Pathologies of The Central Nervous System

In a series of preclinical studies, the anticonvulsant properties of the aqueous and ethanolic extracts of CS and safranal have been observed and. Specifically, it has been demonstrated that CS extracts and safranal counteracted pentylenetetrazol-induced seizures in mice and rats and these effects seem to be mediated by their interaction with the GABAergic and opioids systems [20,21]. Further, both saffron and its active components were found to be protective in preclinical models of Parkinson's disease (PD) and cerebral ischemia [22–25].

The efficacy of saffron and crocins to attenuate memory impairments in preclinical models associated with Alzheimer's disease (AD), cerebral injuries, or schizophrenia is well documented For a review, see [26]. The outcome of clinical trials designed to examine the efficiency of saffron in alleviating memory problems, a common feature of AD, proposes that the effects exerted by CS on cognition, although modest, were similar to those displayed by the reference molecules donepezil and memantine. Importantly, in all human studies conducted, treatment with saffron, in contrast with donepezil and memantine, did not induce noticeable undesired effects [27].

Intensive preclinical research revealed a consistent antidepressant-like effect of saffron and its major constituents crocins and safranal [28]. This antidepressant-like effect of saffron observed in rodents was corroborated by clinical findings. Studies carried out in humans evidenced the efficacy of saffron in the therapy of mild-to-moderate depression [29,30]. In this context, it has been reported that saffron attenuated sexual malfunction in both males and females which was caused by the challenge with the selective serotonin re-uptake inhibitor (SSRI) antidepressant agent fluoxetine [31,32].

Up to now, few studies have been conducted aiming to investigate the potential anti-anxiety effect of CS and its components. In spite of the scant number of studies (preclinical and clinical), the results reported appear promising. Further research is mandatory in order to fully elucidate and establish the anxiolytic profile of saffron and its bioactive components. For review, please see [33].

2.2.3. Pharmacokinetic and Safety Studies

Pharmacokinetic studies revealed that crocins, following oral administration, are not absorbed in the gastrointestinal tract (GIT) but are hydrolyzed to crocetin and in this form are absorbed in the GIT [34,35]. Crocetin is the active metabolite among which crocins exert their beneficial actions. Crocetin reaches the blood circulation and is found to be relatively quickly distributed in all tissues of the human body [36] can be partially conjugated with mono and diglucuronides in the GIT and in the liver [37]. A recent report demonstrated, however, that after oral application also crocins can be absorbed through GIT with poorer bioavailability compared to crocetin [38]. As a whole, either crocins or crocetin when applied orally, display low stability, poor absorption and low bioavailability [39]. Reportedly in this context, it has been evidenced that intraperitoneal or intravenous rather oral administration of saffron and its active components might provide higher levels of absorption and bioavailability [38,40]. In particular, Zhang and colleagues have indicated that intravenous application of crocins in rats did not reveal the presence of crocetin in plasma but solely crocins were detected, eliciting thus that hepatic metabolism of crocins would be insignificant [38]. Further studies are required, however, aiming to clarify this important issue.

Interestingly, it has been shown that crocins despite their high hydrophilic profile, similarly to crocetine [41,42], can cross the blood–brain barrier (BBB) and reach the central nervous system [40]. Concerning safranal, it can be hypothesized that might be able to penetrate the BBB since in a series of studies its anticonvulsant and antidepressant properties have been revealed [20,21,28].

Toxicological investigations performed in rodents that have received saffron extracts shown that the hematological and the biochemical parameters of the animals were not altered by treatment with saffron and remained at physiological levels [43]. In this context, it has been reported that the oral LD_{50} of CS was 20.7 g/kg when was delivered as a decoction in mice [44]. Further research confirmed the good safety profile of CS and its ingredients. Specifically, it has been observed that acute treatment of mice with saffron (up to 3 g, either orally (p.o.) or intraperitoneally (i.p.)) and repeated with crocin (15–180 mg/kg, i.p.) did not affect a series of biochemical, hematological and pathological markers recorded [45].

The outline of human studies confirmed the safe profile of CS extracts and crocin observed in preclinical experiments. In a double-blind, placebo-controlled study, carried out on healthy volunteers, repeated challenge with saffron (200–400 mg/day, for seven consecutive days) did not induce appreciable abnormalities. It caused only some minor consistency clinical and laboratory parameter changes such as hypotension, reduced platelets and bleeding time and increased creatinine and blood urea nitrogen levels [46].

In agreement with the above, are the findings of another clinical trial conducted on healthy participants who received 20 mg/day of crocin for 30 consecutive days. Treatment with crocin did not produce any alteration of various hematological, biochemical, hormonal and urinary parameters recorded [47]. Finally, the challenge with very high doses of saffron (1.2–2 g) in healthy volunteers caused nausea, diarrhea, vomiting, and bleeding [48]. As a whole, saffron and its main bioactive components can be considered as safe natural products displaying very low toxicity.

3. Effects of CS and Its Constituents in Schizophrenia

3.1. Preclinical Studies

Table 1 summarizes the existing literature regarding the effects of crocins on animal models of schizophrenia. Crocins (15–30 mg/kg, acutely) counteracted disruption of non-spatial recognition memory caused by acute administration of the NMDA receptor antagonist ketamine (3 mg/kg, acutely) in rats. This finding strongly proposes the involvement of this bioactive ingredient of CS in schizophrenia-related cognitive impairments. Additionally, crocins (50 mg/kg, acutely) attenuated ketamine (25 mg/kg, acutely)—induced psychotomimetic effects (hypermotility, stereotypies and ataxia) in the rat. Further, in a behavioural procedure mimicking the negative symptoms of schizophrenia (social interaction test), these active components of saffron (50 mg/kg, acutely) were found able to reduce the social isolation-induced by treatment with ketamine (8 mg/kg, sub-chronically) in rats [49].

In agreement with the above, crocins (30 mg/kg, acutely) antagonized disruption of non-spatial recognition memory caused by a single injection of the mixed DA D1/D2 receptor agonist apomorphine (1 mg/kg). By contrast, crocins failed to counteracted spatial recognition memory induced by apomorphine (1 mg/kg, acutely). It has been suggested that this dual action of crocins on recognition memory deficits observed in a dopaminergic model of amnesia might depend to differences in stimuli intensity (higher in non-spatial tasks as compared to spatial tasks) [50].

Table 1. Effects of crocins on preclinical models of schizophrenia.

Scheme	Agent	Dose Range	Route	Behavioral Test	Effect	Reference
Rat	Crocins	15, 30, 50 mg/kg	i.p. acute	ORT	Crocins (15, 30 mg/kg) counteracted ketamine-induced non-spatial recognition memory deficits.	[49]
	Ketamine	3 mg/kg (NORT)	i.p. acute			
	Ketamine	8 mg/kg (SI)	i.p. sub-chronic	SI	Crocins (50 mg/kg) attenuated ketamine-induced social isolation.	[49]
	Ketamine	25 mg/kg (motor activity)	i.p. acute	Motor activity, stereotypies, ataxia	Crocins (50 mg/kg) attenuated ketamine-induced hypermotility, stereotypies and ataxia.	[49]
Rat	Crocins	15, 30, 50 mg/kg	i.p. acute	ORT	Crocins (15, 30 mg/kg) counteracted ketamine-induced non-spatial recognition memory deficits.	[50]
	Apomorphine	1 mg/kg	i.p. acute			
Rat	Crocins	15, 30, 50 mg/kg	i.p. acute	OLT	No effect	[50]
	Apomorphine	1 mg/kg	i.p. acute			
Rat	Crocins	25, 50 mg/kg	i.p. acute	RR, OFT	Crocin (25, 50 mg/kg) counteracted MK-801-induced motor activity deficits.	[51]
	MK-801	1 mg/kg	i.p. acute			
	Crocins	25, 50 mg/kg	i.p. acute	MWM	Crocin (25, 50 mg/kg) counteracted MK-801-induced spatial memory deficits.	[51]
	MK-801	1 mg/kg	i.p. acute			

Abbreviations: *i.p*, intraperitoneally; *MWM*, Morris water maze; *OFT*, open field test; *OLT*, object location task; *ORT*, object recognition task; *RR*, rotarod; *SI*, social interaction.

It has recently been reported that crocin attenuated schizophrenia-like symptoms in a glutamatergic model of this psychiatric disease. In particular, crocin (25 and 50 mg/kg, acutely) attenuated motor disturbances and spatial navigation impairments induced by acute administration of the NMDA receptor antagonist MK-801 (1 mg/kg) in rats [51].

It is important to emphasize that the beneficial effects of crocins, summarized in Table 1, were observed following intraperitoneal application of them in rodents. Intraperitoneal compared to oral route of administration might be of higher utility since it can be avoided the first-pass metabolism and/or gastric hydrolysis and obtain consistent bioavailability profile of the compound (elimination of liver-induced metabolism as well exposure of crocins in a low pH of the stomach [52].

3.2. Clinical Studies

Up to our days, clinical information dealing with a potential anti-schizophrenia efficacy of CS and its bioactive constituents is inconsistent. Only one clinical study was conducted aiming to evaluate the safety and the tolerability of treatment with saffron and crocin in schizophrenia patients. This was a double-blind, placebo-controlled trial and participated 61 schizophrenics. Patients were treated twice daily with saffron or crocin (15 mg) or placebo for 12 consecutive weeks. In agreement with prior reports [27,29,53], the results of this study showed that saffron extracts, safranal and crocin were well-tolerated in schizophrenics [54]. In this context, is important to emphasize that challenge with a saffron aqueous extract (30 mg/day, for 12 weeks) administered in schizophrenics on treatment with olanzapine prevented the metabolic syndrome, a well-known side effect of this atypical neuroleptic [55].

3.3. Potential Mechanism of Action of CS and Its Constituents in Schizophrenia

The exact mechanism(s) through which crocins exert their effects on schizophrenia-like behavior caused by glutamatergic and dopaminergic dysfunction is (are) not yet elucidated. Research is needed aiming to clarify this important issue. That schizophrenia-like effects of NMDA receptor antagonists (e.g., ketamine, MK-801) are related to increased concentrations of glutamate, hypermotility, stereotypy and cognition deficits [56,57] is well-documented. In this context, it has been reported that acute systemic administration of safranal reduced kainic acid-induced increase of extracellular glutamate concentrations in the rat hippocampus [58]. Further, it has been observed that either saffron or crocetin but not crocins partly counteract the NMDA receptor by binding to the phencyclidine

(PCP) binding site of it [59]. The apparent failure of crocins to bind at the NMDA receptor might depend on pharmacokinetic issues, and in particular, their poor intestinal absorption after oral administration in rats [59]. Moreover, it has been shown that CS extracts and crocetin normalized excessive glutamatergic synaptic transmission in rat cortical brain slices [60]. Finally, CS extracts and crocetin were found to display a strong affinity for the sigma (σ)1 receptor [59]. As a whole, these results propose that this decrease of glutamate concentrations by CS and its constituents might be crucial for the beneficial action exerted by crocins on NMDA receptor antagonists-induced psychotomimetic effects and cognitive deficits.

There is poor evidence concerning the mechanism(s) by which crocins could counteract the detrimental effects of apomorphine on non-spatial recognition memory. In this context, it has been reported that apomorphine prevented the induction of long-term potentiation (LTP) which is the electrophysiological correlate of cognition [61], while crocins promote it [62].

Although the pathogenesis of schizophrenia is not yet fully clarified, a possible association with oxidative stress [5,51], inflammation [51,63] and abnormally low concentrations of different neurotrophins as is the brain-derived neurotrophic factor (BDNF) [64] has been suggested. In line with the above, in a series of reports, the pro-oxidative and pro-inflammatory profile either of NMDA receptor antagonists [51,65] or apomorphine [61] has emerged. The potent antioxidant properties of crocins may offer an alternative explanation for the beneficial effects exerted by these bioactive components of saffron in preclinical models of schizophrenia [66–69]. In this context, it has recently been demonstrated that the neuroprotective action of crocins evidenced in a preclinical glutamatergic model of schizophrenia was related to their ability to restore the expression of BDNF and that of the silent information regulator-1 (SIRT-1), a modulator of oxidative stress and inflammation, thus eliciting alleviation of the oxidative stress [51].

4. Conclusions

There is poor available information (either preclinical or clinical) concerning a potential beneficial role for CS and its bioactive constituents in the therapy of schizophrenia. In spite of it, the few preclinical data produced do not lack consistency and are really promising. The latter elicits that future research is mandatory in order to definitively establish if these compounds are suitable candidates and provide a benefit in the therapy of schizophrenia. It is important to underline the clinical efficacy expressed by saffron and its constituents in depression [28–30] and anxiety [33] which are typical features of patients suffering from schizophrenia [70,71] and further emphasize their good safety profile expressed in human studies.

Future research should examine the efficacy of these natural products on preclinical models resembling attentional deficits and extensively evaluate their efficacy on animal models mimicking negative symptoms of this devastating psychiatric disorder. The utilization of other than pharmacological models (e.g., neurodevelopmental, genetic etc.) will be of high value. Finally, in the case of positive preclinical findings, human studies (double-blind, placebo-controlled studies) by recruiting an appropriate number of participants should be conducted in order to evaluate the efficacy of these compounds in schizophrenia. A summary of some future research activities (either preclinical or clinical) is provided in Table 2.

Table 2. Summary of future studies designed to evaluate the role of *Crocus sativus* and its bioactive components in schizophrenia. Key plans.

Preclinical research
Acute vs. repeated drug treatment
Not pharmacological animal models of schizophrenia (genetic, neonatal ventral hippocampal lesions models etc)
Evaluation of the effects of saffron and its constituents in animal models of attentional deficits
Further evaluation of the effects of saffron and its constituents in animal models resembling cognitive impairments and negative symptoms of schizophrenia
Investigation of potential mechanism(s) of action underlying the beneficial effects of saffron and its constituents observed in preclinical studies (molecular, biochemical, neurochemical, electrophysiological studies etc)
Clinical research
Multi-center, double-blind, placebo-controlled studies
Studies of the effects of saffron alone in schizophrenia patients
Studies of the effects of saffron in combination with atypical antipsychotics in schizophrenia patients
Use of broad dose range of *C. sativus*
Appropriate number of participants

Funding: This research received no external fundings.

Data Availability Statement: The data presented in this study are available on request from the corresponding author.

Conflicts of Interest: The author declares no conflict of interest.

References

1. Freedman, R. Schizophrenia. *N. Engl. J. Med.* **2003**, *349*, 1738–1749. [CrossRef]
2. Lewis, D.A.; Lieberman, J.A. Catching up on schizophrenia: Natural history and neurobiology. *Neuron* **2000**, *28*, 1738–1749. [CrossRef]
3. Van Os, J.; Kenis, G.; Rutten, B.P. The environment and schizophrenia. *Nature* **2010**, *468*, 203–212. [CrossRef]
4. Weinberger, D.R. Implications of normal brain development for the pathogenesis of schizophrenia. *Arch. Gen. Psychiatry* **1987**, *44*, 660–669. [CrossRef]
5. Bitanihirwe, B.K.; Woo, T.U. Oxidative stress in schizophrenia: An integrated approach. *Neurosci. Biobehav. Rev.* **2011**, *35*, 878–893. [CrossRef] [PubMed]
6. Steeds, H.; Carhart-Harris, R.L.; Stone, J.M. Drug models of schizophrenia. *Ther. Adv. Psychopharmacol.* **2015**, *5*, 43–58. [CrossRef]
7. Javitt, D.C. Glutamate and schizophrenia: Phencyclidine, N-methyl-D-aspartate receptors, and dopamine-glutamate interactions. *Int. Rev. Neurobiol.* **2007**, *78*, 69–108. [PubMed]
8. Pratt, J.; Winchester, C.; Dawson, N.; Morris, B. Advancing schizophrenia drug discovery: Optimizing rodent models to bridge the translational gap. *Nat. Rev. Drug Discov.* **2012**, *11*, 560–579. [CrossRef]
9. Lewis, D.A.; Pierri, J.; Volk, D.; Melchitzky, D.; Woo, T. Altered GABA neurotransmission and prefrontal cortical dysfunction in schizophrenia. *Biol. Psychiatry* **1999**, *46*, 616–626. [CrossRef]
10. Field, J.R.; Walker, A.G.; Conn, P.J. Targeting glutamate synapses in schizophrenia. *Trends Mol. Med.* **2011**, *17*, 689–698. [CrossRef]
11. Abbott, A. Schizophrenia: The drug deadlook. *Nature* **2010**, *468*, 158–159. [CrossRef]
12. Liakopoulou-Kyriakides, M.; Kyriakidis, D. *Crocus Sativus*-biological active constituents. *Stud. Nat. Prod. Chem.* **2002**, *16*, 293–312.
13. Tarantilis, P.A.; Tsoupras, G.; Polissiou, M. Determination of saffron (*Crocus sativus* L.) components in crude plant extract using high-performance liquid chromatography-UV/Visible photodiode-array detection-mass spectrometry. *J. Chromatogr. A.* **1995**, *699*, 107–118. [CrossRef]
14. Rios, J.L.; Recio, M.C.; Ginger, R.M.; Manz, S. An update review of saffron and its active constituents. *Phytother. Res.* **1996**, *10*, 189–193. [CrossRef]
15. Tarantilis, P.A.; Polissiou, M.; Marnait, M. Separation of picrocrocin, cis-trans-crocins and safranal of saffron using high-performance liquid chromatography with photodiode-array detection. *J. Chromatogr. A* **1994**, *664*, 55–61. [CrossRef]
16. Kanakis, C.D.; Daferera, D.J.; Tarantilis, P.A.; Polissiou, M.G. Qualitative determination of volatile compounds and quantitative evaluation of safranal and 4-hydroxy-2,6,6-trimethyl-1-cyclohexene-1-carboxaldehyde. *J. Agric. Food Chem.* **2004**, *52*, 4515–4521. [CrossRef] [PubMed]
17. Abdullaev, F.I.; Espinosa-Aguirre, J.J. Biomedical properties of saffron and its potential use in cancer therapy and chemoprevention trials. *Cancer Detect. Prev.* **2004**, *28*, 426–432. [CrossRef]

18. Bathaie, S.Z.; Mousavi, S.Z. New applications and mechanisms of action of saffron and its important ingredients. *Crit. Rev. Food Sci. Nutr.* **2010**, *50*, 761–786. [CrossRef]
19. Alavizadeh, S.H.; Hosseinzadeh, H. Bioactivity assessment and toxicity of crocin: A comprehensive review. *Food Chem. Toxicol.* **2014**, *64*, 65–80. [CrossRef]
20. Hosseinzadeh, H.; Khosravan, V. Anticonvulsant effects of aqueous and ethanolic extracts of *Crocus Sativus*, L., stigmas in mice. *Arch. Iran Med.* **2005**, *5*, 44–47.
21. Hosseinzadeh, H.; Sadeghnia, H.R. Protective effect of safranal on pentylenetetrazol-induced seizures in the rat: Involvement of the GABAergic and opioids systems. *Phytomedicine* **2007**, *14*, 256–262. [CrossRef]
22. Ahmad, A.S.; Ansari, M.A.; Ahmad, M.; Saleem, S.; Yousuf, S.; Hoda, M.N.; Islam, F. Neuroprotection by crocin in a hemi-parkinsonian rat model. *Pharmacol. Biochem. Behav.* **2005**, *81*, 805–813. [CrossRef] [PubMed]
23. Hosseinzadeh, H.; Sadeghnia, H.R. Safranal a constituent of Crocus sativus (saffron) attenuated cerebral ischemia-induced oxidative damage in rat hippocampus. *J. Pharm. Pharm. Sci.* **2005**, *8*, 394–399. [PubMed]
24. Hosseinzadeh, H.; Sadeghnia, H.R.; Ghaeni, F.A.; Motamedshariaty, V.S.; Mohajeri, S.A. Effects of saffron (*Crocus sativus* L.) and its active constituent crocin, on recognition and spatial memory after chronic cerebral hypofunction in rats. *Phytother. Res.* **2012**, *26*, 381–386. [CrossRef] [PubMed]
25. Saleem, S.; Ahmad, M.; Ahmad, A.S.; Yousuf, F.; Ansari, M.A.; Khan, M.B.; Ishrat, T.; Islam, F. Effect of Saffron (*Crocus sativus*) on neurobehavioral and neurochemical changes in cerebral ischemia in rats. *J. Med. Food* **2006**, *9*, 246–253. [CrossRef] [PubMed]
26. Pitsikas, N. The effects of Crocus sativus L. and its constituents on memory: Basic studies and clinical applications. *Evid. Based Complement. Alternat. Med.* **2015**, *2015*, 926284. [CrossRef]
27. Akhondzadeh, S.; Shafiee-Sabet, M.; Harirchian, M.H.; Togha, M.; Cheraghmakani, H.; Razeghi, S.; Hejazi, S.S.; Yousefi, M.H.; Alimardani, R.; Jasmshidi, A.; et al. A 22-week, multicentre randomized, double-blind controlled trial of *Crocus sativus* L., in the treatment of mild-to-moderate Alzheimer's disease. *Psychopharmacology* **2010**, *207*, 637–643. [CrossRef]
28. Hosseinzadeh, H.; Karimi, G.; Niapoor, M. Antidepressant effects of *crocus sativus* stigma extracts and its constituents, crocins and safranal in mice. *J. Med. Plants* **2004**, *3*, 48–58.
29. Akhondzadeh, S.; Fallah-Pour, H.; Afkham, K.; Jamshidi, A.H.; Khalighi-Cigaroudi, F. Comparison of *Crocus sativus* L., and imipramine in the treatment of mild to moderate depression: A pilot double-blind, randomized trial. *BMC Complement. Altern. Med.* **2004**, *4*, 12–16. [CrossRef]
30. Noorbala, A.A.; Akhondzadeh, S.; Tahmacebi-Pour, N.; Jamshidi, A.H. Hydro-alcoholic extract of *Crocus sativus* L., versus fluoxetine in the treatment of mild to moderate depression: A double-blind, randomized trial. *J. Ethnopharmacol.* **2005**, *97*, 281–284. [CrossRef]
31. Kashani, L.; Raisi, F.; Saroukhani, S.; Sohrabi, H.; Moddabernia, H.; Nasehi, A.A.; Jamshidi, A.; Ashrafi, M.; Mansouri, P.; Ghaeli, P.; et al. Saffron for treatment of fluoxetine-induced sexual dysfunction in women: Randomized double-blind placebo-controlled study. *Hum. Psychopharmacol.* **2012**, *28*, 54–60. [CrossRef]
32. Modabbernia, A.; Sohrabi, H.; Nasehi, A.A.; Raisi, F.; Saroukhani, S.; Jamshidi, A.; Tabrizi, M.; Ashrafi, M.; Akhonzadeh, S. Effect of saffron on fluoxetine-induced sexual impairment in men: Randomized double-blind placebo-controlled trial. *Psychopharmacology* **2013**, *223*, 381–388. [CrossRef]
33. Pitsikas, N. Assessment of *Crocus sativus* L., and its bioactive constituents as potential anti-anxiety compounds. Basic and clinical evidence. In *Saffron the age-old panacea in a new light*. Sarwat, M., Sumaiya, S., Eds.; Academic Press: Cambridge, MA, USA, 2020; pp. 131–139.
34. Lautenschlager, M.; Sendker, J.; Huwel, S.; Galla, H.J.; Brandt, S.; Dufer, M.; Riehemann, K.; Hensel, A. Intestinal formation of *trans*-crocetin from saffron extract (*Crocus sativus* L.) and in vitro permeation through intestinal and blood brain barrier. *Phytomedicine* **2015**, *22*, 36–44. [CrossRef] [PubMed]
35. Xi, L.; Quian, Z.; Xu, G.; Zheng, S.; Sun, S.; Wen, N.; Sheng, L.; Shi, Y.; Zhang, Y. Beneficial impact of crocin, a carotenoid from saffron, on insulin sensitivity in fructose-fed rats. *J. Nutr. Biochem.* **2007**, *18*, 64–72. [CrossRef] [PubMed]
36. Kanakis, C.D.; Tarantilis, P.A.; Tahmir-Riahi, H.A.; Polissiou, M.G. Crocetin, dimethylcrocetin and safranal, bind human serum albumin: Stability and antioxidative properties. *J. Agric. Food Chem.* **2007**, *55*, 970–977. [CrossRef] [PubMed]
37. Asai, A.; Nakano, T.; Takahashi, M.; Nagao, A. Orally administered crocetin and crocins are absorbed into blood plasma as crocetin and its glucuronide conjugates in mice. *J. Agric. Food Chem.* **2005**, *53*, 7302–7306. [CrossRef]
38. Zhang, Y.; Fei, F.; Zhen, L.; Zhu, X.; Wang, J.; Li, S.; Geng, J.; Sun, R.; Yu, X.; Chen, T.; et al. Sensitive analysis and simultaneous assessment of pharmacokinetic properties of crocin and crocetin after oral administration in rats. *J. Chromatogr. B Analyt. Technol. Biomed. Life Sci.* **2017**, *10*, 1–7. [CrossRef]
39. Puglia, C.; Santonocito, D.; Musumeci, T.; Cardile, V.; Graziano, A.; Salerno, L.; Raciti, G.; Crasci', L.; Panico, A.; Puglisi, G. Nanotechnological approach to increase the antioxidant and cytotoxic efficacy of crocin and crocetin. *Planta Med.* **2018**, *85*, 258–265. [CrossRef]
40. Karkoula, E.; Lemonakis, N.; Kokras, N.; Dalla, C.; Gikas, E.; Skaltsounis, A.L.; Tsarbopoulos, A. Trans-crocin 4 is not hydrolyzed to crocetin following i.p. administration in mice, while it shows penetration through the blood brain barrier. *Fitoterapia* **2018**, *129*, 62–72. [CrossRef]

41. Linardaki, Z.I.; Orkoula, M.; Kokkosis, A.G.; Lamari, F.N.; Margarity, M. Investigation of the neuroprotective action of saffron (*Crocus sativus* L.) in aluminum-exposed adult mice through behavioral and neurobiochemical assessment. *Food Chem. Toxicol.* **2013**, *52*, 163–170. [CrossRef]
42. Yoshino, F.; Yoshida, A.; Umigai, N.; Kubo, K.; Lee, M.C.I. Crocetin reduces the oxidative stress induced reactive oxygen species in the stroke-prone spontaneously hypertensive rats (SHRSPs) brain. *J. Clin. Biochem. Nutr.* **2011**, *49*, 182–187. [CrossRef]
43. Nair, S.C.; Panikkar, B.; Panikkar, K.R. Antitumor activity of saffron. *Cancer Lett.* **1991**, *57*, 109–114. [CrossRef]
44. Abdullaev, F.I. Cancer chemoprotective and tumoricidial properties of saffron (*Crocus sativus* L.). *Exp. Biol. Med.* **2002**, *227*, 20–25. [CrossRef]
45. Hosseinzadeh, H.; Motamedshariaty, V.S.; Sameni, A.K.; Vahabzadeh, M. Acute and sub-acute toxicity of crocin, a constituent of *Crocus sativus* L., (saffron), in mice and rats. *Pharmacologyonline* **2010**, *2*, 943–951.
46. Modaghegh, M.H.; Shahabian, M.; Esmaeli, H.A.; Rajbai, O.; Hosseinzadeh, H. Safety evaluation of saffron (*Crocus sativus*) tablets in healthy volunteers. *Phytomedicine* **2008**, *15*, 1032–1037. [CrossRef] [PubMed]
47. Mohamadpour, A.H.; Ayati, Z.; Parizadeh, M.R.; Rajbai, O.; Hosseinzadeh, H. Safety evaluation of crocin (a constituent of saffron) tablets in healthy volunteers. *Iran, J. Basic Med. Sci.* **2013**, *16*, 39–46.
48. Schmidt, M.; Betti, G.; Hensel, A. Saffron in phytotherapy: Pharmacology and clinical uses. *Wien Med. Wochenschr.* **2007**, *157*, 315–319. [CrossRef] [PubMed]
49. Georgiadou, G.; Grivas, V.; Tarantilis, P.A.; Pitsikas, N. Crocins the active constituents of *Crocus Sativus*, L., counteracted ketamine-induced behavioural deficits in rats. *Psychopharmacology* **2014**, *231*, 717–726. [CrossRef] [PubMed]
50. Pitsikas, N.; Tarantilis, P.A. Crocins, the active constituents of *Crocus sativus* L., counteracted apomorphine-induced performance deficits in the novel object recognition task, but not novel location task, in rats. *Neurosci. Lett.* **2017**, *644*, 37–42. [CrossRef]
51. Sun, X.J.; Zhao, X.; Xie, J.N.; Wan, H. Crocin alleviates schizophrenia-like symptoms in rats by upregulating silent information regulator-1 and brain derived neurotrophic factor. *Compr. Psychiatry* **2020**, *103*, 152209. [CrossRef] [PubMed]
52. Tumer, P.V.; Brabb, T.; Pekow, C.; Vasbinder, M.A. Administration of substances to laboratory animals: Routes of administration and factors to consider. *J. Am. Assoc. Lab. Anim. Sci.* **2011**, *50*, 600–613.
53. Farokhnia, M.; Shafiee-Sabet, M.; Iranpour, N.; Gougol, A.; Yekehtaz, H.; Alimardani, R.; Farsad, F.; Kamalipour, M.; Akhondzadeh, S. Comparing the efficacy and safety of *Crocus sativus* L. with memantine in patients with moderate to severe Alzheimer's disease: A double-blind randomized clinical trial. *Hum. Psychopharmacol.* **2014**, *29*, 351–359. [CrossRef]
54. Mousavi, B.; Bathaie, S.Z.; Fadai, F.; Ashtari, Z.; Ali Beigi, N.; Farhang, S.; Hashempour, S.; Shahhamzei, N.; Heidarzadeh, H. Safety evaluation of saffron stigma (Crocus sativus L.) aqueous extract and crocin in patients with schizophrenia. *Avicenna J. Phytomed.* **2015**, *5*, 413–419.
55. Fadai, F.; Moosavi, B.; Ashtari, Z.; Ali Beigi, N.; Farhang, S.; Hashempour, S.; Shahhamzei, N.; Zahra Bathaie, S. Saffron aqueous extract prevents metabolic syndrome in patients with schizophrenia on olanzapine treatment: A randomized triple blind placebo controlled study. *Pharmacipsychiatry* **2014**, *47*, 156–161. [CrossRef] [PubMed]
56. Moghaddam, B.; Adams, B.; Verma, A.; Daly, D. Activation of glutamatergic transmission by ketamine: a novel step in the pathway from NMDA receptor blockade to dopaminergic and cognitive disruptions associated with the prefrontal cortex. *J. Neurosci.* **1997**, *17*, 2921–2927. [CrossRef] [PubMed]
57. Tricklebank, M.D.; Singh, L.; Oles, R.J.; Preston, C.; Iversen, S.D. The behavioral effects of Mk-801: A comparison with antagonists acting non-competitively and competitively at the NMDA receptor. *Eur. J. Pharmacol.* **1989**, *167*, 127–135. [CrossRef]
58. Hosseinzadeh, H.; Sadeghnia, H.R.; Rahimi, A. Effects of safranal on extracellular hippocampal levels of glutamate and aspartate during kainic acid treatment in anesthetized rats. *Planta Med.* **2008**, *74*, 1441–1445. [CrossRef]
59. Lechtenberg, M.; Schepmann, D.; Niehues, M.; Hellenbrand, M.; Wunsch, B.; Hensel, A. Quality and functionality of saffron: Quality control, species assortment and affinity of extract and isolated saffron compounds to NMDA and σ_1 (Sigma-1) receptors. *Planta Med.* **2008**, *74*, 764–772. [CrossRef]
60. Berger, F.; Hensel, A.; Nieber, K. Saffron extracts and trans-crocetin inhibit glutamatergic synaptic transmission in rat cortical brain slices. *Neuroscience* **2011**, *180*, 238–247. [CrossRef]
61. Arroyo-Garcia, L.E.; Rodriguez-Moreno, A.; Flores, G. Apomorphine effects on hippocampus. *Neural Regen. Res.* **2018**, *13*, 2064–2066.
62. Sugiura, M.; Shoyama, Y.; Saito, H.; Abe, K. Crocin (crocetin di-gentiobiose ester) prevents the inhibitory effect of ethanol on long-term potentiation in the dentate gyrus in vivo. *J. Pharmacol. Exp. Ther.* **1994**, *271*, 703–707.
63. Khandaker, G.M.; Cousins, L.; Deakin, J.; Lennox, R.B.; Yolken, R.; Jones, P.B. Inflammation and immunity in schizophrenia: Implications for pathophysiology and treatment. *Lancet Psychiatry* **2015**, *2*, 258–270. [CrossRef]
64. Rodriguez-Amorim, D.; Rivera-Baltands, T.; Bessa, J.; Sousa, N.; Vallejo-Curto, M.C.; Rodriguez-Jamardo, C.; de las Heras, M.E.; Diaz, R.; Agis-Balboa, R.C.; Olivares, J.M.; et al. The neurobiological hypothesis of neurotrophins in the pathophysiology of schizophrenia: a meta-analysis. *J. Psychiatr. Res.* **2018**, *106*, 43–53. [CrossRef] [PubMed]
65. De Oliveira, L.; Spiazzi, C.M.; Bortolin, T.; Canever, L.; Petronilho, F.; Mina, F.G.; Dal-Pizzol, F.; Quevedoa, J.; Zugno, A.I. Different sub-anesthetic doses of ketamine increase oxidative stress in brain of rats. *Prog. Neuropsychopharmacol. Biol. Psychiatry* **2009**, *33*, 1003–1008. [CrossRef] [PubMed]

66. Naghizadeh, B.; Mansouri, M.T.; Ghorbanzadeh, B.; Farbood, Y.; Sarkaki, A. Protective effects of oral crocin against intracerebroventricular streptozotocin-induced spatial memory deficit and oxidative stress in rats. *Phytomedicine* **2013**, *20*, 537–543. [CrossRef] [PubMed]
67. Ochiai, T.; Soeda, S.; Ohno, S.; Tanaka, H.; Shoyama, Y.; Shimeno, H. Crocin prevent the death of PC-12 cells through sphingomyelinase-ceramide signaling by increasing glutathione synthesis. *Neurochem. Int.* **2004**, *44*, 321–330. [CrossRef]
68. Papandreou, M.A.; Tsachaki, M.; Efthimiopoulos, S.; Cordopatis, P.; Lamari, F.N.; Margarity, M. Memory enhancing effects of saffron in aged mice are correlated with antioxidant protection. *Behav. Brain Res.* **2011**, *219*, 197–204. [CrossRef]
69. Zheng, Y.Q.; Liu, J.X.; Wang, J.N.; Xu, L. Effects of crocin on reperfusion induced oxidative/nitrative injury to cerebral microvessels after global cerebral ischemia. *Brain Res.* **2007**, *1138*, 86–94. [CrossRef]
70. Upthegrove, R.; Marwaha, S.; Birchwood, M. Depression and schizophrenia: Cause, consequence or trans-diagnostic tool? *Schizophr. Bull.* **2016**, *43*, 240–244.
71. Temmingh, H.; Stein, D.J. Anxiety in patients with schizophrenia: Epidemiology and management. *CNS Drugs* **2015**, *29*, 819–832. [CrossRef]

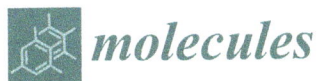

Article

Saffron: Chemical Composition and Neuroprotective Activity

Maria Anna Maggi [1,2,*], Silvia Bisti [3,4] and Cristiana Picco [4,5]

1. Hortus Novus srl, via Campo Sportivo 2, 67050 Canistro, Italy
2. Department of Phyisical and Chemical Sciences, University of L'Aquila, Via Vetoio, 67100 Coppito, Italy
3. Department of Biotecnology and Applied Clinical Sciences, DISCAB, University of L'Aquila, Via Vetoio, 67100 Coppito, Italy; s.bisti@team.it
4. National Institute of Biostructure and Biosystem (INBB), V. le Medaglie D'Oro 305, 00136 Roma, Italy; cristiana.picco@ge.ibf.cnr.it
5. Institute of Biophysics, National Research Council, Via De Marini 6, 16149 Genova, Italy
* Correspondence: m.maggi@hortusnovus.it

Academic Editors: Nikolaos Pitsikas and Konstantinos Dimas
Received: 14 October 2020; Accepted: 25 November 2020; Published: 29 November 2020

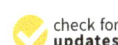

Abstract: *Crocus sativus* L. belongs to the Iridaceae family and it is commonly known as saffron. The different cultures together with the geoclimatic characteristics of the territory determine a different chemical composition that characterizes the final product. This is why a complete knowledge of this product is fundamental, from which more than 150 chemical compounds have been extracted from, but only about one third of them have been identified. The chemical composition of saffron has been studied in relation to its efficacy in coping with neurodegenerative retinal diseases. Accordingly, experimental results provide evidence of a strict correlation between chemical composition and neuroprotective capacity. We found that saffron's ability to cope with retinal neurodegeneration is related to: (1) the presence of specific crocins and (2) the contribution of other saffron components. We summarize previous evidence and provide original data showing that results obtained both "in vivo" and "in vitro" lead to the same conclusion.

Keywords: saffron; crocins; neuroprotective activity; P2X7 receptor; fraction

---

1. Introduction

Saffron is a spice obtained from the dehydrated stigmas of the flower *Crocus sativus Linnaeus*, a member of the family of Iridaceae and probably the result of intensive artificial selection of the *Crocus cartwrightianus*, native in the Island of Crete. Saffron was first grown in Iran, where currently about 90% of the global production comes from [1]. Other producing countries are Spain, Greece, Italy, Morocco, Egypt, Israel, New Zealand, Australia, Pakistan, and India.

The production process of the spice follows a complex procedure that is articulated in several phases: (a) flower collection, (b) separation of the stigmas or cleaning, and (c) drying and conservation. Each of these steps in the production process of saffron is strongly influenced by the traditions present in the area of cultivation while following general guidelines. The different cultures together with the geoclimatic characteristics of the territory determine a different chemical composition that characterizes the final product, making it distinguishable from others. In addition, changes in the preparation procedures might strongly modify the final composition of chemical components. Saffron is one of the most expensive spices in the world, but high costs lead to a high rate of counterfeiting. The scientific community's interest in this product, however, is not limited to guaranteeing its authenticity to the consumer. Advanced pharmacological studies have in fact highlighted its numerous beneficial health effects, including a neuroprotective activity on retinal photoreceptors undergoing/exposed to oxidative stress [2]. Multiple ways of actions have been suggested and widely exploited in microarray experiments [3] and in cellular [4] and animal models [2,5–8]. In addition. interesting data have been obtained in clinical trials with patients affected by either age-related macular degeneration (AMD) or Stargardt [9] and the results are very promising [9–12].

The chemistry of saffron is complex; this spice has primary metabolites, which are ubiquitous in nature, such as carbohydrates, minerals, fats, vitamins, amino acids, and proteins. A large number of compounds belong to different classes of secondary metabolites, products of metabolism not ubiquitous but important for the development or reproduction of the organism, such as carotenoids, monoterpenes, and flavonoids, including mainly anthocyanins [13].

Carotenoids are the most important constituents of the spice, from which it derives its color. They include fat-soluble ones, such as α- and β-carotene, lycopene, and zeaxanthin, and water-soluble ones like the apocarotenoid crocetin ($C_{20}H_{24}O_4$) and crocins, the polyene esters of the mono- and di-glycoside crocetin.

Crocins are a family of carotenoids unusually soluble in water as they are mono- and di-glycosylated esters of the dicarboxylic acid crocetin [14]. They make up 3.5% of the weight of the stigmas in the plant. The glycosidic carotenoids of saffron, like all glycosides, are usually thermally labile and photochemically sensitive, especially in solution. Like their precursor, crocins exist in the two isomeric forms *13-cis* and *all-trans*. There is a great variety of crocins because there are different combinations of carbohydrates that can go to esterify one or both carboxyl groups and both isomeric forms. Although these crocins differ in substituents and in configuration, they are very similar in their chemical-physical properties and in particular polarity. These similarities make their separation and subsequent identification extremely difficult [15–18].

Among the oxidation products of carotenoids, we find two compounds: picrocrocin (monoterpene glycoside) and safranal (cyclic monoterpene aldehyde) that give/are responsible for the spice's bitterness strength and aromatic strength, respectively. According to the most accredited hypothesis, the precursor is considered zeaxanthin, which is broken at both ends by the enzyme CsZCD (*Crocus sativus* zeaxanthin cleavage dioxygenase) to generate the crocetindialdehyde [19], which can be oxidized and esterified by different glucosyltransferases to give the crocins [20], and picrocrocin. Picrocrocin ($C_{16}H_{26}O_7$), which constitutes 3.7% of the weight of the stigma, has been identified only in the genus *Crocus*, of which the only edible spice is *Crocus sativus* L.; therefore, it constitutes the molecular marker of saffron. During the drying process, the β-glucosidase enzyme acts on picrocrocin to release 4-hydroxy-2,6,6-trimethyl-1-cyclohexene-1-carboxyaldehyde (HTCC, $C_{10}H_{16}O_2$) [21]. For dehydration it is transformed into safranal ($C_{10}H_{14}O$). This is present with a percentage of 0.02% in the stigma and is the major component of the volatile fraction of saffron.

The main aim of this paper was to provide evidence of the relationship between the chemical composition of saffron and its neuroprotective activity. Here, we used a consolidated animal model of retinal degeneration to test saffron differing in its chemical components to check whether different saffron preparations might have different efficacy. Experiments involving HPLC analysis and animal treatment were performed in parallel. In addition, we wonder whether all the chemical components of saffron are important in supporting its neuroprotective activities. To test this point we separated two fractions to test crocins and other components separately in both cellular and animal models.

2. Results

2.1. Correlation between Saffron Chemical Composition and Neuroprotective Activity

The saffron samples were analyzed with the chromatographic method described in the previous section. A qualitative identification of the HPLC-DAD chromatographic peaks was performed using literature data, for similar experimental conditions, on the basis of the well-known absorption spectra of the main constituents of saffron, as well as the relative intensities of the peaks and elution order in chromatograms [22–24]. Crocins have characteristic UV-vis spectra, both *trans* and *cis* crocins have a very intense absorption band between 400 and 500 nm, and a further band between 260 and 274 nm, but only *cis* crocins have a relative absorption maximum at 326–327 nm [14,22,24–27]. Since the analytical standards of these molecules are lacking, a method based on the combination of the areas of the HPLC-DAD peaks observed at 440 nm with the coefficients determined by spectrophotometric analysis was used [28] for the quantitative analysis of crocins. The formula used to determine the concentration of crocins is:

$$c\ (\text{mg/g}) = \frac{Mw_i \cdot E^{1\%}_{1\,cm}\,(440\text{ nm}) \cdot A_i}{\varepsilon_{t,c}}, \tag{1}$$

where Mw_i and A_i are the molecular weight and the percentage peak area, respectively, $E^{1\%}_{1\,cm}$ (440 nm) is the coloring strength of the saffron sample, and $\varepsilon_{t,c}$ is the extinction coefficient (89,000 $M^{-1}cm^{-1}$ for *trans*-crocins and 63,350 $M^{-1}cm^{-1}$ for *cis*-crocins).

The results of the experiments carried out by administering different saffron with different contents of crocins to an animal model of retinal-induced degeneration are shown below (Figure 1). Given the high number of tested saffron samples, we concentrated on and quantified the two most abundant crocins: *trans*-crocetin bis (β-D-gentiobiosyl) ester (T1) and *trans*-crocetin (β-D-gentiobiosyl) (β-D-glucosyl) ester (T2).

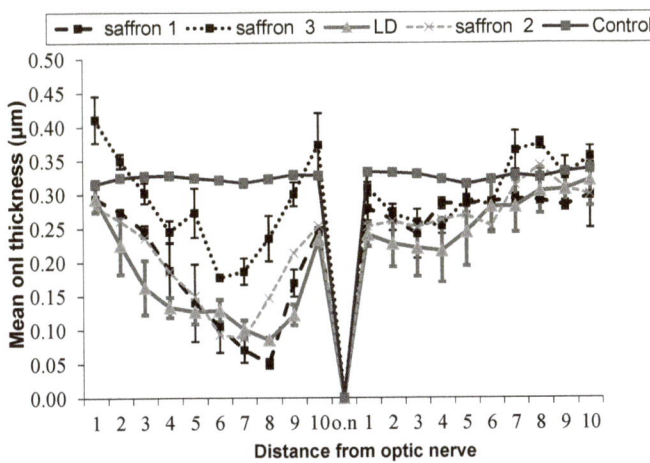

Figure 1. Thickness of the outer nuclear layer (ONL) as a function of the retinal position starting from the dorsal edge of the retina up to the optic nerve entrance and continuing into the ventral retina in 5 experimental groups: healthy animals (control), animals exposed to light damage (LD), and LD animals treated with three different saffron preparations. All animal groups were sacrificed a week after LD. Each point of the graph is the average ±SEM of 5 experiments.

In Figure 1 and Table 1, the comparison between five experimental groups of rats (five animals per group) is shown. In three groups (saffron 1, saffron 2, saffron 3), the degeneration was induced with intense light damage (LD) and saffron with different crocin contents was administered through the diet:

- Group saffron 1: Rats treated with saffron having a content of T1 equal to 13% (mg/g) and T2 equal to 5% (mg/g).
- Group saffron 2: Rats treated with saffron having a content of T1 equal to 14% and T2 equal to 5%.
- Group saffron 3: Rats treated with saffron having a content of T1 equal to 17% and T2 equal to 8%.
- Group LD: Rats untreated but subjected to light damage for 24 h (diseased retina).
- Group control: Healthy animals (healthy retina).

Table 1. Statistical analysis of data performed using Student's *t* test.

	Saffron 1	Saffron 2	Saffron 3	Control	Light Damage
Saffron 1		Not significant	$p < 0.001$	$p < 0.001$	Not significant
Saffron 2	Not significant		$p < 0.001$	$p < 0.001$	Not significant
Saffron 3	$p < 0.001$	$p < 0.001$		$p < 0.005$	$p < 0.001$
Control	$p < 0.001$	$p < 0.001$	$p < 0.005$		$p < 0.001$
Light damage	Not significant	Not significant	$p < 0.001$	$p < 0.001$	

These results show that the neuroprotective activity of saffron depends on the chemical composition of this spice. Looking at Figure 2, it is evident that the ONL of a retina of an animal treated with saffron 3 (neuroprotective saffron) is close in thickness to that of a healthy animal. On the contrary, saffron 1 and 2 (non neuroprotective saffron) do not have neuroprotective activity. The ONL of the two experimental groups 1 and 2 is similar to that of the retina of an animal exposed to LD and untreated. It has to be noted that according to the International Organization for Standardization (ISO) criteria [29] (looking at the coloring strength), all three saffron belong to class I. These results have allowed the filing of an international patent.

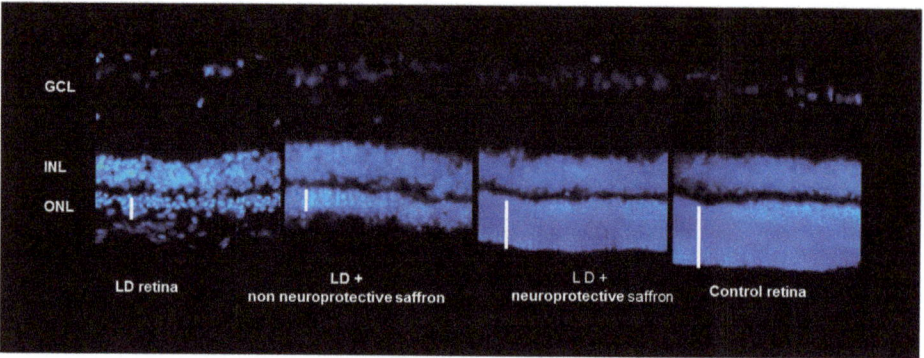

Figure 2. Cross-section of the retina of animals belonging to 4 experimental groups: animals exposed to damage from light not treated with saffron (retinal LD), healthy animals (control retinal), animals exposed to light damage and treated with active saffron (LD+ active saffron), animals exposed to light damage and treated with inactive saffron (LD+ inactive saffron). Images were taken in corresponding dorsal retinal regions. The coloring agent used was bisbenzimide.

2.2. Saffron Components on Cellular Models

To evaluate whether the efficacy of saffron treatment is due to the entire chemical composition of spice or mainly due to specific molecular components [30–32], we separated a saffron extract into two fractions: one containing the most polar active components (kaempferol derivates and picrocrocin) and another containing the crocins, the most apolar molecules. The two fractions were previously tested on an animal model [6].

Here, we report new data on two different cellular models: the photoreceptor-derived mouse 661W cells and the HEK293 cells permanently expressing P2X7R. Recently, we found a novel mechanism of saffron neuroprotection by acting directly on the ionotropic P2X7 receptor (P2X7R) [4]. In Corso et al. (2016) [4], we showed that saffron protects photoreceptors from ATP-induced cytotoxicity.

First, we tested both fractions on photoreceptor-derived mouse 661W cells. These cells are a good model for in vitro experiments on retina since they show the biochemical and cellular properties of retinal photoreceptors and activate the same apoptotic program in response to different stresses. Moreover, they express P2X7R [4]. Figure 3 shows viability measurements on 661W cells stressed with different concentrations of ATP. Cells were incubated with ATP (5 and 10 mM), saffron, crocins, and picocrocins/kaempferol derivates at concentrations of 25 µg/mL for 24 h. As previously observed for saffron [4], both components alone also did not change the cell viability (98%). The stress induced by ATP was concentration dependent, reducing cell viability from 57% to 20% at 5 and 10 mM ATP, respectively. Both fractions, crocins (Cr) and picocrocins/kaempferol derivates (PC/Canf), were able to protect against ATP stress but in a different manner. In particular, Cr was more effective, increasing the viability to 69% and 27%, respectively, at 5 and 10 mM ATP. A smaller but significant protection was also observed in the presence of PC/Canf, which raised the viability to 67% and 23% at 5 and 10 mM ATP. However, both fractions were less effective than the entire saffron extract (77% and 30%). When cells were incubated with ATP and Cr and PC/Canf together, the viability increased compared to the single fractions but less than with saffron alone.

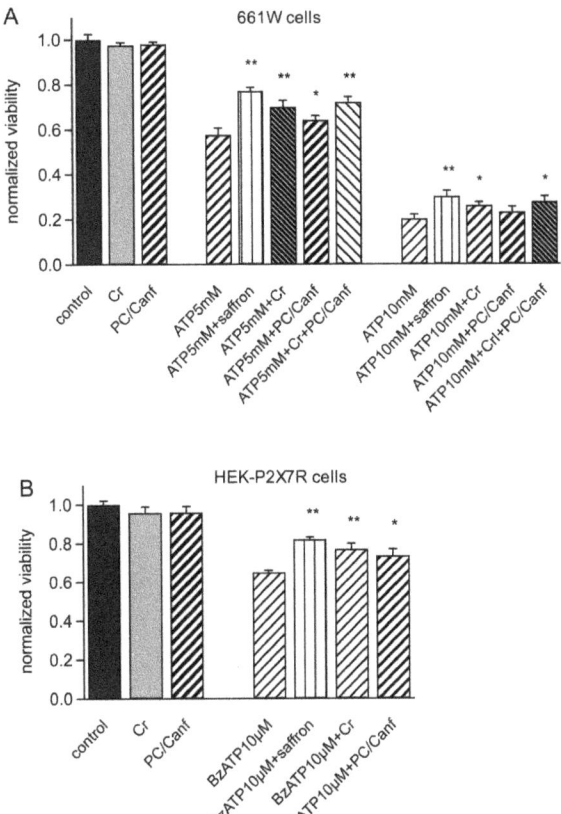

Figure 3. Saffron components increase the viability of 661W and HEK-P2X7R cells. (**A**) Cytotoxic effect in mouse retinal photoreceptor-derived 661W cells induced by application of 5 and 10mM ATP for 24 h and by the co-treatment of ATP saffron, crocins (Cr), picocrocins/kaempferol derivates (PC/Canf) (25 µg/mL). (**B**) Cytotoxicity assay induced on HEK293-P2X7R cells by 10 µM BzATP for 24 h and by the co-treatment of BzATP with 25 µg/mL saffron, Cr, and PC/Canf. Viable cells were counted using an MTT assay (see Materials and Methods) and normalized to control cells. Differences between treatment of ATP and ATP plus saffron and plus the two fractions or BzATP (see Materials and Methods) and BzATP plus saffron and plus the two fractions were significant (* $p < 0.05$, ** $p < 0.01$). Data ± SEM were obtained from triplicates in at least 5 different experiments.

Similar experiments were conducted in HEK293 cells permanently expressing P2X7R to test the effect of the two fractions on the isolated receptor. Viability measurements were obtained from MTT tests in HEK-P2X7R cells incubated for 24 h with saffron or Cr or PC/Canf and the selective agonist 2′(3′)-O-(4-Benzoylbenzoyl)adenosine 5′-triphosphate triethylammonium salt (BzATP). We used 10 μM BzATP to reduce cell viability almost to 60%. As observed for 661W cells, Cr reduced cell mortality more than PC/Canf but less than saffron (Figure 3B).

The P2X7 receptor is characterized by two states of permeability [33]. A common feature of both conductance states is the elevation of free $[Ca^{2+}]_i$, which can reach dramatic levels upon repeated or prolonged application of an agonist. As previously shown, micromolar concentrations of the selective agonist BzATP induced an intracellular calcium elevation in HEK293 cells transfected with the full-length rat P2X7R [4]. Here, we tested the effect of the two fractions in HEK-P2X7R cells loaded with FURA2-AM (Figure 4). First, we verified that both Cr and PC/Canf alone did not change intracellular calcium (Figure 4A, inserts in lower panels). On the contrary, when cells were exposed to 3 μM BzATP, the typical biphasic calcium response with a rapid and a slow $[Ca^{2+}]_i$ rise was observed (Figure 4A, upper left). Finally, cells were exposed to the same concentration of BzATP in the presence of 25 μg/mL Cr and subsequently in the presence of 25 μg/mL PC/Canf. As shown, the two components of saffron produced different effects on the $[Ca^{2+}]_i$ response evoked by BzATP application; crocins reduced the $[Ca^{2+}]_i$ rise, similar to that observed with saffron while picocrocins did not. Moreover, crocins slowed the kinetics of the calcium response as previously found in the presence of saffron [4] and confirmed in the second panel of Figure 4. Vice versa, when cells were exposed to fraction 2, the rise component of the calcium response induced by BzATP was slightly accelerated.

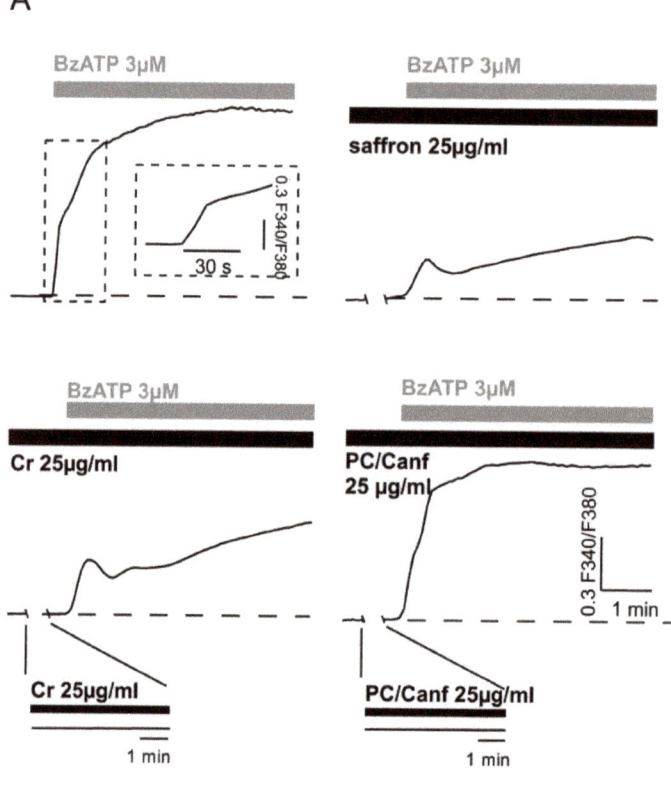

Figure 4. *Cont.*

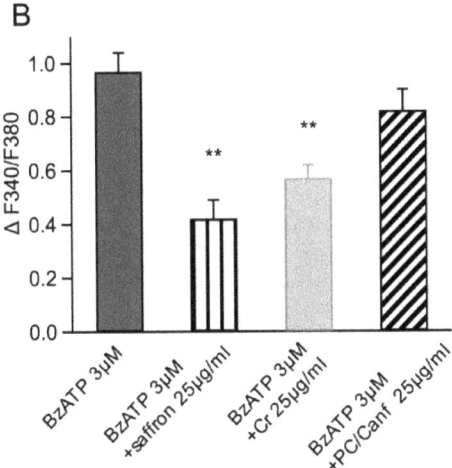

Figure 4. Effect of saffron components on the BzATP-induced $[Ca^{2+}]_i$ elevation in HEK293-P2X7R cells. (**A**) Representative traces of the fluorescence ratio, indicative of $[Ca^{2+}]_i$ variation, in response to application of 3 µM BzATP alone (first trace) or to application of BzATP plus 25 µg/mL saffron (second trace), 25 µg/mL crocins (Cr) (third trace), and 25 µg/mL picocrocins/canferols (PC/Canf) (fourth trace). In each experiment, saffron and both fractions were applied 5 min before the application of BzATP. As observed from the insert, the exposure to Cr or PC/Canf alone did not induce any variation of the trace. Horizontal bars indicate the time period of saffron, Cr and PC/Canf (black bars), and BzATP (grey bars) applications. (**B**) The histogram reports the quantitative analysis of $[Ca^{2+}]_i$ variation elicited by BzATP plus saffron, Cr and PC/Canf. Differences between BzATP and BzATP plus saffron or Cr were significant (** $p < 0.01$), while with PC/Canf no. Data ± SEM were obtained from 44, 61, 44, and 39 cells in the presence of BzATP, plus saffron, plus Cr, and plus PC/Canf, respectively.

2.3. Metabolites of Saffron in Animal Tissues

An open problem is to understand how saffron metabolites reach the various tissues after oral intake. This paper shows the results of analyzed saffron metabolites in different tissues in animal models and blood and urine in AMD patients. Here, we report the data discussed but not shown in a previous paper [5]. We provide evidence of the presence of saffron metabolites only in degenerating retinas. We used 15 animals treated with saffron and LD and 5 control animals treated with saffron without damage. All animals were sacrificed in the morning under the same conditions, saffron was administered through drinking water, and the daily dose was dissolved in the volume of water consumed in 24 h.

Chromatographic analysis of the collected samples revealed the following: in all plasma samples, we found crocetin, while no traces of saffron metabolites were found in other tissue samples, except for degenerating retinas (in 7 of 15 animals, traces of the two main crocins the trans-crocetin bis (β-D-gentiobiosyl) ester and trans-crocetin(β-D-gentiobiosyl)(β-D-glucosyl) ester). The results are shown in Figure 5. We did not find any metabolite (crocetin and/or crocins) in the retina of healthy animals.

In addition to animal tissue samples, we analyzed the blood and urine of two patients with AMD, who were treated with saffron for over a year and three healthy volunteers, who took saffron for two weeks at the same dose of the patients (20 mg/die) (data not shown). Samples were taken two hours after the intake of the morning saffron pill. The most interesting aspect is that crocetin was found only in the samples of healthy volunteers; on the contrary, nothing was found in the blood and urine samples of the patients.

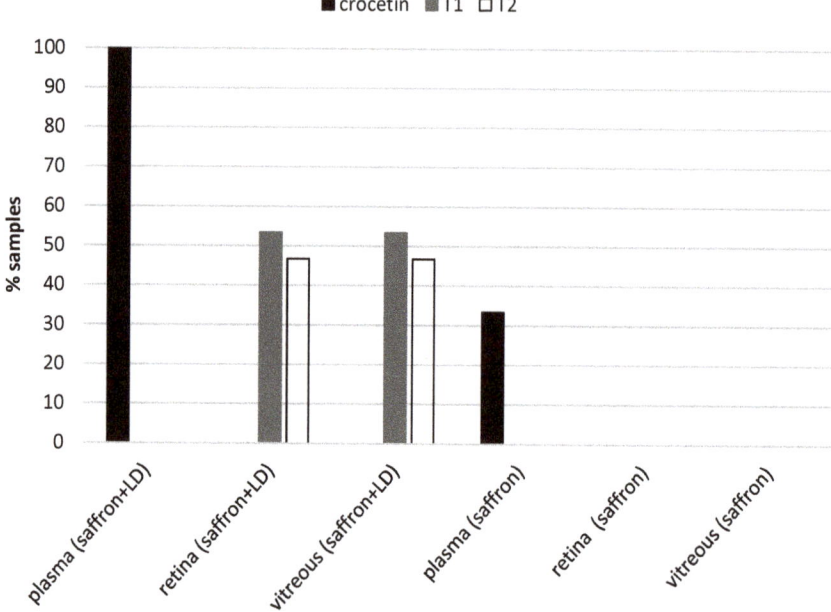

Figure 5. Presence of the main metabolites of saffron: crocetin, trans-crocetin bis (β-D-gentiobiosyl) ester (T1) and trans-crocetin (β-D-gentiobiosyl) (β-D-glucosyl) ester (T2), in the different tissues analyzed. Crocetin is present in plasma samples from animals treated with and without LD, while the two most abundant crocins of saffron are present only in retinal and vitreous samples in about 50% of animals treated and exposed to light damage.

3. Discussion

Saffron is an ancient spice whose beneficial properties have been known for a long time. In the past years, our laboratory has focused the attention on its ability to protect against neurodegeneration, in particular age-related macular degeneration (AMD) and Stargardt. By using different approaches from in vitro to in vivo experiments, also on patients, we found different mechanisms of action of this spice. However, to date, our comprehension is not yet complete. This is probably due to the complexity of the chemical components present in the stigmas of this spice. The composition of the constituents is like a "digital fingerprint" for each saffron sample and provides information on its geographical origin. Is it possible that these different components give different efficacies to protect photoreceptors from stress? To answer this question, we correlated the chemical components of different saffron with their neuroprotective capacity. In particular, we concentrated on the carotenoids, crocins and crocetin, both showing antioxidant properties and which may also suppress the activation of proinflammatory pathways [34–36]. We found that the composition of crocins was important for saffron neuroprotection. Only a saffron sample with a particular concentration of *trans*-crocetin bis (β-D-gentiobiosyl) ester (T1) and trans-crocetin (β-D-gentiobiosyl) (β-D-glucosyl) ester (T2) was able to protects retinal neurons from light damage (Figures 1 and 2). It should be noted that the difference between "neuroprotective" saffron and "non neuroprotective" saffron is due to the small percentage in the crocins concentration. Looking at chromatograms, it is not possible to appreciate the difference in the contents of crocins. It should be noted that we were able to determine the relationship between neuroprotective saffron activity and chemical composition only through experiments conducted in parallel between the chemical characterization of saffron used and an animal model. Experiments performed in vitro confirmed these results: the screening of different saffron on two cellular models stressed by ATP indicated that the "neuroprotective" saffron increased cell viability and decreased calcium entrance significantly, while the "non neuroprotective" saffron did not (data not shown).

Given the importance of the crocin composition to obtain a "good efficient saffron", it is legitimate to ask whether crocins alone are able to reproduce the effects obtained by the whole spice.

Therefore, two fractions, picocrocin/kaempferol derivates and crocins, were isolated from the stigmas of saffron and parallel experiments were carried out on 661W and HEK-P2X7R cells. The first cellular model was derived from retinal tumors of a transgenic mouse line and showed biochemical and cellular properties of photoreceptors, while the P2X7 receptor has been proposed as a potential therapeutic target in Central Nervous System (CNS) diseases [37,38]. In particular, high levels of extracellular ATP in the retina could be the cause of retinal neurodegeneration [39–41]. Previously, saffron was found to act directly on this receptor [3]; therefore, we also asked if specific saffron fractions conserved this characteristic. In both cellular models, the presence of crocins was important for protection from stress induced by ATP (Figure 3). The fraction containing picocrocin and kaempferol derivates was still able to increase cell viability but with less significance. However, both fractions appeared less effective than total saffron: even in the presence of the two fractions, cell viability did not reach the same values obtained with saffron. Moreover, FURA2 experiments showed that crocins were able to reduce ATP-evoked calcium entry while the fraction picocrocin and kaempferol derivates did not (Figure 4). These data strongly suggest that crocins, together with other yet unidentified saffron compounds, directly target P2X7 receptors, inhibiting their activity, which may be a primary cause for their protective effects against ATP-induced cell mortality (Figure 3). Similar effects were previously observed in an LD animal model [6], where the ability of saffron and its different chemical components to reduce the neuroinflammatory response in the retina was evaluated by the quantification of the number of microglia cells. As observed from in vitro experiments, saffron in stigmas had a strong neuroprotective activity. The fraction containing crocins showed neuroprotective effects, although with greater variability; the fraction containing kaempferol derivates and picrocrocin reduced the number of cells of the microglia in the retina but with less significance. All these data highlight the importance of crocins in the neuroprotection of the retina; however, they clearly point out that the single component or different components together were not able to reproduce the effect obtained with the whole saffron extract and confirmed the complexity of its way of action. These results are not surprising, since the two fractions, although representative of the chemical composition of saffron, are obtained by specific extraction methods that may miss certain compounds of the spice.

Different studies have examined the toxicity of saffron. From in vivo studies, saffron has very low toxicity for doses of up to 1.5 g per day, while at high doses, it causes illness: daily doses ≥ 5 g can induce intestinal bleeding [42]. Ayatollahi et al. (2013) [43] excluded side effects in 60 healthy volunteers related to a treatment with saffron (doses ranging from 200 to 400 mg) for 7 days. Accordingly, it is possible to affirm with confidence that in our case, the treatment with saffron showed no side effects at least at the dose used in humans, considering that patients were treated with amounts 10–20 times lower (20 mg/die).

Several studies conducted in mice and rats showed that the metabolic fate of crocetin and crocins is very different from the one of other C40 carotenoids [44,45]. The orally administered crocins are not detectable in the plasma of rats [44], and its concentration does not tend to accumulate after repeated doses of oral crocins. As for humans, it seems that crocins are absorbed very quickly compared to other carotenoids and that they are eliminated within 8 hours. [46]. Our data indicated that crocins and crocetin were present in the retina of LD animals while in healthy animals, saffron metabolites were found only in the plasma; no traces of crocins and crocetin were present in the retina of healthy animals (Figure 5). The most likely hypothesis is that crocins may be resynthesized from crocetin. Crocetin might reach the retina only as a result of damage of the blood-brain barrier [5]. These data were confirmed by the analysis of the blood and urine samples of patients with AMD and healthy volunteers. Crocetin was found only in the samples of healthy volunteers and not in patients. From the results of this study, it is reasonable to think that only patients with AMD quickly process saffron metabolites [47]. Further experiments are necessary to exploit this interesting point as this is only a suggestion.

Saffron appears to have high potential for the treatment of neurodegenerative diseases. Altogether, the results obtained both "in vivo" and "in vitro" support the hypothesis of multiple and integrated ways of action able to cope with neurodegenerative processes. One possibility might be that saffron globally activates tissue resilience, as it has been recently hypothesized [48]. This complex action might be supported by the integrated activity of the entire molecular composition of saffron with a very precise chemical profile.

4. Materials and Methods

4.1. Chemical Analysis of Saffron

We used an HPLC method and spectrophotometric analysis to analyze saffron stigmas, from different regions (Abruzzo, Tuscany, Sardinia, Umbria and Sicily) and from foreign countries (Morocco, Iran, Greece, India, New Zealand, Tasmania, Egypt, and Spain).

Sample preparation for spectrophotometric analysis was carried out according to the procedure ISO-3632 [29], but saffron and solvent amounts were reduced proportionally. About 50 mg of saffron stigma were gently ground in a mortar. In total, 10 mg of powdered sample were suspended in a 20 mL volumetric flask filled with 18 mL of distilled water; the suspension was kept under magnetic stirring for 1 h in the dark and finally diluted to 20 mL. The spectrophotometric measurement was carried out on a suitable aliquot of aqueous extract after a 10 fold dilution and filtration on a 0.45 µM Whatman Spartan 13/0.2 RC (Whatman, GE Healthcare Life Sciences, Little Chalfont, UK) cellulose filter. The UV-vis spectra were acquired in the 200–700 nm range with a Cary 50 Probe (Agilent Techologies, Santa Clara, CA, USA) spectrophotometer using a 1 cm pathway quartz cuvette and pure water for blank correction. The spectra were recorded with a 1 nm resolution. Chromatographic analysis was done using method II of the paper [49].

4.2. Animal Model

The Italian Ministry of Health (authorization number 83/96-A of 29/11/1996) authorized the experiments on animals. In addition, all procedures were in line with the ARVO Statement for the Use of Animals in Ophthalmic and Vision Research and were approved by the local Ethical Committee of University of L'Aquila. We followed the protocol extensively reported in Maccarone et al. (2008) [2] for both light-induced damage treatment and histological analysis.

4.2.1. Light Damage (LD)

Sprague-Dawley adult albino rats (2 months old) born and raised in our colony at 5 lux mean luminance were moved singularly into a cage with cold-white fluorescent lights placed at the top and at the bottom to ensure an iso-luminance environment (1000 lux) inside the cage. The litter was removed from the cage to prevent rats from hiding their eyes from the light. Light exposure started at the beginning of the day phase in the animal house, therefore immediately after the 12 hours of darkness. Animals were consecutively exposed to 1000 lux light for 24 hours, and immediately after, they were placed back into normal cages and returned to normal conditions.

4.2.2. Saffron Treatment

The animals belonging to the "LD + saffron" group were treated with saffron to test neuroprotection. Stigmas of saffron (previously tested for their chemical composition) were dissolved in water to obtain a suspension, and 1 mg/kg was offered daily to rats, for 7 days before the light damage. Saffron treatment uninterruptedly continued during the whole recovery period up to the sacrifice of the animals (7 days after LD).

4.2.3. Immunohistochemistry and Morphological Evaluation by Quantitative Histology

One week after bright light exposure, the eyes were enucleated and fixed in 4% paraformaldehyde for 1 hour, washed in 0.1 M phosphate-buffered saline (PBS, pH 7.4), and cryoprotected by immersion in 15% sucrose overnight. Eyes were embedded in optimum cutting temperature (OCT) compound (TissueTek; Qiagen, Valencia, CA, USA), snap frozen in liquid nitrogen/isopentane, and cryosectioned at 20 µM. Sections were collected on gelatin- and poly-L-lysine-coated slides. Sections were three 5-minute washed in PBS and counterstaining with DNA-specific label, bisbenzamide (Hoechst) 1:10,000, for 1 minute at room temperature (RT) to measure the thickness of the photoreceptor layer. The outer nuclear layer (ONL) thickness was measured starting at the dorsal edge along the vertical meridian crossing the optic nerve. Measurements were reported at 1-mm intervals (each point was the mean of four measurements at 250 µM intervals). In each retina, we measured two sections. Images were taken using a confocal microscope (Nikon, Tokyo, Japan) and fluorescence microscope (Nikon).

4.3. Solid-Phase Extraction (SPE)

Saffron extract was separated into two fractions: one containing the most polar active components (kaempferol derivates and picrocrocin) and another containing the crocins, the most apolar molecules.

The separation of the different chemical components of saffron was carefully managed with the following solid-phase extraction (SPE) procedure: saffron sample (40 mg) was suspended in 40 mL of a 50/50 CH_3OH/H_2O v/v mixture, under magnetic stirring for 1 hour in the dark. Subsequently, it was centrifuged at 1000 rpm for 5 minutes and the supernatant was dried in a vacuum distiller (rotavapor: 30 °C, 150 rpm). The dry sample was dissolved in a volume of 20 mL of deionized water. The sample was passed through an appropriate SPE C18 cartridge (ISOLUTE with 1 g of stationary phase). The extraction steps were:

1. Conditioning: 2 × 5 mL Hexane 2 × 5 mL Methanol (alternating).
2. Loading: 15 mL of extract 40 mg recovered in 20 mL H_2O.
3. Elution A: 2 × 1 mL H_2O-EtOH (75:25).
4. Elution B: 2 × 1 mL EtOH (100%).

With elution A, we obtained the fraction characterized by the presence of kaempferol derivates and picrocrocin, and with elution B, we obtained the fraction constituted by *trans* and *cis* crocins. The entire extraction procedure was repeated simultaneously at least three times for each kind of tested sorbent material.

The two fractions were characterized by an HPLC system used for saffron analysis. After the HPLC analysis, the fractions were dried with a vacuum dryer to remove ethanol and were dissolved in water for animal treatment [2].

We evaluated the effect of two main saffron components, crocins (fraction 1) and picocrocins/kaempferol derivates (fraction 2), on two cellular models.

4.4. Cell Cultures

The mouse retinal photoreceptor-derived 661W cell line (kindly provided by Dr. Muayyad Al-Ubaidi (University of Oklahoma Health Sciences Center, OK, USA)) was cultured in Dulbecco minimum essential medium supplemented with 10% FBS, 10% L-glutamine, 100 units/mL penicillin, and 100 µg/mL streptomycin (Gibco). Human embryonic kidney cell line HEK293 stably transfected with a pcDNA3 plasmid containing the full-length rat P2X7-GFP cDNA was maintained in Dulbecco's modified Eagle's medium/NutrientMixture F-12 Ham supplemented with 10% FBS, 5 mg/mL gentamycin, and 200 mM glutamine.

4.4.1. Viability Assay

Confluent cells were seeded in 96-well culture plates at a density of 5×10^3 cells/well. After 24 h, cells were incubated with saffron and two fractions of saffron, crocins and picocrocins/kaempferol derivates at a concentration of 25 µg/mL alone and with different concentrations of ATP or 2′(3′)-O-(4-Benzoylbenzoyl)adenosine 5′-triphosphate triethylammonium salt (BzATP). Cell viability was assessed 24 hours after cell treatment by measuring the reduction of 3-(4,5-dimethylthiazol-2-yl)-2,5diphenyltetrazolium bromide (MTT) (Sigma-Aldrich). The absorption at 570 nm was measured using a FLUOstar Omega micro-plate reader.

4.4.2. Intracellular Calcium Measurements

Intracellular calcium measurements $[Ca^{2+}]_i$ were performed by using the fluorescent Ca^{2+} indicator fura-2 AM. Cells were loaded with 5 µM fura-2 AM dissolved in extracellular solution with 0.1% of pluronic acid to improve dye uptake, for 45 minutes at 37 °C. The cell coverslip was placed on the stage of an inverted fluorescence microscope Nikon TE200 (Nikon, Tokyo, Japan) equipped with a dual excitation fluorometric calcium imaging system (Hamamatsu, Sunayama-Cho, Japan). Cells were excited at 340 and 380 nm at a sampling rate of 0.5 Hz, and fluorescence emission, measured at 510 nm, was acquired with a digital CCD camera (Hamamatsu C4742-95-12ER). The external standard solution was composed of (in mM) 135 NaCl, 5.4 KCl, 1 $CaCl_2$, 5 Hepes, and 10 glucose at pH 7.3. The fluorescence ratio F340/F380 was used to monitor $[Ca^{2+}]_i$ changes. Monochromator settings, chopper frequency, and data acquisition were controlled by a dedicated software (Aquacosmos/Ratio U7501-01, Hamamatsu).

Data were analyzed using IgorPro (Wavemetrics. Portland, Oregon). Results are presented as mean ± standard error of at least 4 independent experiments. Statistical analysis was performed using student's *t* test or one-way ANOVA to compare the different data sets. Differences were regarded as statistically significant for * $p < 0.05$ and ** $p < 0.01$.

4.5. Tissue Analysis for Saffron Metabolites

We analyzed saffron metabolites in different tissues in both animal models and in blood and urine of AMD patients. We used an animal model with induced photoreceptor degeneration [2], treated with saffron through the diet at a dose of 5 mg/kg for a week. As an experimental control group, we used animals without degeneration treated with saffron. The analyzed samples of tissue were retina, plasma, urine, kidney, and liver. Plasma and urine samples from healthy volunteers and AMD patients who took saffron for over a year were analyzed. The samples were analyzed using the solid-phase extraction procedure (SPE) of Yamauchi et al. (2011) [30]. The different tissues were combined with 2.0 mL of methanol, then centrifuged (3000 rpm, 10 minutes) and subjected to the extraction procedure. The various eluates were analyzed with the following HPLC system: Sinergy 4 µM Fusion-RP column (250 × 150 nm, Phenomenex), photodiode array detector (DAD, 210–500 nm, Waters) [5].

Author Contributions: Conceptualization: C.P., S.B., M.A.M. Data analysis and investigation: C.P., M.A.M. Writing original draft preparation: C.P., S.B., M.A.M. Writing review and editing: C.P., S.B., M.A.M. All authors have read and agreed to the published version of the manuscript.

Funding: Institutional fundings (CNR) and Hortus Novus srl. Sponsors.had no role in study design, data collection and analysis, decision to publish, or preparation of the manuscript.

Acknowledgments: We wish to remember our esteemed colleague Mario Nobile, who left us untimely, and acknowledge his valuable contribution to these studies. We thank Francesca Quartino for technical assistance on cell cultures. We thank researchers, postgraduates, Ph.D. students and students from Bisti's lab. We thank Joachim Scholz-Starke for the critical revision of the manuscript.

Conflicts of Interest: S. Bisti and M. A. Maggi are inventors of the following international patent.: "Compositions based on saffron for the prevention and/or treatment of degenerative eye disorders", 2015 (W02015/145316) and is owned by Hortus Novus srl, to which is linked a mark (Repron TM) that attests the quality of ophthalmic saffron. S.B. holds a non-remunerative relationship with Hortus Novus srl.

References

1. Serrano-Díaz, J.; Sanchez, A.M.; Martínez-Tomé, M.; Winterhalter, P.; Alonso, G.L. Flavonoid Determination in the Quality Control of Floral Bioresidues from *Crocus sativus* L. *J. Agric. Food Chem.* **2014**, *62*, 3125–3133. [CrossRef]
2. Maccarone, R.; Di Marco, S.; Bisti, S. Saffron Supplement Maintains Morphology and Function after Exposure to Damaging Light in Mammalian Retina. *Investig. Opthalmol. Vis. Sci.* **2008**, *49*, 1254–1261. [CrossRef]
3. Natoli, R.; Zhu, Y.; Valter, K.; Bisti, S.; Eells, J.; Stone, J. Gene and noncoding RNA regulation un-derly-ing photoreceptor protection: Microarray study of dietary antioxidant saffron and photobi-omodulation in rat retina. *Mol. Vis.* **2010**, *16*, 1801–1822.
4. Corso, L.; Cavallero, A.; Baroni, D.; Garbati, P.; Prestipino, G.; Bisti, S.; Nobile, M.; Picco, C. Saffron reduces ATP-induced retinal cytotoxicity by targeting P2X7 receptors. *Purinergic Signal.* **2016**, *12*, 161–174. [CrossRef]
5. Bisti, S.; Maccarone, R.; Falsini, B. Saffron and retina: Neuroprotection and pharmacokinetics. *Vis. Neurosci.* **2014**, *31*, 355–361. [CrossRef] [PubMed]
6. Bisti, S.; Di Marco, S.; Maggi, M.A.; Di Paolo, M.; Piccardi, M.; Falsini, B. Saffron Shifts the Degenera-tive and Inflammatory Phenotype in Photoreceptor Degeneration. In *Saffron the Age-Old Panacea in a New Light*; Elsevier: Amsterdam, The Netherlands, 2020; Chapter 14.
7. Maccarone, R.; Rapino, C.; Zerti, D.; Di Tommaso, M.; Battista, N.; Di Marco, S.; Bisti, S.; Maccarrone, M. Modulation of Type-1 and Type-2 Cannabinoid Receptors by Saffron in a Rat Model of Retinal Neurodegeneration. *PLoS ONE* **2016**, *11*, e0166527. [CrossRef] [PubMed]
8. Di Marco, S.; Carnicelli, V.; Franceschini, N.; Di Paolo, M.; Piccardi, M.; Bisti, S.; Falsini, B. Saffron: A Multitask Neuroprotective Agent for Retinal Degenerative Diseases. *Antioxidants* **2019**, *8*, 224. [CrossRef] [PubMed]
9. Piccardi, M.; Fadda, A.; Martelli, F.; Marangoni, D.; Magli, A.; Minnella, A.M.; Bertelli, M.; Di Marco, S.; Bisti, S.; Falsini, B. Antioxidant Saffron and Central Retinal Function in ABCA4-Related Stargardt Macular Dystrophy. *Nutrients* **2019**, *11*, 2461. [CrossRef] [PubMed]
10. Falsini, B.; Piccardi, M.; Minnella, A.; Savastano, M.C.; Capoluongo, E.; Fadda, A.; Balestrazzi, E.; Maccarone, R.; Bisti, S. Influence of Saffron Supplementation on Retinal Flicker Sensitivity in Early Age-Related Macular Degeneration. *Investig. Opthalmol. Vis. Sci.* **2010**, *51*, 6118–6124. [CrossRef] [PubMed]
11. Heitmar, R.; Brown, J.E.; Kyrou, I. Saffron (*Crocus sativus* L.) in Ocular Diseases: A Narrative Review of the Existing Evidence from Clinical Studies. *Nutrients* **2019**, *11*, 649. [CrossRef] [PubMed]
12. Piccardi, M.; Marangoni, D.; Minnella, A.M.; Savastano, M.C.; Valentini, P.; Ambrosio, L.; Capoluongo, E.D.; Maccarone, R.; Bisti, S.; Falsini, B. A Longitudinal Follow-Up Study of Saffron Supplementation in Early Age-Related Macular Degeneration: Sustained Benefits to Central Retinal Function. *Evid. Based Complement. Altern. Med.* **2012**, *2012*. [CrossRef] [PubMed]
13. Bathaie, S.Z.; Farajzade, A.; Hoshyar, R. A review of the chemistry and uses of crocins and crocetin, the carotenoid natural dyes in saffron, with particular emphasis on applications as colorants including their use as biological stains. *Biotech. Histochem.* **2014**, *89*, 401–411. [CrossRef]
14. Lozano, P.; Castellar, M.; Simancas, M.; Iborra, J.L. A quantitative high-performance liquid chromatographic method to analyse commercial saffron (*Crocus sativus* L.) products. *J. Chromatogr. A* **1999**, *830*, 477–483. [CrossRef]
15. Rubert, J.; Lacina, O.; Zachariasova, M.; Hajslova, J. Saffron authentication based on liquid chromatography high resolution tandem mass spectrometry and multivariate data analysis. *Food Chem.* **2016**, *204*, 201–209. [CrossRef] [PubMed]
16. Han, J.; Wanrooij, J.; Van Bommel, M.; Quye, A. Characterisation of chemical components for identifying historical Chinese textile dyes by ultra high performance liquid chromatography photodiode array electrospray ionisation mass spectrometer. *J. Chromatogr. A* **2017**, *1479*, 87–96. [CrossRef]
17. Moras, B.; Loffredo, L.; Rey, S. Quality assessment of saffron (*Crocus sativus* L.) extracts via UHPLC-DAD-MS analysis and detection of adulteration using gardenia fruit extract (Gardenia jasminoides Ellis). *Food Chem.* **2018**, *257*, 325–332. [CrossRef]
18. D'Archivio, A.A.; Di Donato, F.; Foschi, M.; Maggi, M.A.; Ruggieri, F. UHPLC Analysis of Saffron (*Crocus sativus* L.): Optimization of Separation Using Chemometrics and Detection of Minor Crocetin Esters. *Molecules* **2018**, *23*, 1851. [CrossRef]

19. Bouvier, F.; Suire, C.; Mutterer, J.; Camara, B. Oxidative Remodeling of Chromoplast Carotenoids: Identi-fication of the carotenoid dioxygenase CsCCD and CsZCD genes involved in *Crocus secondary* metab-olite biogenesis. *Plant Cell* **2003**, *15*, 47–62. [CrossRef]
20. Moraga Ángela, R.; Nohales, P.F.; Pérez, J.A.F.; Gómez-Gómez, L. Glucosylation of the saffron apocarotenoid crocetin by a glucosyltransferase isolated from *Crocus sativus* stigmas. *Planta* **2004**, *219*, 955–966. [CrossRef]
21. Himeno, H.; Sano, K. Synthesis of Crocin, Picrocrocin and Safranal by Saffron Stigma-like Structures Proliferated in Vitro. *Agric. Biol. Chem.* **1987**, *51*, 2395–2400. [CrossRef]
22. Carmona, M.; Zalacain, A.; Sanchez, A.M.; Novella, A.J.L.; Alonso, G.L. Crocetin Esters, Picrocrocin and Its Related Compounds Present in *Crocus sativus* Stigmas and Gardenia jasminoides Fruits. Tentative Identification of Seven New Compounds by LC-ESI-M S. *J. Agric. Food Chem.* **2006**, *54*, 973–979. [CrossRef] [PubMed]
23. Cossignani, L.; Urbani, E.; Simonetti, M.S.; Maurizi, A.; Chiesi, C.; Blasi, F. Characterisation of secondary metabolites in saffron from central Italy (Cascia, Umbria). *Food Chem.* **2014**, *143*, 446–451. [CrossRef] [PubMed]
24. Tarantilis, P.A.; Tsoupras, G.; Polissiou, M. Determination of saffron (*Crocus sativus* L.) components in crude plant extract using high-performance liquid chromatography-UV-visible photodiode-array detection-mass spectrometry. *J. Chromatogr. A* **1995**, *699*, 107–118. [CrossRef]
25. Lech, K.; Witowska-Jarosz, J.; Jarosz, M. Saffron yellow: Characterization of carotenoids by high performance liquid chromatography with electrospray mass spectrometric detection. *J. Mass Spectrom.* **2009**, *44*, 1661–1667. [CrossRef] [PubMed]
26. Koulakiotis, N.S.; Pittenauer, E.; Halabalaki, M.; Tsarbopoulos, A.; Allmaier, G. Comparison of different tandem mass spectrometric techniques (ESI-IT, ESI- and IP-MALDI-QRTOF and vMALDI-TOF/RTOF) for the analysis of crocins and picrocrocin from the stigmas of *Crocus sativus* L. *Rapid Commun. Mass Spectrom.* **2012**, *26*, 670–678. [CrossRef]
27. Li, N.; Lin, G.; Kwan, Y.W.; Min, Z.-D. Simultaneous quantification of five major biologically active ingredients of saffron by high-performance liquid chromatography. *J. Chromatogr. A* **1999**, *849*, 349–355. [CrossRef]
28. Sanchez, A.M.; Carmona, M.; Zalacain, A.; Carot, J.M.; Jabaloyes, J.M.; Alonso, G.L.; Carmona, M. Rapid Determination of Crocetin Esters and Picrocrocin from Saffron Spice (*Crocus sativus* L.) Using UV-Visible Spectrophotometry for Quality Control. *J. Agric. Food Chem.* **2008**, *56*, 3167–3175. [CrossRef]
29. ISO 3632-2. *Saffron (Crocus sativus L.) Part 2 (Test Methods)*; International Organization for Stand-Ardiza-Tion Genève: Genève, Switzerland, 2010.
30. Yamauchi, M.; Tsuruma, K.; Imai, S.; Nakanishi, T.; Umigai, N.; Shimazawa, M.; Hara, H. Crocetin prevents retinal degeneration induced by oxidative and endoplasmic reticulum stresses via inhibition of caspase activity. *Eur. J. Pharmacol.* **2011**, *650*, 110–119. [CrossRef]
31. Ohno, Y.; Nakanishi, T.; Umigai, N.; Tsuruma, K.; Shimazawa, M.; Hara, H. Oral administration of crocetin prevents inner retinal damage induced by N-methyl-d-aspartate in mice. *Eur. J. Pharmacol.* **2012**, *690*, 84–89. [CrossRef]
32. Fernández-Sánchez, L.; Lax, P.; Esquiva, G.; Martín-Nieto, J.; Pinilla, I.; Cuenca, N. Safranal, a Saffron Constituent, Attenuates Retinal Degeneration in P23H Rats. *PLoS ONE* **2012**, *7*, e43074. [CrossRef]
33. Surprenant, A.; Rassendren, F.; Kawashima, E.; North, R.A.; Buell, G. The Cytolytic P2Z Receptor for Extracellular ATP Identified as a P2X Receptor (P2X7). *Science* **1996**, *272*, 735–738. [CrossRef] [PubMed]
34. Giaccio, M. Crocetin from Saffron: An Active Component of an Ancient Spice. *Crit. Rev. Food Sci. Nutr.* **2004**, *44*, 155–172. [CrossRef] [PubMed]
35. Poma, A.; Fontecchio, G.; Carlucci, G.; Chichiricco, G. Anti-Inflammatory Properties of Drugs from saffron crocus. *Anti Inflamm. Anti-Allergy Agents Med. Chem.* **2012**, *11*, 37–51. [CrossRef] [PubMed]
36. Sung, Y.-Y.; Kim, H.K. Crocin Ameliorates Atopic Dermatitis Symptoms by down Regulation of Th2 Response via Blocking of NF-κB/STAT6 Signaling Pathways in Mice. *Nutrients* **2018**, *10*, 1625. [CrossRef] [PubMed]
37. Sperlágh, B.; Vizi, E.S.; Wirkner, K.; Illes, P. P2X7 receptors in the nervous system. *Prog. Neurobiol.* **2006**, *78*, 327–346. [CrossRef] [PubMed]
38. Housley, G.D.; Bringmann, A.; Reichenbach, A. Purinergic signaling in special senses. *Trends Neurosci.* **2009**, *32*, 128–141. [CrossRef] [PubMed]
39. Puthussery, T.; Fletcher, E. Extracellular ATP induces retinal photoreceptor apoptosis through activation of purinoceptors in rodents. *J. Comp. Neurol.* **2009**, *513*, 430–440. [CrossRef]

40. Vessey, K.A.; Jobling, A.; Greferath, U.; Fletcher, E. The Role of the P2X7 Receptor in the Retina: Cell Signalling and Dysfunction. *Biol. Mammary Gland* **2011**, *723*, 813–819. [CrossRef]
41. Zhang, X.; Laties, A.M.; Mitchell, C.H. Stimulation of P2X7 Receptors Elevates Ca2+ and Kills Retinal Ganglion Cells. *Investig. Opthalmol. Vis. Sci.* **2005**, *46*, 2183–2191. [CrossRef]
42. Schmidt, M.V.; Betti, G.; Hensel, A. Saffron in phytotherapy: Pharmacology and clinical uses. *Wien. Med. Wochenschr.* **2007**, *157*, 315–319. [CrossRef]
43. Ayatollahi, H.; Javan, A.O.; Khajedaluee, M.; Shahroodian, M.; Hosseinzadeh, H. Effect of *Crocus sativus* L. (Saffron) on Coagulation and Anticoagulation Systems in Healthy Volunteers. *Phytother. Res.* **2013**, *28*, 539–543. [CrossRef] [PubMed]
44. Xi, L.; Qian, Z.; Du, P.; Fu, J. Pharmacokinetic properties of crocin (crocetin digentiobiose ester) following oral administration in rats. *Phytomedicine* **2007**, *14*, 633–636. [CrossRef] [PubMed]
45. Asai, A.; Nakano, T.; Takahashi, M.; Nagao, A. Orally Administered Crocetin and Crocins Are Absorbed into Blood Plasma as Crocetin and Its Glucuronide Conjugates in Mice. *J. Agric. Food Chem.* **2005**, *53*, 7302–7306. [CrossRef] [PubMed]
46. Umigai, N.; Murakami, K.; Ulit, M.; Antonio, L.; Shirotori, M.; Morikawa, H.; Nakano, T. The pharmacokinetic profile of crocetin in healthy adult human volunteers after a single oral administration. *Phytomedicine* **2011**, *18*, 575–578. [CrossRef] [PubMed]
47. Kanakis, C.D.; Tarantilis, P.A.; Tajmir-Riahi, H.A.; Polissiou, M.G. Crocetin, Dimethylcrocetin, and Safranal Bind Human Serum Albumin: Stability and Antioxidative Properties. *J. Agric. Food Chem.* **2007**, *55*, 970–977. [CrossRef] [PubMed]
48. Stone, J.; Mitrofanis, J.; Johnstone, D.M.; Falsini, B.; Bisti, S.; Adam, P.; Nuevo, A.B.; George-Weinstein, M.; Mason, R.; Eells, J. Acquired Resilience: An Evolved System of Tissue Protection in Mammals. *Dose-Rsponse* **2018**, *16*, 1–40. [CrossRef]
49. D'Archivio, A.A.; Giannitto, A.; Maggi, M.A.; Ruggieri, F. Geographical classification of Italian saffron (*Crocus sativus* L.) based on chemical constituents determined by high-performance liquid-chromatography and by using linear discriminant analysis. *Food Chem.* **2016**, *212*, 110–116. [CrossRef]

Sample Availability: Samples of the compounds are available from the authors.

Publisher's Note: MDPI stays neutral with regard to jurisdictional claims in published maps and institutional affiliations.

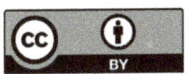

© 2020 by the authors. Licensee MDPI, Basel, Switzerland. This article is an open access article distributed under the terms and conditions of the Creative Commons Attribution (CC BY) license (http://creativecommons.org/licenses/by/4.0/).

Article

The GABA$_A$-Benzodiazepine Receptor Antagonist Flumazenil Abolishes the Anxiolytic Effects of the Active Constituents of *Crocus sativus* L. Crocins in Rats

Nikolaos Pitsikas [1,*] and Petros A. Tarantilis [2]

1. Department of Pharmacology, Faculty of Medicine, School of Health Sciences, University of Thessaly, Biopolis, Panepistimiou 3, 415-00 Larissa, Greece
2. Laboratory of Chemistry, Department of Food Science and Human Nutrition, School of Food and Nutritional Sciences, Agricultural University of Athens, 118-55 Athens, Greece; ptara@aua.gr
* Correspondence: npitsikas@med.uth.gr; Tel.: +30-2410-685535; Fax: +30-2410-685552

Academic Editor: Derek J. McPhee
Received: 6 November 2020; Accepted: 28 November 2020; Published: 30 November 2020

Abstract: Anxiety is a chronic severe psychiatric disorder. Crocins are among the various bioactive components of the plant *Crocus sativus* L. (Iridaceae) and their implication in anxiety is well-documented. However, which is the mechanism of action underlying the anti-anxiety effects of crocins remains unknown. In this context, it has been suggested that these beneficial effects might be ascribed to the agonistic properties of these bioactive ingredients of saffron on the GABA type A receptor. The current experimentation was undertaken to clarify this issue in the rat. For this research project, the light/dark and the open field tests were used. A single injection of crocins (50 mg/kg, i.p., 60 min before testing) induces an anti-anxiety-like effect revealed either in the light-dark or open field tests. Acute administration of the GABA$_A$-benzodiazepine receptor antagonist flumazenil (10 mg/kg, i.p., 30 min before testing) abolished the above mentioned anxiolytic effects of crocins. The current findings suggest a functional interaction between crocins and the GABA$_A$ receptor allosteric modulator flumazenil on anxiety.

Keywords: crocins; flumazenil; anxiety; rat

1. Introduction

Anxiety is a serious psychiatric disease. Various forms of this psychiatric disorder, such as generalized anxiety disorder (GAD), specific phobias (agoraphobia, social phobia, etc.), post-traumatic stress disorder (PTSD), obsessive-compulsive disorder (OCD) and panic disorder have been described. Common features of all these disorders are temporary worry and exaggerated fear [1].

Although a conspicuous number of pharmacological approaches are actually used aiming to alleviate the symptoms of this psychiatric pathology [f.i., benzodiazepines, partial agonists of the serotonergic 5-HT$_{1A}$ receptor, selective serotonin reuptake inhibitors (SSRIs)] different types of anxiety do not respond satisfactorily to these medications [2]. Additionally, these medications are often associated to severe side effects [3].

Based on the above, there is a mandatory necessity to unfold novel molecules for the therapy of this severe psychiatric disease [4]. Among the various alternative approaches for the treatment of anxiety symptoms, the involvement of the extracts of the stigmas of *Crocus sativus* L. (saffron) and its bioactive constituents as potential anti-anxiety agents has recently been proposed [5].

Crocus sativus L. (Iridaceae) is a plant cultivated in many countries all around the world including Iran, India, Italy, Spain and Greece. Its product is the well-known spice saffron. Saffron is the dried red stigmas of the flower. The main substances of saffron are crocins, picrocrocin and safranal. Crocins, glucosyl esters of crocetin, are water-soluble carotenoids and are responsible for its characteristic color. Picrocrocin, glycoside of safranal, is responsible for the bitter taste of the spice and is precursor of safranal. Safranal, the main component of the distilled essential oil, is a monoterpene aldehyde, responsible for its characteristic aroma [6,7].

The stigmas of C. sativus L. (saffron) are used in folk medicine as an anticatarrhal, eupeptic, expectorant and emmenagogue [8]. Contemporary preclinical pharmacological studies have demonstrated that saffron's crude extracts and purified chemicals possess anti-tumor effects, display anti-inflammatory properties and counteract atherosclerosis and hepatic damage [8]. Additionally, the outcome of various preclinical and clinical studies suggest a promising effect of saffron and its bioactive constituents in different pathologies of the central nervous system including depression, schizophrenia, memory disorders and anxiety [5].

Specifically, crocins were found to display anxiolytic effects in different behavioral procedures assessing anxiety either in rats [9,10] or mice [11]. However, the mechanism of action underlying the anti-anxiety effects of crocins is not yet elucidated.

Consistent experimental evidence proposes that the anxiolytic effects of benzodiazepines are mediated by their agonistic action on the $GABA_A$ receptor [12]. In this context, it has been observed that some other flavonoids isolated from plants express an affinity for the benzodiazepine binding site at the $GABA_A$ receptor [13,14]. It has been reported that crocins enhance the anti-epileptic properties of diazepam [15] while the anti-convulsant action of safranal seems to be mediated by its agonistic action on the $GABA_A$ receptor [16].

Based on the above, it can be hypothesized that the $GABA_A$ receptor might be a potential target of anxiolytic effects of crocins. The current study was designed to examine this issue. Consequently, the anxiolytic-like effects of crocins in the rat were challenged with the benzodiazepine receptor antagonist, flumazenil. The light/dark box and open field tests were the behavioral paradigms used for this evaluation. The light/dark test is a behavioral procedure that is based on the innate aversion of rodents to strongly illuminated zones and the conflicting tendency of rodents to explore new spaces [17]. The open field test implies an encounter of the rodent with new open spaces and trigger behavioral and physiological reactions associated to anxiety [18].

2. Results

2.1. Experiment 1: Effects of Acute Administration of Crocins and Flumazenil on Rats' Performance in the Light/Dark Test

Data are illustrated in Figure 1. Analysis of the first entry into to the dark chamber (Figure 1A) and the number of transitions between the two compartments data (Figure 1B) did not evidence a statistically significant main effect either of flumazenil or of crocins or a statistically significant interaction between crocins and flumazenil. Analysis of the total time spent in the light chamber data revealed a statistically significant main effect of flumazenil [$F(1,31) = 10.24$, $p = 0.003$], of crocins [$F(1,31) = 10.52$, $p = 0.003$] and a significant flumazenil x crocins interaction [$F(1,31) = 15.02$, $p < 0.001$]. The post-hoc analysis conducted on these data showed that rats treated with vehicle + crocins (50 mg/kg) spent more time in the lit chamber of the apparatus with respect to the vehicle + vehicle, flumazenil (10 mg/kg) + vehicle and flumazenil (10 mg/kg) + crocins (50 mg/kg) groups ($p < 0.05$, Figure 1C).

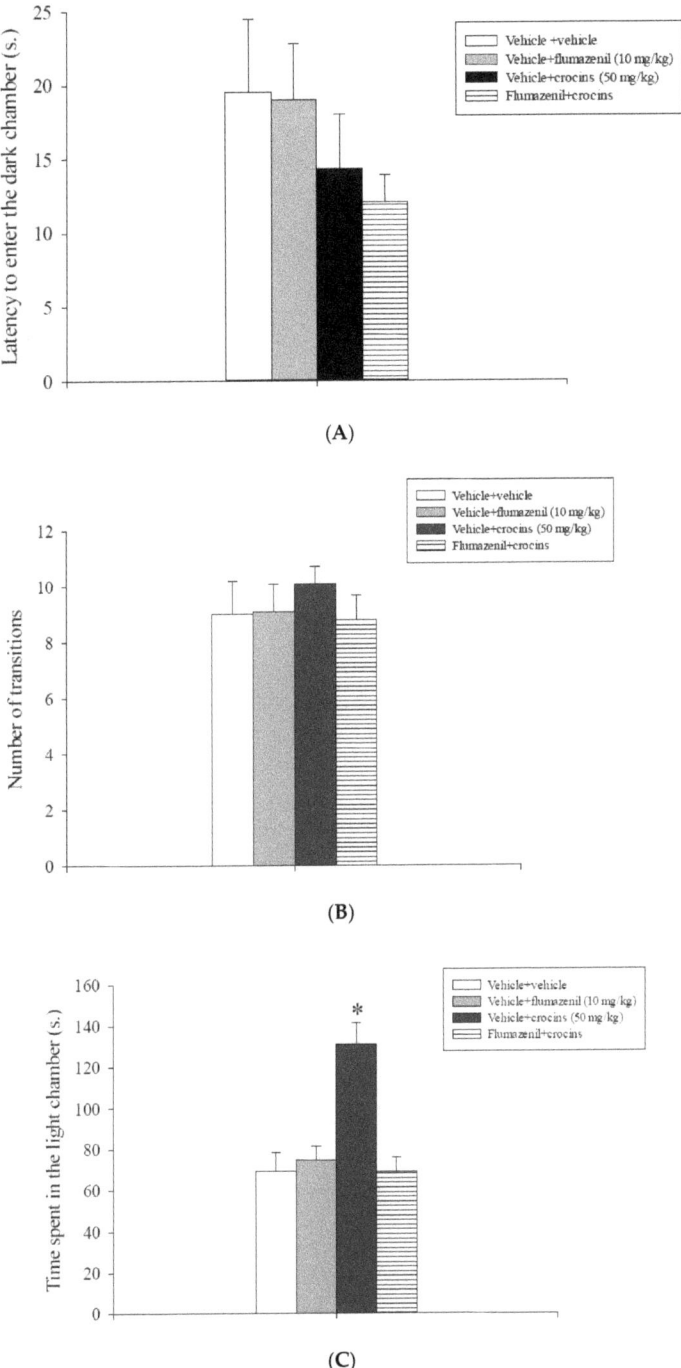

Figure 1. Light/dark box test. Crocins and flumazenil were injected intraperitoneally 60 and 30 min respectively before testing. The graphic illustrates the means ± S.E.M. of 8 rats per experimental group. (**A**) Latency to enter the dark chamber. (**B**) Number of transitions. (**C**) Time spent in the light chamber. * $p < 0.05$ vs. all the other groups.

2.2. Experiment 2: Effects of Acute Administration of Crocins and Flumazenil on Rats' Performance in the Open Field Test

Data are illustrated in Table 1. The effects of acute treatment either with flumazenil or crocins did not affect the number of squares crossed, the rearing and grooming episodes. Interestingly, a main effect of flumazenil [$F(1,31) = 12.5, p = 0.001$], of crocins [$F(1,31) = 9.7, p = 0.004$] and a statistically significant interaction between flumazenil and crocins [$F(1,31) = 15.65, p < 0.001$] was evidenced with regard to the time consumed in the central zone of the arena. The post-hoc comparisons showed that rats that received crocins (50 mg/kg) + vehicle spent more time in the central area of the open field apparatus compared to all the other treatment groups ($p < 0.05$).

Table 1. Effects of acute treatment with crocins and flumazenil on rats' performance in the open field test (n = 8 rats per group).

Treatment	Number of Squares Crossed	Number of Rearings	Time Spent in the Central Zone (s.)	Grooming Duration (s.)
Vehicle + vehicle	96 ± 5.5	29.4 ± 4	7.8 ± 2.3	10.8 ± 2.1
Flumazenil (10 mg/kg) + vehicle	107.3 ± 6.3	32 ± 1.4	9.3 ± 2.1	9.4 ± 1.7
Crocins (50 mg/kg) + vehicle	94.4 ± 4	29 ± 1.5	21.1 ± 1.7 *	7.8 ± 0.8
Flumazenzil + crocins	99.6 ± 4.9	32.8 ± 2.5	8.5 ± 0.7	9.9 ± 0.5

Crocins and flumazenil were injected intraperitoneally 60 or 30 min before testing respectively. The values are mean ± SEM. * $p < 0.05$ vs. all the other groups.

3. Discussions

The light/dark test has been shown to reliably predict the anxiolytic- and anxiogenic-like effects of drugs in rodents [17]. This test has the advantages of being quick and easy to use without prior training of the animals and neither food nor water deprivation is required [19]. Transitions in this test are considered an index of activity/exploration because habituation over time is seen with this measure, whereas the time spent in each compartment reflects aversion/attraction [20].

The open field test is a typical behavioral paradigm of anxiety evaluating neophobia. In this behavioral procedure either mice or rats usually manifest fear for open spaces. Therefore, the amount of time consumed in the central zone of the apparatus reflects an anxiety state [18].

The objective of the current study was to examine whether or not the $GABA_A$-benzodiazepine receptor is involved in the anti-anxiety properties of crocins.

In agreement with previous results of ours, crocins induced anxiolytic-like effects in rats [9,10]. In particular, crocins (50 mg/kg) administered 60 min before testing, in rats augmented the time consumed in the aversive (lit) compartment of the apparatus (light/dark box) and the time consumed in the central zone of the open field arena as compared with all the other experimental groups. It is the first time, to our knowledge, that the anti-anxiety effects of crocins were observed in the open field test. Further, the current findings are in line with prior reports in which the aqueous extracts of saffron and crocin were found to reduce stress-induced anorexia [11] in mice and diminish anxiety symptoms assessed in the elevated plus maze test and freezing behavior in rats [21].

The $GABA_A$-benzodiazepine receptor antagonist flumazenil blocked the anxiolytic effects of crocins in both anxiety procedures tested. Flumazenil on its own was inactive either in the light/dark or in the open field test. The results here exposed propose that the anxiolytic effects of crocins may be mediated by their interaction with the benzodiazepine binding site on the $GABA_A$ receptor.

Chemicals that influence general activity may alter rodents' performance in anxiety tests because of changes in motoric activity that are unrelated to any anxiogenic- or anxiolytic effects of the compound. The results here presented cannot be ascribed to a potential action exerted by both crocins and flumazenil on general activity because the number of transitions between the two different compartments in the light/dark box test and the number of squares crossed and number of rearing events registered in the open field test did not vary among the different treatment groups.

Our results are in contrast with a recent study in which flumazenil was found unable to reverse the effects of crocins on anxiety [22]. Important differences however, underlie this discrepancy. In the present study, crocins (50 mg/kg) were injected 60 min before testing and displayed their anxiolytic profile in agreement with previous studies [9,10]. Further, flumazenil was injected at the dose of 10 mg/kg, 30 min before testing. On the contrary, in the study by Ceremuga and colleagues [22] the treatment schedule of compounds was different to that used in our study. Specifically, crocins (50 mg/kg, 30 min before testing) failed to induce an anti-anxiety effect while flumazenil was administered at a lower dose and at different time point (3 mg/kg, 10 min before testing) and did not affect crocins performance.

It is well-documented that flumazenil counteracted the anxiolytic effects also of non-benzodiazepine compounds (f.i., 5-HT$_{1A}$ receptor agonists and 5-HT$_3$ receptor antagonists). This suggests that the GABA$_A$-benzodiazepine receptor may be a common downstream component of different neurochemical systems modulating anxiety states [23].

The observed reversal of the effects of flumazenil on crocins anxiolytic effects corroborates the hypothesis of crocins acting directly or indirectly on the GABA$_A$-benzodiazepine receptor. A direct interaction of crocins with the GABA$_A$ receptor complex might involve their action on Cl$^-$ conductance. An indirect action of crocins might reside on the modulation of metabolism or regulation of GABA release. Research is mandatory in order to evaluate this hypothesis.

The GABA type A receptor is a pentameric ligand-gated chloride channel constituted of distinct classes of subunits ($\alpha1$–$\alpha6$, $\beta1$–$\beta3$, $\gamma1$–$\gamma3$, δ, ϵ, θ, π and $\rho1$–$\rho3$). This receptor is a molecular target for various classes of benzodiazepine-site ligands. It has been suggested that binding to the $\alpha2$ subunit is crucial for the anxiolytic effects of benzodiazepines [24]. Thus, by utilizing appropriate ligands it will be of interest to investigate whether or not the anxiolytic effects of crocins might be mediated by their interaction with the $\alpha2$ subunit of the GABA$_A$ receptor. In line with the above, additional studies should be performed aiming to elucidate if the anti-anxiety effects displayed by crocins can be mediated also by other types of receptors related to GABAergic, serotonergic or to glutamatergic system.

In summary, the present results suggest that the GABA$_A$-benzodiazepine receptor complex might modulate crocins' beneficial effects on anxiety. The current findings also indicate a functional interaction between crocins and the benzodiazepine ligand site.

4. Materials and Methods

4.1. Drugs

Crocins used in the current experimentation were derived from the same batch of plant material (saffron) and the same purification procedure, extraction and separation. Our plant material was kindly offered by the Cooperative of Saffron, Krokos, Kozani, Greece.

Crocins were isolated from the red dried stigmas of *C. sativus* using a slightly modified method described previously [25]. They were purified from stigmas after successive and exhaustive extraction by: (a) petroleum ether 40–60 °C; (b) diethyl ether (Et$_2$O) and (c) methanol (MeOH) 80% using ultrasound assisted extraction. The ultrasound extraction was performed in a Sonorex, Super RK 255H type (300 mm × 150 mm × 150 mm internal dimensions) ultrasound water bath (indirect sonication), at the fixed frequency of 35 kHz. The temperature of the sonicated water was 25 °C. Procedures (a) and (b) took place in order for the stigmas to be free the final extract from the presence of unwanted compounds such as lipids, safranal and picrocrocin. The methanol extract after evaporation (condensed to dryness) under vacuum at room temperature, provided crocins, which are dark red powder residue. Crocins are unusual water-soluble carotenoids (glucosyl esters of crocetin). The chemical profile of crocins has been well documented in previous studies [7,26–28] and we evaluated the quality of the fresh prepared extract used in this study. The major component is a digentiobiosyl ester of crocetin [29]. The purity of crocins was 85% (by HPLC). Crocins were dissolved in saline (NaCl 0.9%). The dose of crocins (50 mg/kg) which induced the highest anti-anxiety properties under to our experimental conditions was selected based on previous findings [9,10]. Specifically, in a previous study designed to test at which concentration crocins might display an anti-anxiety it has been demonstrated that crocins were effective as anxiolytic agents at 50 but not at 15 or 30 mg/kg [9].

Flumazenil (Sigma, St. Louis, MO, USA) was dissolved in saline containing 0.1% Tween 80. The dose of flumazenil (10 mg/kg) was selected based on previous studies [30,31] and our unpublished observations. In those studies [30,31] flumazenil reversed the anxiolytic effects of different potential anti-anxiety agents as are the g-hydroxybutyrate, a product of GABA metabolism and MGS0039, a selective group II metabotropic glutamate receptor antagonist.

All drug solutions were freshly prepared on the day of testing and were administered intraperitoneally (i.p.) in a volume of 1 mL/kg. For all studies, control animals received isovolumetric amounts of the specific vehicle solutions.

4.2. Animals

Independent groups of naive male (3-month-old) Wistar rats (Hellenic Pasteur Institute, Athens, Greece) weighing 250–300 g were used. The animals were housed in Makrolon cages (47.5 cm length × 20.5 cm height × 27 cm width), three per cage in a regulated environment (21 ± 1 °C; 50–55% relative humidity; 12-h/12-h light/dark cycle, lights on at 07.00 h) with free access to food and water.

The procedures that involved animals and their care were in accordance with international guidelines and national (Animal Act, P.D. 160/91) and international laws and policies (EEC Council Directive 86/609, JL 358, 1, 12 December 1987). Experiments were approved by the local committee (Prefecture of Larissa, Greece, protocol number 255200/1 October 2020).

4.3. Behavior

4.3.1. Light/Dark Test

The light/dark box apparatus consisted of a wooden box (48 cm length × 24 cm height × 27 cm width) divided into two equal-size chambers by a barrier that contained a doorway (10 cm height × 10 cm width). One of the chambers was painted black and was covered with a lid and the other chamber was painted white and illuminated with a 60-W light bulb placed 40 cm above the upper edge of the apparatus. Testing was conducted in agreement to a prior report [32]. In brief, on the test day, animals were moved to the obscured test room and remained in their home cages for 2 h. Subsequently, the rats were positioned in the middle of the lit chamber, facing away from the dark chamber. Animals were allowed to freely move the test apparatus for 5 min. The latency to enter (with all four paws) the dark chamber, number of transitions and time spent in the light and dark compartments were registered.

4.3.2. Open Field Test

The test apparatus consisted of a dark arena made of Plexiglas (70 cm length × 50 cm height × 70 cm width). The open field was divided-by black lines-into 16 squares of 17.5×17.5 cm^2. The central four squares were defined as the central area, in which rats' behavior was considered as a measure of anxiety [18]. The test was conducted in agreement to previous reports [32,33]. On the test day, the rats were moved to the dimly illuminated (20 lux) test room and remained their home cages for 2 h. Subsequently, each rat was positioned in the same corner of the apparatus and its behavior was registered for 5 min. The parameters recorded were: (a) the total time spent in the central area of the open field arena as defined by all forepaws being in the central four squares of the apparatus, (b) the number of squares crossed (which reflects horizontal activity), (c) the number of rearing episodes (which reflects vertical activity, defined as raising both forepaws above the floor while balancing on hind limbs) and (d) the duration of self-grooming episodes.

4.4. Experimental Protocol

Daily testing was carried out between 9:00 AM and 3:00 PM during the light phase of the light/dark cycle. To avoid the presence of olfactory traces, all the apparatuses (light/dark box and open field apparatus) were intensively cleaned with 20% ethanol and then wiped with dry paper after each animals' performance.

Animals' behavior in the light/dark and open field tests was video-recorded. Data evaluation was performed by an experimenter who was not involved in the experimental protocol.

4.4.1. Experiment 1: Effects of Acute Challenge with Crocins and Flumazenil on Animals' Performance in the Light/Dark Test

Animals were randomly divided into four experimental groups with 8 rats per group as follows: vehicle (NaCl 0.9%) + vehicle (NaCl 0.9% containing 0.1% Tween 80); vehicle (NaCl 0.9% containing 0.1% Tween 80) + flumazenil (10 mg/kg); vehicle (NaCl 0.9%) + crocins (50 mg/kg) and flumazenil (10 mg/kg) + crocins (50 mg/kg). Control rats were treated with the vehicle 60 and 30 min i.p. respectively before testing. Crocins and flumazenil were injected 60 and 30 min respectively before testing.

4.4.2. Experiment 2: Effects of Acute Challenge with Crocins and Flumazenil on Animals' Performance in the Open Field Test

The same experimental design used in experiment 1 was applied for experiment 2.

4.5. Statistical Analysis

Data are expressed as mean ± S.E.M. Data were analyzed using the two-way analysis of variance (ANOVA). The factors were flumazenil and crocins. Post-hoc comparisons between treatment means were made with the Tukey's post-hoc test. Values of $p < 0.05$ were considered statistically significant.

Author Contributions: Conceptualization, N.P.; methodology, N.P. and P.A.T.; formal analysis, N.P. and P.A.T.; investigation, N.P.; data curation, N.P.; writing-original draft preparation, N.P. and P.A.T. All authors have read and agreed to the published version of the manuscript.

Funding: This research was funded by the Research Committee of the University of Thessaly (grant number 5490) to Nikolaos Pitsikas.

Conflicts of Interest: The authors declare no conflict of interest.

References

1. Steimer, T. The biology of fear-and anxiety-related behaviors. *Dialogues Clin. Neurosci.* **2002**, *28*, 123–137.
2. Hammer, M.B.; Robert, S.; Fruech, B.S. Treatment-resistant posttraumatic stress disorder: Strategies for intervention. *CNS Spectr.* **2004**, *9*, 740–752. [CrossRef] [PubMed]
3. Cryan, J.F.; Sweeney, F.F. The age of anxiety: Role of animal models of anxiolytic action in drug discovery. *Br. J. Pharmacol.* **2011**, *164*, 1129–1161. [CrossRef] [PubMed]
4. Gorman, J.M. New molecule targets for antianxiety interventions. *J. Clin. Psychiatry* **2003**, *64*, 28–35.
5. Pitsikas, N. Constituents of saffron (*Crocus sativus* L.) as potential candidates for the treatment of anxiety disorders and schizophrenia. *Molecules* **2016**, *21*, 303. [CrossRef]
6. Kanakis, C.D.; Daferera, D.J.; Tarantilis, P.A.; Polissiou, M.G. Qualitative determination of volatile compounds and quantitative evaluation of safranal and 4-hydroxy-2,6,6-trimethyl-1-cyclohexene-1-carboxaldehyde. *J. Agric. Food Chem.* **2004**, *52*, 4515–4521. [CrossRef]
7. Tarantilis, P.A.; Tsoupras, G.; Polissiou, M. Determination of saffron (*Crocus sativus* L.) components in crude plant extract using high-performance liquid chromatography-UV/Visible photodiode-array detection-mass spectrometry. *J. Chromatogr.* **1995**, *699*, 107–118. [CrossRef]
8. Rios, J.L.; Recio, M.C.; Ginger, R.M.; Manz, S. An update review of saffron and its active constituents. *Phytother. Res.* **1996**, *10*, 189–193. [CrossRef]
9. Pitsikas, N.; Boultadakis, A.; Georgiadou, G.; Tarantilis, P.A.; Sakellaridis, N. Effects of the active constituents of *Crocus sativus*, L., crocins, in an animal model of anxiety. *Phytomedicine* **2008**, *15*, 1135–1139. [CrossRef]

10. Georgiadou, G.; Tarantilis, P.A.; Pitsikas, N. Effects of the active constituents of *Crocus sativus* L., crocins in an animal model of obsessive-compulsive disorder. *Neurosci. Lett.* **2012**, *528*, 27–30. [CrossRef]
11. Halatei, B.S.; Khosravi, M.; Sahrei, H.; Golmanesch, L.; Zardooz, H.; Jalili, C.; Ghoshoomi, H. Saffron (*Crocus sativus*) aqueous extract and its constituent crocin reduces stress-induced anorexia in mice. *Phytother. Res.* **2011**, *25*, 1833–1838. [CrossRef] [PubMed]
12. Shekhar, A. GABA receptors in the region of the dorsomedial hypothalamus of rats mediate anxiety in the elevated plus-maze test. I. Behavioral measures. *Brain Res.* **1993**, *627*, 9–16. [CrossRef]
13. Ai, J.; Dekermendjian, K.; Wang, X.; Nielsen, M.; Witt, M.R. 6-methylflavone, a benzodiazepine receptor ligand with antagonistic properties on rat brain and human recombinant GABA(A) receptors in vitro. *Drug Dev. Res.* **1997**, *41*, 99–106. [CrossRef]
14. Marder, M.; Estiu, G.; Blanch, L.B.; Viola, H.; Wasowski, C.; Medina, J.H.; Paladini, A.C. Molecular modelling and QSAR analysis of the interaction of flavone derivatives with the benzodiazepine binding site of the GABA(A) receptor complex. *Bioorg. Med. Chem.* **2001**, *9*, 323–335. [CrossRef]
15. Tamaddonfard, E.; Gooshchi, N.H.; Seiednejard-Yamchi, S. Central effect of crocin on penicillin-induced epileptiform activity in rats. *Pharmacol. Rep.* **2012**, *64*, 94–101. [CrossRef]
16. Hosseinzadeh, H.; Sadeghnia, H.R. Protective effect of safranal on pentylenetetrazol-induced seizures in the rat: Involvement of GABAergic and opioids systems. *Phytomedicine* **2007**, *14*, 256–262. [CrossRef]
17. Crawley, J.N.; Goodwin, F.K. Preliminary report of a simple animal behavior for the anxiolytic effect of benzodiazepines. *Pharmacol. Biochem. Behav.* **1980**, *13*, 167–170. [CrossRef]
18. Prut, L.; Belzung, C. The open field as a paradigm to measure the effects of drugs on anxiety-like behaviours: A review. *Eur. J. Pharmacol.* **2003**, *463*, 3–33. [CrossRef]
19. Bourin, M.; Hascoet, M. The mouse light/dark box test. *Eur. J. Pharmacol.* **2003**, *463*, 55–65. [CrossRef]
20. Belzung, C.; Misslin, R.; Vogel, E.; Dodd, R.H.; Chapouthier, G. Anxiogenic effects of methyl-β-carboline-carboxylate in a light/dark choice situation. *Pharmacol. Biochem. Behav.* **1987**, *28*, 29–33. [CrossRef]
21. Mokhtari-Hashtjini, M.; Pirzad-Jahromi, G.; Meftahi, G.H.; Esmaeili, D.; Javidnazar, D. Aqueous extract of saffron administration along with amygdala deep brain stimulation promoted alleviation of symptoms in post-traumatic stress disorder (PTSD) in rats. *Avicenna J. Phytomed.* **2018**, *8*, 358–369. [PubMed]
22. Ceremuga, T.E.; Ayala, M.P.; Ryan, W.C.; Chun, S.M.; DeGroot, J.M.; Henson, D.T.; Randall, S.A.; Stanley, L.H.; Beaumont, D.M. Investigation of the anxiolytic and antidepressant effects of crocin, a compound from saffron (*Crocus sativus L*), in the male Sprague-Dawley rat. *AANA J.* **2018**, *86*, 225–233. [PubMed]
23. Assie', M.B.; Chopin, P.; Stenger, A.; Palmier, C.; Briley, M. Neuropharmacology of a new potential anxiolytic compound, F2692,1-3X-trifluoromethyl phenyl. 1,4-dihydro-3-amino-4-oxo-6-methyl pyridazine: 1 Acute and in vivo effects. *Psychopharmacology* **1993**, *110*, 13–18. [CrossRef] [PubMed]
24. Uusi-Oukari, M.; Korpi, E.R. Regulation of GABAA receptor subunit expression by pharmacological agents. *Pharmacol. Rev.* **2010**, *62*, 97–135. [CrossRef]
25. Kanakis, C.D.; Tarantilis, P.A.; Tajmir-Riahi, A.; Polissiou, M.G. DNA interaction with saffron's secondary metabolites safranal, crocetin and dimethylcrocetin. *DNA Cell. Biol.* **2007**, *26*, 63–70. [CrossRef]
26. Carmona, M.; Zalacain, A.; Sanchez, A.M.; Novella, J.L.; Alonso, G.L. Crocetin esters, picrocrocin and its related compounds present in *Crocus sativus* stigmas and *Gardenia jasminoides* fruits. Tentative identification of seven new compounds by LC-ESI-MS. *J. Agric. Food Chem.* **2006**, *54*, 973–979. [CrossRef]
27. Mohajeri, S.A.; Hosseinzadeh, H.; Keyhanfar, F.; Aghamohammadian, J. Extraction of crocin from saffron (*Crocus sativus*) using molecularly imprinted polymer solid-phase extraction. *J. Sep. Sci.* **2010**, *33*, 2302–2309. [CrossRef]
28. Karkoula, E.; Angelis Koulakiotis, N.S.; Gikas, E.; Halabalaki, M.; Tsarbopoulos, A.; Skaltsounis, A.L. Rapid isolation and characterization of crocins, picrocrocin and crocetin from saffron using centrifugal partition chromatography and LC-MS. *J. Sep. Sci* **2018**, *41*, 4105–4114. [CrossRef]
29. Del Campo, C.P.; Carmona, M.; Maggi, L.; Kanakis, C.D.; Anastasaki, E.G.; Tarantilis, P.A.; Polyssiou, M.G.; Alonso, G.L. Effects of mild temperature conditions during dehydration procedures on saffron quality parameters. *J. Sci. Food Agric.* **2010**, *90*, 719–725. [CrossRef]
30. Schmidt-Mutter, C.; Pain, L.; Sandner, G.; Gobaille, S.; Maitre, M. The anxiolytic effect of g-hydroxybutyrate in the elevated plus maze is reversed by the benzodiazepine receptor antagonist, flumazenil. *Eur. J. Pharmacol.* **1998**, *342*, 21–27. [CrossRef]

31. Stachowicz, K.; Wierońska, J.; Domin, H.; Chaki, S.; Pilc, A. Anxiolytic-like activity of MGS0039, a selective group II mGlu receptor antagonist, is serotonin and GABA-dependent. *Pharmacol. Rep.* **2011**, *63*, 880–887.
32. Grivas, V.; Markou, A.; Pitsikas, N. The metabotropic glutamate 2/3 receptor agonist LY379268 induces anxiety-like behavior at the highest dose tested in two rat models of anxiety. *Eur. J. Pharmacol.* **2013**, *715*, 105–110. [CrossRef] [PubMed]
33. Kalouda, T.; Pitsikas, N. The nitric oxide donor molsidomine induces anxiolytic-like behaviour in two different rat models of anxiety. *Pharmacol. Biochem. Behav.* **2015**, *138*, 111–116. [CrossRef] [PubMed]

Sample Availability: Samples of crocins and flumazenil are available from the authors.

Publisher's Note: MDPI stays neutral with regard to jurisdictional claims in published maps and institutional affiliations.

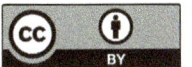

© 2020 by the authors. Licensee MDPI, Basel, Switzerland. This article is an open access article distributed under the terms and conditions of the Creative Commons Attribution (CC BY) license (http://creativecommons.org/licenses/by/4.0/).

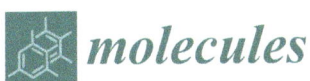

Article

Crocins, the Bioactive Components of *Crocus sativus* L., Counteract the Disrupting Effects of Anesthetic Ketamine on Memory in Rats

Nikolaos Pitsikas [1,*] and Petros A. Tarantilis [2]

[1] Department of Pharmacology, Faculty of Medicine, School of Health Sciences, University of Thessaly, Biopolis, Panepistimiou 3, 415-00 Larissa, Greece
[2] Laboratory of Chemistry, Department of Food Science and Human Nutrition, School of Food and Nutritional Sciences, Agricultural University of Athens, 115-27 Athens, Greece; ptara@aua.gr
* Correspondence: npitsikas@med.uth.gr; Tel.: +30-2410-685-535; Fax: +30-2410-685-552

Abstract: Consistent experimental evidence suggests that anesthetic doses of the non-competitive *N*-methyl-D-aspartate (NMDA) receptor antagonist ketamine cause severe memory impairments in rodents. Crocins are among the various bioactive ingredients of the plant *Crocus sativus* L., and their implication in memory is well-documented. It has not yet been elucidated if crocins are able to attenuate the memory deficits produced by anesthetic ketamine. The present study was undertaken aiming to clarify this issue in the rat. For this aim, the object recognition, the object location and the habituation tests, reflecting non-spatial recognition memory, spatial recognition memory and associative memory, respectively, were utilized. A post-training challenge with crocins (15–30 mg/kg, intraperitoneally (i.p.), acutely) counteracted anesthetic ketamine (100 mg/kg, i.p.)-induced performance impairments in all the above-mentioned behavioral memory paradigms. The current findings suggest that crocins modulate anesthetic ketamine's amnestic effects.

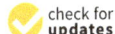

Keywords: crocins; anesthetic ketamine; memory; rat

1. Introduction

Ketamine is a drug largely utilized in clinical and veterinary medicine due to its important anesthetic and analgesic properties [1,2]. Ketamine binds to the phencyclidine (PCP) binding site within the pore of the channel of the *N*-methyl-D-aspartate (NMDA) receptor and exerts its effects as a non-competitive antagonist [3]. Exposure to a low-dose range of ketamine (sub-anesthetic doses) induces schizophrenia-like symptoms, including memory impairments, both in humans and rodents [2].

By contrast, anesthetic doses of ketamine cause an anesthetic state called "dissociative anesthesia" characterized by severe sensory loss and analgesia, and does not depress the cardiovascular or the respiratory system, but disrupts cognition [4,5]. Regarding the latter, it has been demonstrated that a challenge with anesthetic ketamine disrupted rodents' anterograde memory [6], memory consolidation [7] and recall of previous information [8,9]. Based on the complexity of the behavioral paradigm used and in agreement with clinical findings [10], 72 h are required for the recovery of memory in rats that receive anesthetic doses of ketamine [6]. Anesthetic ketamine's adverse behavioral effects are ascribed to its inhibitory action on the NMDA receptor [11] and on the extracellular signal-regulated kinase (ERK) signal transduction pathway [12]. Additionally, anesthetic ketamine promotes the overexpression of the transcriptional marker c-fos [13] and oxidative stress [14].

Crocus sativus L. is a plant cultivated in many countries all around the world including Iran, India, Italy, Spain and Greece. The spice saffron is its product. Saffron is the dried red stigmas of the flower. The major components of saffron are crocins, picrocrocin and safranal. [15,16].

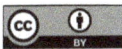

The stigmas of *C. sativus* L. are used in traditional medicine as an anti-catarrhal, eupeptic, expectorant and emmenagogue [17]. Modern pharmacological studies have demonstrated that saffron's crude extracts and purified chemicals possess anti-tumor and anti-inflammatory properties, counteract atherosclerosis and hepatic damage [17], and exert a beneficial action in different pathologies of the central nervous system including depression, schizophrenia and anxiety [18].

In line with the above, a conspicuous number of preclinical and clinical studies propose the involvement of crocins in cognition [19]. Crocins, glycosyl esters of crocetin, are water-soluble carotenoids. It has recently been shown that crocins, despite their highly hydrophilic profile, are capable of penetrating the blood–brain barrier and reaching the central nervous system following intraperitoneal administration in mice [20]. In this context, it has been demonstrated that crocins attenuated the schizophrenia-like behavioral deficits, including cognitive impairments, induced by sub-anesthetic doses of ketamine in rats [21]. In particular, crocins counteracted the disruption of non-spatial recognition memory caused by sub-anesthetic ketamine in a procedure reflecting the modulation of post-training memory components (the storage and/or retrieval of information) [21]. Several lines of evidence suggest that the beneficial effects exerted by crocins on memory might be related to their strong anti-oxidant properties [22,23].

Little is known at present regarding if and how crocins are able to attenuate the cognitive deficits caused by the administration of anesthetic doses of ketamine in animals. In spite of its well-documented amnestic effects, anesthetic ketamine increases cerebral blood flow and metabolism in spontaneously breathing patients and does not influence intracranial pressure [24], and it did not induce neurodegeneration in the developing brain [25]. Due to these interesting properties, ketamine is the anesthetic of choice in specific situations such as patients with compromised hemodynamic profiles or suffering from asthma [24] and in pediatrics [25]. Thus, compounds that might be able to attenuate the cognition problems associated with the administration of anesthetic ketamine might be of high utility in clinical practice.

Furthermore, it has not yet been elucidated if crocins can attenuate the cognitive deficits induced by anesthetic doses of ketamine related to types of memory other than non-spatial recognition memory (e.g., spatial recognition memory and associative memory) and modulate mnemonic components other than the storage and retrieval of information (e.g., the acquisition of information).

Taking the above into account, the aim of our research was to test the efficiency of crocins in attenuating the usual memory problems expressed by rats that have received anesthetic ketamine. For these studies, the object recognition task (ORT), the object location task (OLT) and the habituation test (HT) were used. The ORT and OLT measure non-spatial [26] and spatial recognition memory [27], respectively, while the HT is a non-associative learning task [28].

2. Results

In line with prior results, the righting reflex was lost in rats within 8 min, and anesthesia was extinguished in all groups of rats that received ketamine within 30 min, independently of the pharmacological treatment [6,9,29,30].

2.1. Experiment 1: Effects of Acute Challenge with Crocins and Anesthetic Ketamine on Animals' Performance in the ORT

The evaluation of the discrimination index D data evidenced a statistically significant main effect of ketamine ($F(1,47) = 25.2$, $p < 0.001$), a statistically significant main effect of crocins ($F(2,47) = 4.6$, $p = 0.016$) and a significant ketamine x crocins interaction ($F(2,47) = 8.4$, $p < 0.001$). Post hoc comparisons showed that the ketamine + vehicle group displayed an inferior index D with respect to all the other experimental groups, including the ketamine + 15 mg/kg crocins and ketamine + 30 mg/kg crocins groups ($p < 0.05$; Figure 1A).

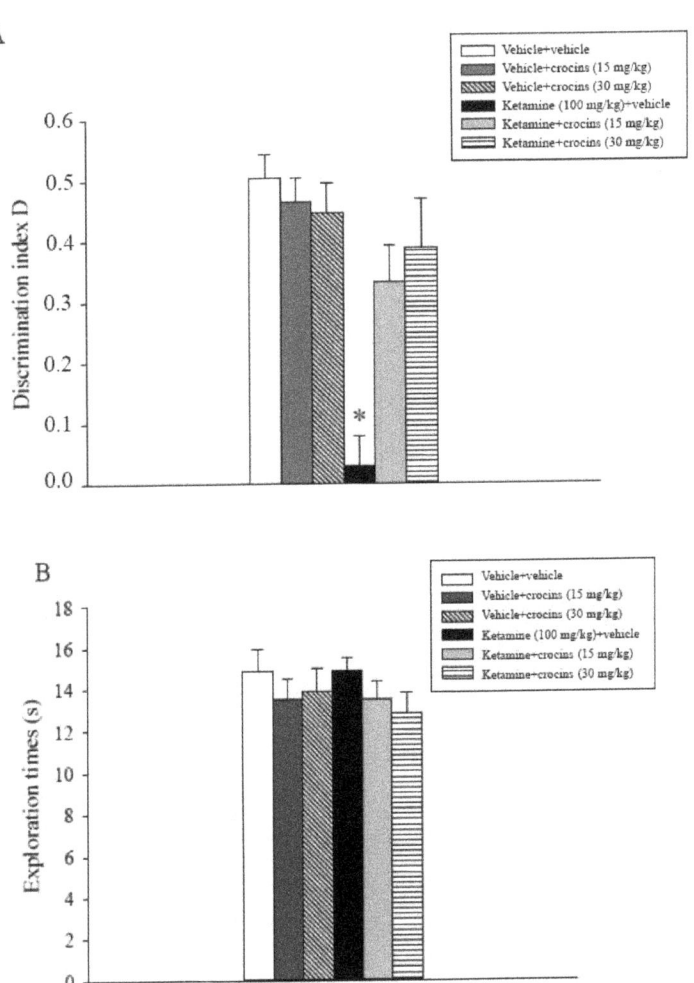

Figure 1. Object recognition task. The histogram represents the mean ± S.E.M. of 8 rats per treatment group. (**A**) Discrimination index D performance expressed by various groups of rats during the choice phase (T2). * $p < 0.05$ vs. all the other groups including the ketamine + crocins (15 mg/kg) and ketamine + crocins (30 mg/kg) groups. (**B**) Total exploration times.

Assessment of the exploratory activity data obtained for the various groups of rats during the choice phase (T2) did not show significant effects of ketamine, crocins or their combination (Figure 1B). The results indicate that treatment with crocins alleviated the disruption of non-spatial recognition memory caused by anesthetic ketamine.

2.2. Experiment 2: Effects of Acute Challenge with Crocins and Anesthetic Ketamine on Animals' Performance in the OLT

Discrimination index D index data analysis showed a statistically significant main effect of ketamine ($F(1,47) = 27.99$, $p < 0.001$), a statistically significant main effect of crocins ($F(2,47) = 4.06$, $p = 0.024$) and a significant interaction between ketamine and crocins ($F(2,47) = 4.09$, $p = 0.024$). Subsequent post hoc comparisons indicated that the ketamine- and vehicle-treated rats displayed a significantly inferior index D with respect to all the other populations of rats, including the ketamine + 15 mg/kg crocins and ketamine + 30 mg/kg crocins groups ($p < 0.05$; Figure 2A).

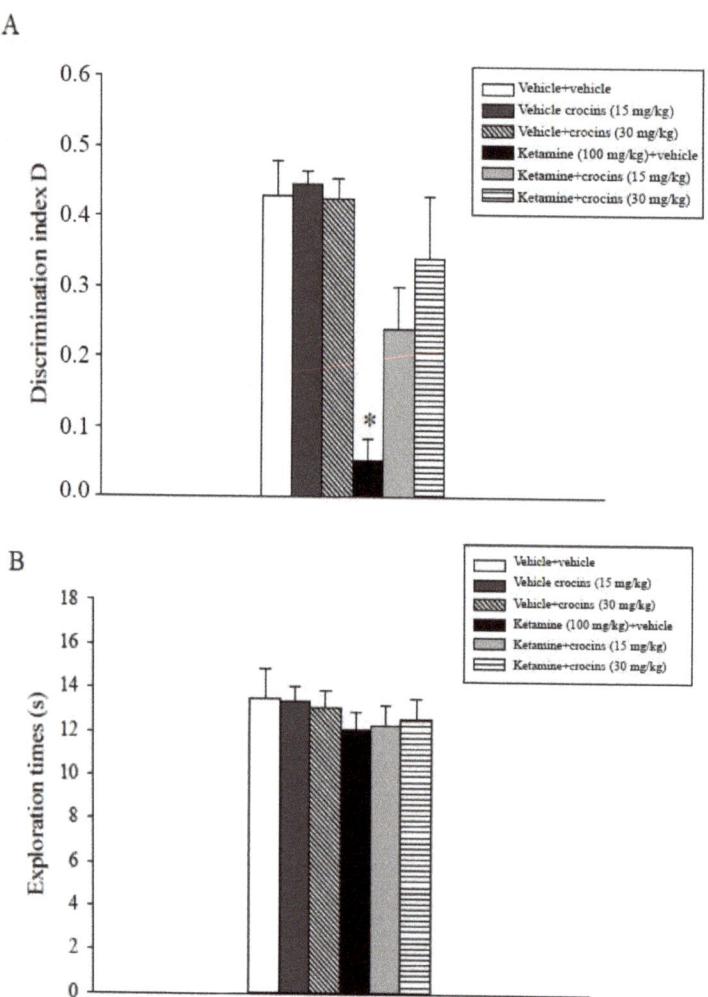

Figure 2. Object location task. The histogram represents the mean ± S.E.M. of 8 rats per treatment group. (**A**) Discrimination index D performance expressed by different groups of rats during T2. * $p < 0.05$ vs. all the other groups including the ketamine + crocins (15 mg/kg) and ketamine + crocins (30 mg/kg) groups. (**B**) Total exploration times.

Assessment of the exploratory activity data obtained for the various groups of rats during the choice phase (T2) did not show significant effects of ketamine, crocins or their combination (Figure 2B). The results indicate that crocins counteracted anesthetic ketamine-induced spatial recognition memory deficits.

2.3. Experiment 3: Effects of Acute Challenge with Crocins and Anesthetic Ketamine on Animals' Performance in the HT

The HT results are reported in Figure 3. Overall analysis of the number of rearings revealed an effect of crocins ($F(1,63) = 12.3$, $p < 0.001$) and of trials ($F(1,63) = 18.8$, $p < 0.001$) but not an effect of ketamine or an interaction between ketamine, crocins and trials. A post hoc analysis carried out on these data indicated that the vehicle + vehicle, vehicle + crocins and ketamine + crocins groups but not the ketamine + vehicle group expressed significantly lower numbers of rearing episodes during Day 2 with respect to their performance during Day 1 ($p < 0.05$).

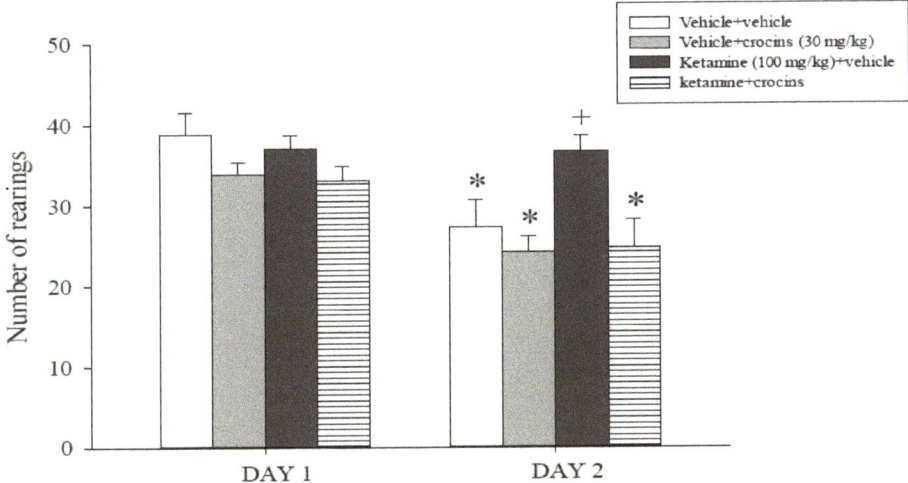

Figure 3. Habituation test. The histogram represents the mean ± S.E.M. of 8 rats per treatment group. * $p < 0.05$ vs. the same groups of rats on Day 1; + $p < 0.05$ vs. all the other groups on Day 2.

A two-way ANOVA test conducted on results related to rats' performance during Day 1 did not evidence any effect either of ketamine or of crocins or an interaction ketamine x crocins. Conversely, evaluation of the Day 2 data showed a main effect of crocins ($F(1,31) = 5.9$, $p = 0.022$) but not an effect of ketamine or an interaction between ketamine and crocins. Post hoc comparisons showed that the ketamine + vehicle group displayed a significantly higher number of rearings compared to all the other experimental groups, including the ketamine + 15 mg/kg crocins and ketamine + 30 mg/kg crocins groups ($p < 0.05$).

The high number of rearing episodes displayed by the ketamine + vehicle-treated rats is an indication of an impairing effect caused by anesthetic ketamine on the associative learning abilities of the rats. The reduction of it by crocins suggests that this bioactive component of saffron counteracted the disruption of associative memory induced by anesthetic ketamine.

3. Discussion

According to previous reports, anesthetic ketamine impaired rodents' performance in either the ORT [6,9,29,30] or OLT [6], two procedures reflecting non-spatial and spatial recognition memory, respectively. Interestingly, for the first time to our knowledge, anesthetic ketamine also disrupted the performance of animals in the HT, a behavioral paradigm assessing associative learning [28].

An acute challenge with crocins (15–30 mg/kg) counteracted the impairing effects caused by anesthetic ketamine on cognition evidenced in the above-reported behavioral paradigms. A per se effect of crocins was not revealed. In both recognition memory studies (ORT and OLT) and in the associative learning experiment (HT), retention was assessed 24 h after the training trial. This means that the effects of the compounds were revealed in procedures assessing long-term memory. Concerning the ORT and OLT, the chemicals were injected immediately after the sample phase. This suggests that ketamine and crocins might have acted on post-training memory components (the storage and/or retrieval of information). Conversely, in the habituation test, the compounds were administered 24 h before the training trial. The latter implies that the compounds could critically have exerted their effects on the encoding of information, although possible effects on the consolidation and retrieval of information can also be considered.

The present results provide new information with respect to previous findings of ours in which crocins were found to be able to attenuate the non-spatial recognition memory deficits produced by sub-anesthetic ketamine [21]. Specifically, in the present experiments, crocins counteracted anesthetic ketamine's amnestic effects in different behavioral paradigms, reflecting non-spatial recognition but also spatial recognition and associative memory, respectively. Moreover, the current findings suggest that crocins modulated the memory disturbances induced by anesthetic ketamine in procedures evaluating not only the storage and retrieval but also the acquisition of information.

The compounds were administered peripherally. It cannot be ruled out, therefore, that unspecific factors (e.g., sensorimotor or motivational) might have influenced rats' performance in the various memory tasks. It has been shown, however, that the exploratory levels displayed by animals either in the ORT and OLT during the retention trial (Day 2) and the number of rearing episodes expressed by rats during the training trial (Day 1) in the HT were not different among the various experimental groups. This pattern of results, thus, suggests that the implication of non-specific factors in the effects of anesthetic ketamine and crocins on animals' cognitive performance can probably be excluded.

The mechanism(s) underlying anesthetic ketamine's adverse effects, has (have) been, at least partially, attributed to its inhibitory effect on the NMDA receptor. It has been demonstrated that anesthetic ketamine inhibits glutamatergic neurotransmission by reducing glutamate release and suppressing axonal conduction, polysynaptic potential and cell excitability [31,32]. Anesthetic ketamine seems to reduce NMDA-mediated responses by two distinct mechanisms: (a) anesthetic concentrations of ketamine seem to block the open channel of the NMDA receptor and thereby decrease the mean channel-open time, and (b) reducing the frequency of channel opening through an allosteric mechanism [33]. A recent report has indicated that cognitive impairments induced by anesthetic ketamine might be dependent on its suppressing effects on astrocyte-mediated slow inward current (SIC) synchronization [34].

There is also evidence that alternative target sites, such as the $GABA_A$ and the nicotinic cholinergic receptor, might be implicated in the amnestic effects of anesthetic ketamine. In this context, it has been reported that the potential interaction of ketamine with the $GABA_A$-benzodiazepine receptor [29] and the α7 sub-unit of the nicotinic acetylcholine receptor [30] might also be involved in anesthetic ketamine's amnestic action.

The mechanism(s) through which crocins reversed anesthetic ketamine's impairing action on memory is (are) not yet elucidated and is (are) still a matter of investigation. In this context, it has been shown that saffron extracts and crocetin (the hydrolysis product of crocins) but not crocins partly antagonize the NMDA receptor by binding to the PCP binding site of it. In addition, both chemicals display an affinity for the sigma (σ) 1 receptor [35]. This apparent failure of crocins to bind at the NMDA receptor might depend on pharmacokinetic issues and, in particular, their poor intestinal absorption after oral administration in the rat [35].

Another study confirmed the above-mentioned antagonistic effects of saffron and crocetin on the NMDA receptor since both molecules reduced glutamatergic transmission in rat cortical brain slices [36]. Importantly, this partial blocking of the NMDA receptor might be critical for the presumed therapeutic effects of saffron and its bioactive constituents [35].

Furthermore, it has been reported that anesthetic ketamine interferes with the ERK signal transduction pathway since it has been shown that the inhibition of ERK by anesthetic ketamine underlies the memory impairments observed in the young rat [12]. Interestingly, it has recently been shown that crocins were able to reverse memory deficits caused by a challenge with hyoscine and normalized ERK levels in the rat hippocampus [37].

Anesthetic ketamine was also found to induce the overexpression of the transcription marker c-fos, which is an index of neuronal damage [13]. By contrast, in a series of studies, the beneficial action of saffron and crocins against cognitive dysfunctions, a typical feature of neurodegenerative diseases such as Alzheimer's disease, or cerebral ischemia has been revealed [38]. In particular, crocins (injected intraperitoneally) were found to exert an inhibitory action on acetylcholinesterase activity [39] and demonstrated efficacy in counteracting β-amyloid (Aβ)-induced cognitive deficits [40] and c-fos overexpression in rats [41]. In this context, it has been revealed that the oral administration of crocins conferred neuroprotection in a rat model of cerebral ischemia [42].

A correlation between anesthetic ketamine and oxidative stress has also been proposed. It has been demonstrated that anesthetic ketamine impaired mitochondrial function and potentiated superoxide dismutase activity in the rat brain [14]. Regarding this latter issue, the well-known anti-oxidant properties of crocins may provide an alternative explanation for the findings reported here. Specifically, the oral or intraperitoneal administration of crocins attenuated memory deficits caused either by streptozotocin or chronic stress and enhanced anti-oxidant activity in rodents [22,23].

Collectively, it can be hypothesized that the partial antagonistic affinity of saffron and crocetin for the NMDA receptor, and the beneficial role played by crocins in the ERK pathway and c-fos expression along with their potent anti-oxidant properties might be critical for counteracting the amnestic effects of anesthetic ketamine.

The present work has some limitations. The current results might be considered preliminary and are limited to behavioral findings. Further research (e.g., molecular, biochemical and electrophysiological studies) is required to elucidate the mechanism(s) of action underlying crocins' anti-amnestic effects.

In summary, the present results show, for the first time to our knowledge, that a bioactive constituent of saffron (crocins) exerts a modulatory role on anesthetic ketamine's amnestic effects. The findings reported here might be of importance since ketamine is largely utilized in clinical and veterinary medicine in anesthesia and perioperative analgesia.

4. Materials and Methods

4.1. Animals

Different populations of male (3-month-old) Wistar rats (Hellenic Pasteur Institute, Athens, Greece) weighing 250–300 g were used for each experiment. The rats were housed in Makrolon cages (47.5 cm length × 20.5 cm height × 27 cm width), with three per cage, in a standard environment (21 ± 1 °C; 50–55% relative humidity; 12 h/12 h light/dark cycle, lights on at 7 a.m.) with access to food and water ad libitum.

The experiments that involved animals and their care were conducted in accordance with international guidelines and national (Animal Act, P.D. 160/91) and international laws and policies (EEC Council Directive 86/609, JL 358, 1, 12 December 1987). The present study was approved by the local committee (Prefecture of Larissa, Greece, protocol number 255200/1 October, 2020).

4.2. Behavior

4.2.1. Object Recognition Task (ORT)

The ORT assesses non-spatial recognition memory abilities in rodents. This paradigm lacks a reward, and it is based on the spontaneous exploratory behavior of rodents [26]. The test apparatus consisted of a dark open box made of Plexiglas (80 cm length × 50 cm height × 60 cm width) that was illuminated by a 60 W light suspended 60 cm above the box. The light intensity was equal in the different parts of the apparatus. The objects to be discriminated (in triplicate) were made of glass, plastic or metal, and were in three different shapes—metallic cubes, glass pyramids and plastic cylinders 7 cm high—and could not be displaced by rats.

The ORT was performed as described previously [6]. Briefly, during the week before undertaking the testing, the animals were handled twice a day for 3 consecutive days. Before testing, the rats were allowed to explore the empty apparatus for 2 min for 3 consecutive days. During testing, a session that consisted of two trials was conducted. During the "sample" trial (T1), two identical samples (objects) were positioned in two opposite corners of the apparatus in a casual fashion, 10 cm away from the sidewalls. A rat was gently positioned in the center of the arena and allowed to inspect the two similar objects. After the sample phase (T1), the rat went back to its home cage, and an intertrial interval (ITI) followed. Subsequently, the "choice" trial (T2) was conducted. During T2, a novel object substituted one of the objects presented during T1. The animals, thus, were re-exposed to two objects: a copy of the familiar (F) object and the novel (N) object. All the combinations and positions of the objects were counterbalanced to reduce the potential bias due to preferences for specific places or objects.

Directing the nose toward the object at a distance no more of 2 cm and/or touching the object with the nose was considered exploratory behavior. Turning around or sitting on the object was not considered exploratory behavior. The total time spent by the rats exploring the two identical objects (F1 and F2) during the sample phase (T1) and the total time spent exploring the two different objects (F and N) during the choice trial (T2) were manually recorded by using a stopwatch. The discrimination between F and N during T2 was measured by comparing the time spent exploring the familiar object with the time spent exploring the novel object. Because the exploratory time may be influenced by differences in the total exploratory activity, a discrimination index (D) representing the preference for the new as opposed to familiar object was calculated as follows: $D = N - F/N + F$, where N is the exploration time for the novel object, F is that for the familiar object and N+F is the total exploration time for both objects during T2 [43]. Correct recognition was shown by rats consistently spending more time inspecting a novel object than the familiar one during T2 [26].

4.2.2. Object Location Task (OLT)

The OLT is a version of the ORT that evaluates spatial recognition memory. This task assesses the ability of rodents to discriminate the novelty of the object locations but not the objects themselves because the testing arena is already familiar to the animals [27]. The testing arena was that utilized in the ORT. The apparatus was placed in a large observation room and was surrounded with external large and typical objects (cues) to assist the animals to successfully perform the test. These cues were kept in a fixed position for the entire testing period. The objects were the same objects as in the ORT.

The OLT was performed as described elsewhere [27,44]. Briefly, during the week before undertaking testing, the animals were handled twice daily for 3 consecutive days. Before testing, the rats were allowed to explore the empty apparatus for 2 min for 3 consecutive days. During testing, a session that consisted of two trials was carried out. During the "sample" trial (T1), two identical samples (objects) were positioned in two opposite corners of the apparatus in a casual fashion, 10 cm away from the sidewalls. A rat was gently positioned in the center of the arena and allowed to inspect the two similar objects. After the sample phase (T1), the rat went back to its home cage, and an intertrial interval (ITI) followed. Subsequently, the "choice" trial (T2) was conducted. During T2, one of the two similar objects was relocated to a different position (new location (NL)), while the other object remained in the same position (familiar location (FL)) as in the sample phase (T1). Thus, the two objects were now in diagonal corners. All the combinations and positions of the objects were counterbalanced to reduce the potential bias due to preferences for specific places or objects.

The definition of exploration is described above in the object recognition protocol. The time spent by the rats exploring each object during T1 and T2 was manually recorded with a stopwatch. The discrimination between the FL and NL during T2 was measured by comparing the time spent exploring the object in the FL with the time spent exploring the object in the NL. Because the exploratory time may be influenced by differences in the total exploratory activity, a discrimination index (D) representing the preference for the new as opposed to familiar object position was calculated as follows: $D = NL - FL/NL + FL$, where NL is the exploration time for the object in the novel position, FL is that for the object in the familiar location and NL + FL is the total exploration time for both objects during T2 [43]. Correct recognition is shown by rats spending consistently more time inspecting the novel place of the object than the familiar one during the choice trial T2 [26].

4.2.3. Habituation Test (HT)

The retention of a habituation to a novel environment reflects a non-associative, non-aversive form of learning. It can be quantified by the number of rearing episodes expressed by rodents in each test trial. A decrement in rearing episodes during the retention trial is considered to be an index of the intact non-associative memory abilities of rodents [28]. The apparatus consisted of a box made of Plexiglas (41 cm length × 33 cm height × 41 cm width). The test was performed as described previously [28]. Each animal was placed into the test arena, and the number of rearing episodes was recorded for 5 min. During testing, a session that consisted of two 5 min trials was performed. An intertrial period of 24 h was utilized.

In all the above-reported behavioral procedures, in order to avoid the presence of olfactory traces, devices and objects (where necessary) were washed with a solution containing 20% alcohol following each trial and then dried with sanitary towels.

4.3. Drugs

The crocins used in the current experiments were derived from the same batch of plant material (saffron) and the same purification procedure, extraction and separation. Our plant material was kindly offered by the Cooperative of Saffron, Krokos, Kozani, Greece.

The crocins were isolated from the red dried stigmas of C. sativus using a slightly modified method described previously [45]. They were purified from the stigmas after successive and exhaustive extraction with (a) petroleum ether at 40–60 °C, (b) diethyl ether (Et$_2$O) and (c) 80% methanol (MeOH) using ultrasound-assisted extraction. The ultrasound extraction was performed in a Sonorex, Super RK 255H type (300 × 150 × 150 mm internal dimensions) ultrasound water bath (indirect sonication), at a fixed frequency of 35 kHz. The temperature of the sonicated water was 25 °C. Procedures (a) and (b) took place in order for the stigmas to be free of the picrocrocin and safranal, respectively. The methanol extract, after evaporation (condensed to dryness) under vacuum at room temperature, provided crocins, which were dark red powder residue. Crocins are unusual water-soluble carotenoids (glucosyl esters of crocetin). The major component is a digentiobiosyl ester of crocetin (approximately 60% of the total crocins) [46]. The chemical profile of crocins has been well documented in previous studies [14,47–49], and we evaluated the quality of the fresh prepared extract used in this study. The purity of the crocins was 85% (according to HPLC., Figure 4).

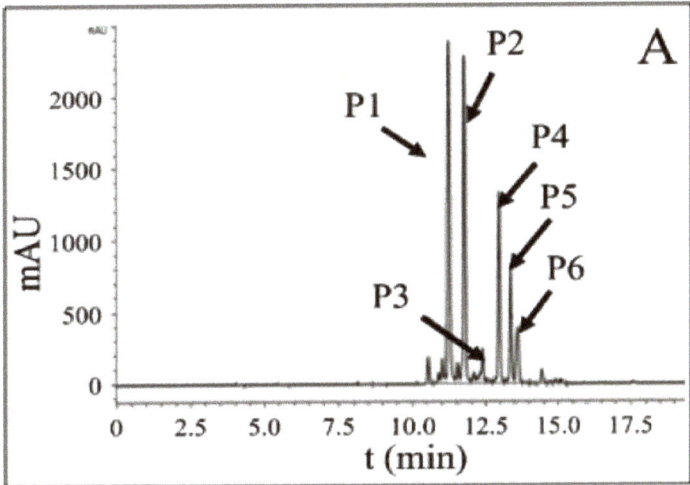

Figure 4. Cont.

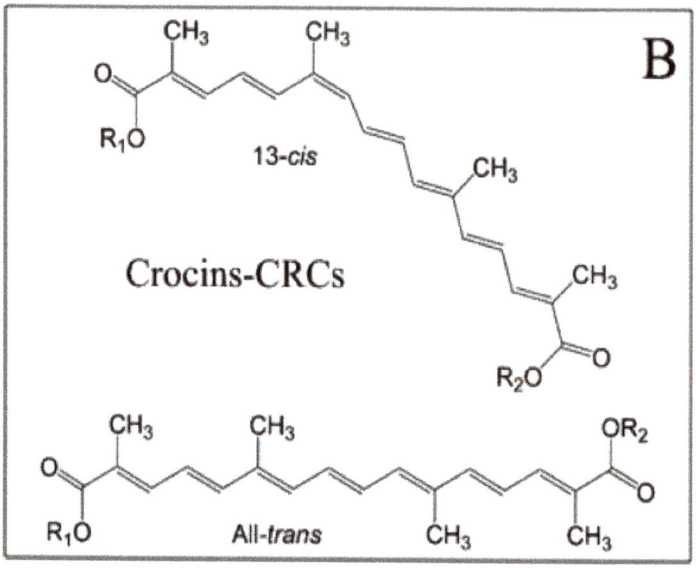

Figure 4. Chromatogram of crocin extract at 440 nm and structures of crocins. Identification of crocins according to HPLC analysis was performed, comparing the UV-vis spectra and the retention times (tR) of the peaks with literature data and MS data. The identified peaks presented are as follows: P1: trans-4GG, P2: trans 3Gg, P3: trans 2gg, P4: cis4 GG, P5: trans 2G, P6: cis crocin (**A**). The most abundant were trans-crocin 4 and trans-crocin 3. Nomenclature of crocins was based on the proposal of Carmona et al., i.e., the first part describes the cis/trans form of the aglycon part, followed by the total number of sugar moieties (glycose monomers), and finally, the type of sugar in each part of the crocin structure is indicated. Namely, G refers to gentiobiose and g, to glucose (2) (**B**).

The crocins were dissolved in saline (NaCl 0.9%) and were administered intraperitoneally (i.p.). The doses of crocins (15 and 30 mg/kg) were selected based on previous findings [21].

Ketamine hydrochloride (Sigma, St Louis, MO, USA) was dissolved in saline and administered i.p. at the anesthetic dose of 100 mg/kg [6].

All drug solutions were freshly prepared on the day of testing and were administered i.p. in a volume of 1 mL/kg. For all studies, control animals received isovolumetric amounts of the specific vehicle solutions.

4.4. Experimental Protocol

Given the fact that the hypothermic properties of ketamine exert a protective effect on rats' recognition memory [6], the different groups of animals received treatment in a "warm" (25 °C) room to avoid hypothermia and remained there under these conditions for 2 h, starting immediately after injection [6,9,29,30]. Testing was carried out under standard environmental conditions (21 °C) 24 h after treatment, when a complete recovery of animals' sensorimotor functions was achieved [6–9,29,30]. The experimental protocol is summarized in Figure 5.

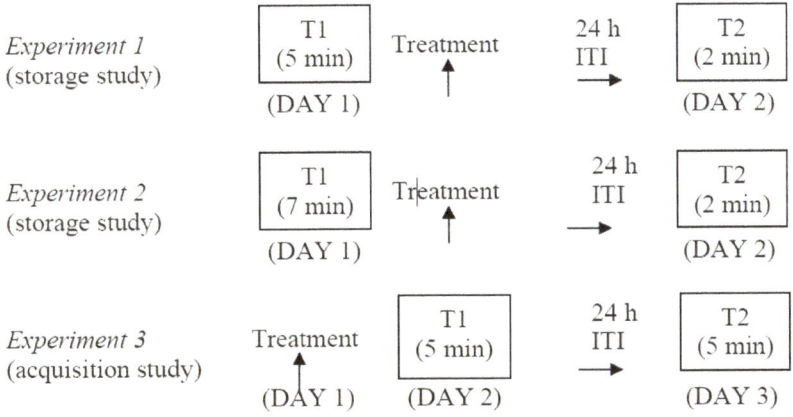

T1: first trial; T2: second trial; ITI: intertrial interval

Figure 5. Summary of the experimental protocol.

An *anesthetic state* was defined as the loss of the righting reflex and movement. The animals' behavior was video recorded. Data evaluation was subsequently performed by an experimenter who was unaware of the pharmacological treatment of each subject.

4.4.1. Experiment 1: Effects of Acute Challenge with Crocins and Anesthetic Ketamine on Animals' Performance in the ORT

Animals were randomly divided into six experimental groups with 8 rats per group as follows: vehicle + vehicle; vehicle + crocins (15 mg/kg); vehicle + crocins (30 mg/kg); vehicle + ketamine (100 mg/kg); ketamine (100 mg/kg) + crocins (15 mg/kg); ketamine (100 mg/kg) + crocins (30 mg/kg). Appropriate treatment was performed immediately after the training (sample) trial T1. The crocins were administered 5–10 s after the vehicle or ketamine.

In this study, the duration of the sample trial T1 was increased from 2 to 5 min, since under this condition, it has been shown that control rats' non-spatial recognition memory abilities can be preserved for 24 h, while the duration of the choice phase remained unchanged (2 min) [29,30].

4.4.2. Experiment 2: Effects of Acute Challenge with Crocins and Anesthetic Ketamine on Animals' Performance in the OLT

Animals were randomly divided into six experimental groups with 8 rats per group as follows: vehicle + vehicle; vehicle + crocins (15 mg/kg); vehicle + crocins (30 mg/kg); vehicle + ketamine (100 mg/kg); ketamine (100 mg/kg) + crocins (15 mg/kg); ketamine (100 mg/kg) + crocins (30 mg/kg). Appropriate treatment was performed immediately after the training (sample) trial T1. The crocins were administered 5–10 s after the vehicle or ketamine.

In this study, the duration of the sample trial T1 was increased from 2 to 7 min, since under this condition, it has been shown that control rats' spatial recognition memory abilities can be preserved for 24 h, while the duration of the choice phase remained unchanged (2 min) (our unpublished observations).

4.4.3. Experiment 3: Effects of Acute Challenge with Crocins and Anesthetic Ketamine on Animals' Performance in the HT

Animals were randomly divided into four experimental groups with 8 rats per group as follows: vehicle + vehicle; vehicle + crocins (30 mg/kg); vehicle + ketamine (100 mg/kg); ketamine (100 mg/kg) + crocins (30 mg/kg). Appropriate treatment was performed 24 h before starting the training (sample) trial T1. The crocins were administered 5–10 s after the vehicle or ketamine.

4.5. Statistical Analysis

Data are expressed as mean ± S.E.M. The data of Experiments 1 and 2 were analyzed using two-way analysis of variance (ANOVA). The factors were crocins and ketamine. Experiment 3's data were analyzed using three-way ANOVA with the between-subjects factors crocins and ketamine and the within-subjects factor trials. Further analyses were carried out separately for each trial (day) using the two-way ANOVA test. The factors were crocins and ketamine. Post hoc comparisons between the treatment means were made using Tukey's t-test. Values of $p < 0.05$ were considered statistically significant [50].

Author Contributions: Conceptualization, N.P.; methodology, N.P. and P.A.T.; formal analysis, N.P. and P.A.T.; investigation, N.P.; data curation, N.P.; writing—original draft preparation, N.P. and P.A.T. All authors have read and agreed to the published version of the manuscript.

Funding: This research was funded by the Research Committee of the University of Thessaly (grant number 5490) to Nikolaos Pitsikas.

Institutional Review Board Statement: The protocol of the experiment was previously approved by Local Ethical Committee for research involving animals (protocol number 255200/1 October, 2020).

Informed Consent Statement: Not applicable.

Data Availability Statement: The data presented in this study are available on request from the corresponding author.

Conflicts of Interest: The authors declare no conflict of interest.

Sample Availability: Samples of crocins and ketamine are available from the authors.

References

1. Javitt, D.C.; Zukin, R.S. Recent advances in the phencyclidine model of schizophrenia. *Am. J. Psychiatry* **1991**, *148*, 1301–1308.
2. Krystal, J.H.; Karper, L.P.; Seibyl, J.P.; Freeman, G.K.; Delaney, R.; Bremne, J.D.; Heninger, G.R.; Bowers, M.B.; Charney, D.S. Subanesthetic effects of the noncompetitive NMDA antagonist, ketamine, in humans. Psychotomimetic, perceptual, cognitive and neuroendocrine responses. *Arch. Gen. Psychiatry* **1994**, *51*, 199–214. [CrossRef] [PubMed]
3. Avis, N.A.; Burton, N.R.; Berry, S.C.; Lodge, D. The dissociative anesthetics ketamine and phencyclidine selectively reduce excitation of central mammalian neurons by N-methyl-D-aspartate. *Br. J. Pharmacol.* **1983**, *79*, 565–575.
4. Corssen, G.; Domino, E.F. Dissociative anesthesia: Further pharmacological studies and first clinical experience with the phencyclidine derivative CI-581. *Anesth. Analg.* **1966**, *45*, 29–40. [CrossRef]
5. Okon, T. Ketamine: An introduction for the pain and palliative medicine physician. *Pain Physician* **2007**, *10*, 493–500.
6. Pitsikas, N.; Boultadakis, A. Pre-training administration of anesthetic ketamine differentially affects rats' spatial and non-spatial recognition memory. *Neuropharmacology* **2009**, *57*, 1–7. [CrossRef] [PubMed]
7. Wang, J.H.; Fu, Y.; Wilson, F.A.W.; Ma, Y.Y. Ketamine affects memory consolidation: Differential effects in T-maze and passive avoidance paradigms in mice. *Neuroscience* **2006**, *140*, 993–1002. [CrossRef] [PubMed]
8. Gerlai, R.; McNamara, A. Anesthesia induced retrograde amnesia is ameliorated by ephrinA5-IgG in mice: EphA receptor tyrosine kinases are involved in mammalian memory. *Behav. Brain Res.* **2000**, *108*, 133–143. [CrossRef]
9. Boultadakis, A.; Pitsikas, N. Anesthetic ketamine impairs rats' recall of previous information. The nitric oxide synthase inhibitor N-nitro-L-arginine methylester antagonizes this ketamine-induced recognition memory deficit. *Anesthesiology* **2011**, *114*, 1345–1353. [CrossRef]
10. Morgan, C.J.; Mofeez, A.; Brandner, B.; Bromley, L.; Curran, H.V. Acute effects of ketamine on memory systems and psychotic symptoms in healthy volunteers. *Neuropsychopharmacology* **2004**, *29*, 208–218. [CrossRef]
11. Irifune, M.; Shimizu, T.; Nomoto, M. Ketamine-induced anesthesia involves the N-methyl-D-aspartate receptor-channel complex in mice. *Brain Res.* **1992**, *596*, 1–9. [CrossRef]
12. Peng, S.; Zhang, Y.; Zhang, J.; Wang, H.; Ren, B. Effect of ketamine on ERK expression in hippocampal neural cell and the ability of learning behavior in minor rats. *Mol. Biol. Rep.* **2010**, *7*, 3137–3142. [CrossRef] [PubMed]
13. Nakao, S.; Nagata, A.; Miyamoto, E.; Masuzawa, M.; Shingu, K. Inhibitory effect of profolol on ketamine-induced c-Fos expression in the rat posterior cingulate and retrosplenial cortices is mediated by $GABA_A$ receptor activation. *Acta Anesthesiol. Scand.* **2003**, *47*, 284–290. [CrossRef] [PubMed]
14. Venancio, C.; Felix, L.; Almeida, V.; Coutinho, J.; Antunes, L.; Peixoto, F.; Summavielle, T. Acute ketamine impairs mitochondrial function and promotes superoxide dismutase activity in the rat brain. *Anesth. Analg.* **2015**, *120*, 320–328. [CrossRef] [PubMed]

15. Kanakis, C.D.; Daferera, D.J.; Tarantilis, P.A.; Polissiou, M.G. Qualitative determination of volatile compounds and quantitative evaluation of safranal and 4-hydroxy-2,6,6-trimethyl-1-cyclohexene-1-carboxaldehyde. *J. Agric. Food Chem.* **2004**, *52*, 4515–4521. [CrossRef] [PubMed]
16. Tarantilis, P.A.; Tsoupras, G.; Polissiou, M. Determination of saffron (*Crocus sativus* L.) components in crude plant extract using high-performance liquid chromatography-UV/Visible photodiode-array detection-mass spectrometry. *J. Chromatogr.* **1995**, *699*, 107–118. [CrossRef]
17. Rios, J.L.; Recio, M.C.; Ginger, R.M.; Manz, S. An update review of saffron and its active constituents. *Phytother Res* **1996**, *10*, 189–193. [CrossRef]
18. Pitsikas, N. Constituents of saffron (*Crocus sativus* L.) as potential candidates for the treatment of anxiety disorders and schizophrenia. *Molecules* **2016**, *21*, 303. [CrossRef]
19. Pitsikas, N. The effects of Crocus sativus L. and its constituents on memory: Basic studies and clinical applications. *Evid. Based Complement. Alternat. Med.* **2015**, *2015*, 926284. [CrossRef]
20. Karkoula, E.; Lemonakis, N.; Kokras, N.; Dalla, C.; Gikas, E.; Skaltsounis, A.L.; Tsarbopoulos, A. Trans-crocin 4 is not hydrolyzed to crocetin following i.p. administration in mice, while it shows penetration through the blood brain barrier. *Fitoterapia* **2018**, *129*, 62–72. [CrossRef]
21. Georgiadou, G.; Grivas, V.; Tarantilis, P.A.; Pitsikas, N. Crocins the active constituents of *Crocus Sativus* L., counteracted ketamine-induced behavioural deficits in rats. *Psychopharmacology* **2014**, *231*, 717–726. [CrossRef] [PubMed]
22. Ghadrdoost, B.; Vafaei, A.; Rashidy-Pour, A.; Hajisoltani, R.; Bandegi, A.R.; Motamedi, F.; Haghighi, S.; Sameni, H.R.; Pahlvan, S. Protective effect of saffron extracts and its active constituent crocin against oxidative stress and spatial learning and memory deficits induced by chronic stress in rats. *Eur. J. Pharmacol.* **2011**, *667*, 222–229. [CrossRef] [PubMed]
23. Naghizadeh, B.; Mansouri, M.T.; Ghorbanzadeh, B.; Farbood, Y.; Sarkaki, A. Protective effects of oral crocin against intracerebroventricular streptozotocin-induced spatial memory deficit and oxidative stress in rats. *Phytomedicine* **2013**, *20*, 537–543. [CrossRef] [PubMed]
24. Himmelseher, S.; Durieux, M.E. Revising a dogma: Ketamine for patients with neurological injury? *Anesth. Analg.* **2005**, *101*, 524–534. [CrossRef] [PubMed]
25. Xiang, Q.; Tan, L.; Zhao, Y.; Wang, J.; Luo, A. Ketamine: The best partner for isoflurane in neonatal anesthesia? *Med. Hypoth.* **2008**, *71*, 868–871. [CrossRef] [PubMed]
26. Ennaceur, A.; Delacour, J. A new one-trial test for neurobiological studies of memory in rats. 1. Behavioral data. *Behav. Brain Res.* **1988**, *31*, 47–59. [CrossRef]
27. Ennaceur, A.; Neave, N.; Aggleton, J.P. Spontaneous object recognition and object location memory in rats: The effects of lesions in the cingulated cortices, the medial prefrontal cortex, the cingulum bundle and the fornix. *Exp. Brain Res.* **1997**, *113*, 509–519. [CrossRef]
28. Vianna, M.R.M.; Alonso, M.; Vila, H.; Quevedo, J.; de Paris, F.; Furman, M.; Levi de Stein, M.; Medina, J.H.; Izquierdo, I. Role of hippocampal signaling pathways in long-term memory formation of a nonassociative learning task in the rat. *Learn. Mem.* **2000**, *7*, 333–340. [CrossRef]
29. Lafioniatis, A.; Bermperian, V.C.; Pitsikas, N. Flumazenil but not bicuculline counteract the impairing effects of anesthetic ketamine on recognition memory in rats. Evidence for a functional interaction between the GABA$_A$-benzodiazepine receptor and ketamine? *Neuropharmacology* **2019**, *148*, 87–95. [CrossRef]
30. Pitsikas, N. The nicotinic α7receptor agonist GTS-21 but not the nicotinic α4β2 receptor agonist ABT-418 attenuate the disrupting effect of anesthetic ketamine on recognition memory. *Behav. Brain Res.* **2020**, *393*, 112778. [CrossRef]
31. Yamakura, T.; Chavez-Noriega, L.E.; Harris, R.A. Subunit-dependent inhibition of human neuronal nicotinic acetylcholine receptors and other ligand-gated ion channels by dissociative anesthetics ketamine and dizocilpine. *Anesthesiology* **2000**, *92*, 1144–1153. [CrossRef] [PubMed]
32. Buggy, D.J.; Nicol, B.; Rowbotham, D.J.; Lambert, D.G. Effects of intravenous anesthetic agents on glutamate release. *Anesthesiology* **2000**, *92*, 1067–1073. [CrossRef] [PubMed]
33. Orser, B.A.; Pennefather, P.S.; MacDonald, J.F. Multiple mechanisms of ketamine blockade of N-methyl-D-aspartate receptors. *Anesthesiology* **1997**, *86*, 903–917. [CrossRef] [PubMed]
34. Zhang, Y.; Wu, S.; Xie, L.; Yu, S.; Zhang, L.; Liu, C.; Zhou, W.; Yu, T. Ketamine within effective range inhibits glutamate transmission from astrocytes to neurons and disrupts synchronization of astrocytes SICs. *Front. Cell Neurosci.* **2019**, *13*, 240. [CrossRef] [PubMed]
35. Lechtenberg, M.; Schepmann, D.; Niehues, M.; Hellenbrand, N.; Wunsch, B.; Hensel, A. Quality and functionality of saffron: Quality control, species assortment, and affinity of extract and isolated saffron compounds to NMDA and σ_1 (Sigma-1) receptors. *Planta Med.* **2008**, *74*, 764–772. [CrossRef]
36. Berger, F.; Hensel, A.; Nieber, K. Saffron extract and trans-crocetin inhibit glutamatergic synaptic transmission in rat cortical brain slices. *Neuroscience* **2011**, *180*, 238–247. [CrossRef]
37. Adabizadeh, M.; Mehri, S.; Rajabpour, M.; Abnous, K.; Rashedinia, M.; Hosseinzadeh, H. The effects of crocin on spatial memory impairment induced by hyoscine: Role of NMDA, AMPA, ERK, and CaMKII proteins in rat hippocampus. *Iran J. Basic Med. Sci.* **2019**, *22*, 601–609.

38. Saeedi, M.; Rashidi-Pour, A. Association between chronic stress and Alzheimer's disease: Therapeutic effects of saffron. *Biomed. Pharmacother.* **2021**, *133*, 110995. [CrossRef]
39. Geromichalos, G.D.; Lamari, F.N.; Papandreou, M.A.; Trafalis, D.T.; Margarity, M.; Papageorgiou, A.; Sinakos, Z. Saffron as a source of novel acetylcholinesterase inhibitors: Molecular docking and in vitro enzymatic studies. *J. Agric. Food Chem.* **2012**, *60*, 6131–6138. [CrossRef]
40. Papandreou, M.A.; Kanakis, C.D.; Polisssiou, M.G.; Efthimiopoulos, S.; Cordopatis, P.; Margarity, M.; Lamari, F.N. Inhibitory activity of amyloid-β aggregation and antioxidant properties of *Crocus sativus* extract and its crocins constituents. *J. Agric. Food Chem.* **2006**, *54*, 8762–8768. [CrossRef]
41. Hadipour, M.; Kaka, G.; Bahrami, F.; Meftahi, G.H.; Jahromi, G.P.; Mohammadi, A.; Sahraei, H. Crocin improved amyloid beta induced long-term potentiation and memory deficits in the hippocampal CA1 neurons in freely moving rats. *Synapse* **2018**, *72*, e22026. [CrossRef] [PubMed]
42. Yuan, Y.; Shan, X.; Men, W.; Zhai, H.; Qiao, X.; Geng, L.; Li, C. The effects of crocin on memory, hippocampal acetylcholine level, and apoptosis, in a rat model of cerebral ischemia. *Biomed. Pharmacother.* **2020**, *130*, 110543. [CrossRef] [PubMed]
43. Cavoy, A.; Delacour, J. Spatial but not object recognition is impaired by aging in rats. *Physiol. Behav.* **1993**, *53*, 527–530. [CrossRef]
44. Pitsikas, N. Effects of scopolamine and L-NAME on rats' performance in the object location test. *Behav. Brain Res.* **2007**, *179*, 294–298. [CrossRef]
45. Kanakis, C.D.; Tarantilis, P.A.; Tajmir-Riahi, A.; Polissiou, M.G. DNA interaction with saffron's secondary metabolites safranal, crocetin, and dimethylcrocetin. *DNA Cell. Biol.* **2007**, *26*, 63–70. [CrossRef]
46. Del Campo, C.P.; Carmona, M.; Maggi, L.; Kanakis, C.D.; Anastasaki, E.G.; Tarantilis, P.A.; Polyssiou, M.G.; Alonso, G.L. Effects of mild temperature conditions during dehydration procedures on saffron quality parameters. *J. Sci. Food Agric.* **2010**, *90*, 719–725. [CrossRef]
47. Carmona, M.; Zalacain, A.; Sanchez, A.M.; Novella, J.L.; Alonso, G.L. Crocetin esters, picrocrocin and its related compounds present in *Crocus sativus* stigmas and Gardenia jasminoides fruits. Tentative identification of seven new compounds by LC-ESI-MS. *J. Agric. Food Chem.* **2006**, *54*, 973–979. [CrossRef]
48. Mohajeri, S.A.; Hosseinzadeh, H.; Keyhanfar, F.; Aghamohammadian, J. Extraction of crocin from saffron (*Crocus sativus*) using molecularly imprinted polymer solid-phase extraction. *J. Sep. Sci.* **2010**, *33*, 2302–2309. [CrossRef]
49. Karkoula, E.; Angelis Koulakiotis, N.S.; Gikas, E.; Halabalaki, M.; Tsarbopoulos, A.; Skaltsounis, A.L. Rapid isolation and characterization of crocins, picrocrocin, and crocetin from saffron using centrifugal partition chromatography and LC-MS. *J. Sep. Sci.* **2018**, *41*, 4105–4114. [CrossRef]
50. Kirk, R.E. *Experimental Design: Procedures for the Behavioral Science*; Brooks/Cole: Belmont, CA, USA, 1968.

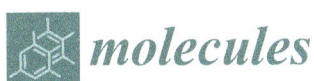 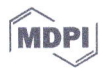

Article

Antianhedonic and Antidepressant Effects of Affron®, a Standardized Saffron (*Crocus Sativus* L.) Extract

Laura Orio, Francisco Alen *, Antonio Ballesta, Raquel Martin and Raquel Gomez de Heras

Department of Psychobiology and Behavioral Sciences Methods, Faculty of Psychology, Complutense University of Madrid, 28223 Madrid, Spain; lorio@psi.ucm.es (L.O.); aj.ballesta@ucm.es (A.B.); rmarti14@ucm.es (R.M.); rgomezhe@psi.ucm.es (R.G.d.H.)
* Correspondence: falenfar@ucm.es

Academic Editor: Nikolaos Pitsikas
Received: 25 May 2020; Accepted: 7 July 2020; Published: 15 July 2020

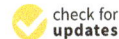

Abstract: Anxiety and depression have high prevalence in the general population, affecting millions of people worldwide, but there is still a need for effective and safe treatments. Nutritional supplements have recently received a lot of attention, particularly saffron. Thus, several pre-clinical studies support a beneficial role for bioactive compounds, such as saffron, in anxiety and depression. Here we used an animal model of depression based on social isolation to assess the effects of affron®, a standardized saffron extract containing ≥3.5% of total bioactive compounds safranal and crocin isomers. Affron® was administered both through the oral and the intraperitoneal routes, and several tasks related to anxiety and depression, such as the elevated plus maze, the forced swimming test or the sucrose preference test, were assessed. These tasks model key features of depressive states and anxious states relating to fear, behavioral despair or anhedonia, the lack of motivation and/or pleasure from everyday activities, respectively. Animals receiving oral affron® displayed behaviors congruent with improvements in their anxious/depressive state, showing the enhanced consumption of a sweet solution, as well as an increase in certain escape responses in the forced swimming test. Our data support a beneficial role for oral saffron in anxious/depressive states.

Keywords: saffron; affron®; depression; anxiety; antioxidant

1. Introduction

Anxiety and depression are widely acknowledged as psychiatric disorders of global concern that could compromise human welfare [1], thus, the two conditions often co-exist; between 40% and 60% of patients with a common mental health disorder meet criteria for both anxiety and depression [2,3]. According to the World Health Organization data, there is high prevalence for depression and anxiety, affecting more than 300 million people worldwide, and they include the mixed depressive and anxiety disorder in their International Classification of Diseases [4]. These two conditions share common risk factors and many symptoms that can be regarded as existing on a spectrum of the disorder [5].

Mood alterations, including clinical depression, range from non-clinical low mood to major depression [6–8]. This low mood can include many of the symptoms characteristic of depression, such as sadness, crying, fatigue, pessimism, changes in appetite, changes in sleep patterns and anhedonia [6,7,9]. Currently there is no pharmacological treatment for low mood, and prescription medications are not only deemed inappropriate but also ineffective [10,11].

The conventional management of depression and anxiety disorders includes cognitive behavioral therapy, pharmacotherapy or electroconvulsive therapy [8,12]. However, despite the availability of numerous classes of drugs for the treatment, full remission of disease symptoms has remained elusive. Nevertheless, the clinical use of these drugs is limited by their characteristic side effects and poor tolerability profile [13]. Several natural compounds are being considered for their possible role in the treatment of mood disorders, including saffron, St John's wort, tryptophan and omega-3 fatty acids, among others [14–16].

Saffron dried stigmas from *Crocus sativus* L. are conventionally used as a spice, textile dye or even as a perfume, due to its organoleptic properties. In addition, it is also widely known in traditional medicine for eye problems, headaches, genitourinary complications and other illnesses in different cultures [17–20]. The quality of saffron is determined by its secondary metabolites, such as picrocrocin, which is responsible for the bitter taste, safranal, which is related to saffron aroma, and crocins, which provide the color [21–23]. These compounds, mainly safranal and crocin isomers, as well as their metabolic derivate, crocetin, are related to antioxidant [24,25], anxiolytic [26,27], neuroprotective [28], anti-inflammatory [29–31] antidepressant [32–34] and anti-Alzheimer properties, which have been proven in several clinical trials [35].

As with most psychiatric disorders, the etiopathology of depression appears to be complex and multifactorial, including genetic, social and mood regulation mechanisms, among others. Alterations in neurotransmitter levels, including the abnormal regulation of cholinergic, catecholaminergic (noradrenergic or dopaminergic), glutamatergic and serotonergic (5-HT) neurotransmission have been observed in depressed patients [36]. Neuroendocrine dysregulation may also be a factor, with emphasis on three axes: hypothalamic–pituitary–adrenal and hypothalamic–pituitary–thyroid [37]. A molecular imbalance, characterized by increased levels of oxidative stress and low antioxidant status, has also been observed in patients with depression [38]. This would favor the appearance of immune responses and a pro-inflammatory environment, thus contributing to the pathology of depression [39]. Recently the relation between alterations in neuroplasticity and depression has received considerable attention. The term refers to the ability of the neural system to adapt to the internal and external stimuli and to respond adaptively to future stimuli. Neuroplasticity is of key significance in the brain's adaptation to stress, which may underlie various psychiatric disorders, such as depression, post-traumatic stress disorder, etc., and is the basis of the so-called neuroplasticity theory, which suggests a decrease in neuroplasticity in the hippocampus and prefrontal cortex in depressed patients, as well as a decrease in the concentration of neurotrophic factors, such as brain-derived neurotrophic factor (BDNF), in subjects with depression. According to this theory, antidepressants would elevate the concentration of neurotrophic factors and improve neuroplasticity in the hippocampus and PFC [40].

Kell and colleagues found positive effects in subjects self-reporting low mood but not diagnosed with depression or another mood disorder and who were otherwise healthy [33]. Additionally, there is also growing evidence supporting the antidepressant and anxiolytic effects of saffron in humans suffering from depression and anxiety. Thus, saffron extracts can relieve the severity of symptoms of depression and the effect of saffron extracts resemble those of tricyclic (TCA), Selective Serotonin Reuptake Inhibitors (SSRI) and Selective Noradrenaline Reuptake Inhibitors antidepressants in depressed patients [41,42]. Saffron extracts, when administered in combination with pharmacological antidepressants, were also shown to improve some scores related to depression, even in subjects who had been using the antidepressants with no improvement [43]. In this case, the affron® dose used was 14 mg b.i.d.

The active principles contained in saffron extracts, which account for the active antidepressants, are basically safranal and crocin isomers [44–46]. However, there is a wide variety of presentations that do not control the content of these bioactive molecules, making it very difficult to compare commercial brands in terms of pharmacological effectiveness. The safety and efficacy of safranal and crocin bioactive components have been described elsewhere, showing an exceptionally low toxicity, with an LD50 for normal cells of 20.7 g/kg [47]. In living animals, doses of the ethanolic extract up to 5 g/kg did not produce any demonstrable acute toxic effects in mice, and thus saffron is considered to have practically no acute toxic effect [48]. In our experiment, affron®, a standardized extract from Spanish *C. sativus* stigmas, was used.

Although there are a number of favorable clinical studies regarding the effects of affron® on the modulation of the symptoms of depression and anxiety in humans [43,49–59], it is necessary to observe

2. Results and Discussion

2.1. Effects of Affron® in the Elevated Plus Maze Test

Affron® was shown to be equally as ineffective either orally administered or by the intraperitoneal route. A one-way ANOVA showed that neither dose of affron® (200 mg/kg p.o. and 50 mg/kg ip) produced changes in any of the anxiety-related parameters (time spent in the open arms and number of entries into open arms of the EPM) ($p > 0.05$, not significant (ns)). Bonferroni's post hoc test confirmed that no statistically significant differences existed between treated and placebo groups ($p > 0.05$, ns) in acute and chronic treatments. No differences were observed for the time in open arms variable in any of the groups, as shown in Figure 1C,D. Values represent the mean ± SEM ($n = 10$ animals per group).

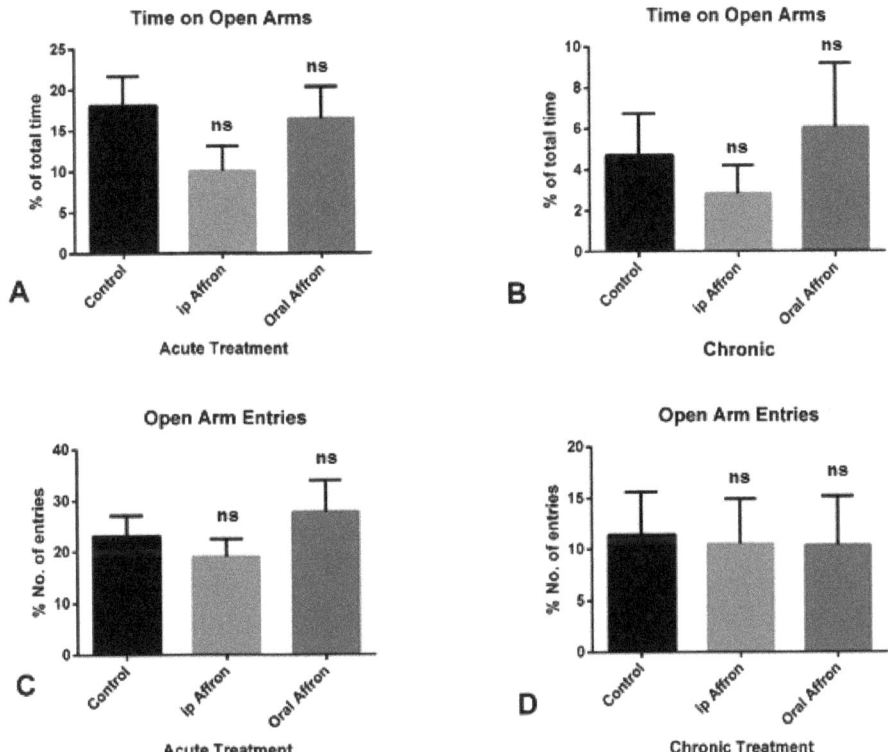

Figure 1. Effects of affron in the Elevated Plus Maze. (**A,B**): Percentage of time spent in open arms over the total in the acute and chronic treatment groups, respectively. (**C,D**): Percentage of entries in the open arms in the acute and chronic treatment, respectively. No significant effects were found between any of the groups in any condition (ns). The tests were administered on day one of treatment and on day 21 for the chronic group, 30 min after drug administration.

2.2. Effects of Affron® in the Forced Swimming Test

A one-way ANOVA revealed that affron® (200 mg/kg, oral) administered 30 min before the FST significantly increased swimming time [F (2.27) = 7.37, $p < 0.01$], as shown in Figure 2A] but had no impact on climbing time or immobility time (ns) (data not shown). The post-hoc Bonferroni's test showed that affron®, given at a dose of 200 mg/kg significantly increased the time of swimming in the oral group compared to the control and ip groups ($p < 0.05$ and $p < 0.01$, respectively). Concerning the antidepressant-like activity of affron®, after 20 days of treatment, an increase in climbing time was observed in the oral group [$F (2,27) = 4.91, p < 0.05$], as shown in Figure 2D. A one-way ANOVA did not find any statistically significant difference in the rest of the variables (ns); however, affron® treatment, both oral and intraperitoneal, tended to decrease immobility time compared to the control group, which led to a possible antidepressant effect of this compound, as shown in Figure 2D. The post hoc test revealed a significant increase in climbing time in the oral group compared with the control group ($p < 0.05$), but there were no significant differences in the remaining groups (ns).

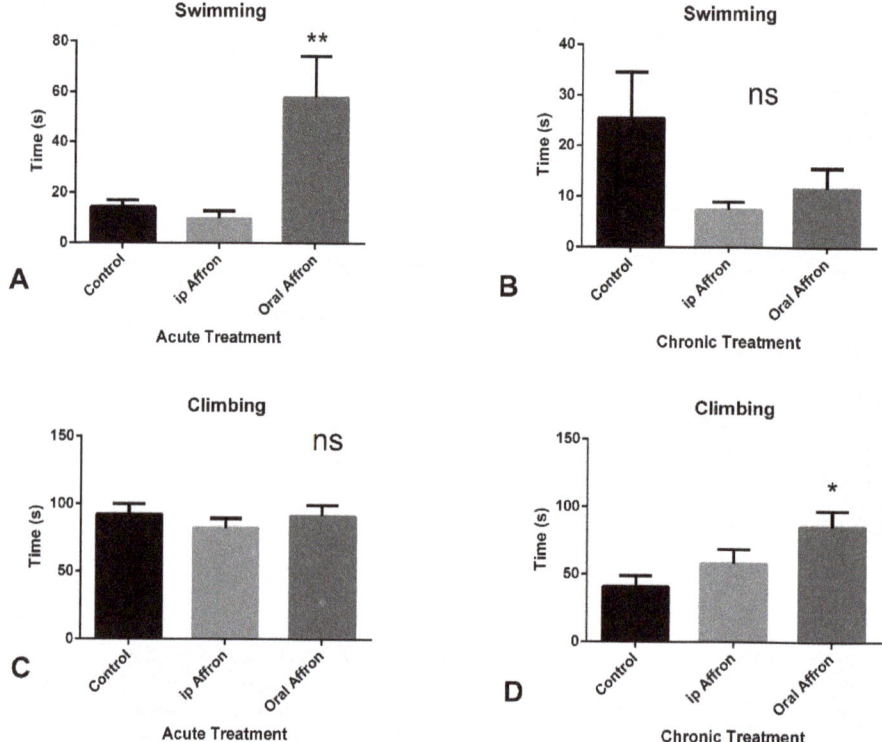

Figure 2. (**A,B**): Average time spent in immobility or swimming in the Porsolt test in animals receiving either an acute or a chronic treatment with affron through the intraperitoneal (gray column) or the oral (black column) route, respectively (** $p < 0.01$). (**C,D**): Average time climbing in the acute and chronic treatments, respectively (* $p < 0.05$; ns = Non Significant). The tests were administered on day one of treatment and on day 21 for the chronic group, 40 min after drug administration.

2.3. Effects of affron® in the Sucrose Preference Test

Repeated-measures two-way ANOVA found an overall interaction between time and treatments [$F (6,78) = 12.30, p < 0.0001$] and main effects of time [$F (3,78) = 318.7, p < 0.0001$] and treatment [$F (2,26) = 19.20, p < 0.0001$]. Subsequent analysis revealed that, as reflected in Figure 3, after an hour, a significant increase in the sucrose preference was found in the oral group with respect to the intraperitoneal group ($p < 0.05$), but there were no differences between the oral and intraperitoneal groups compared to the control group (ns). Statistically significant differences were observed in the 3 h measure in sucrose consumption between the oral group with respect to the control and intraperitoneal groups ($p < 0.0001$), but there was no difference between the control and the intraperitoneal groups (ns).

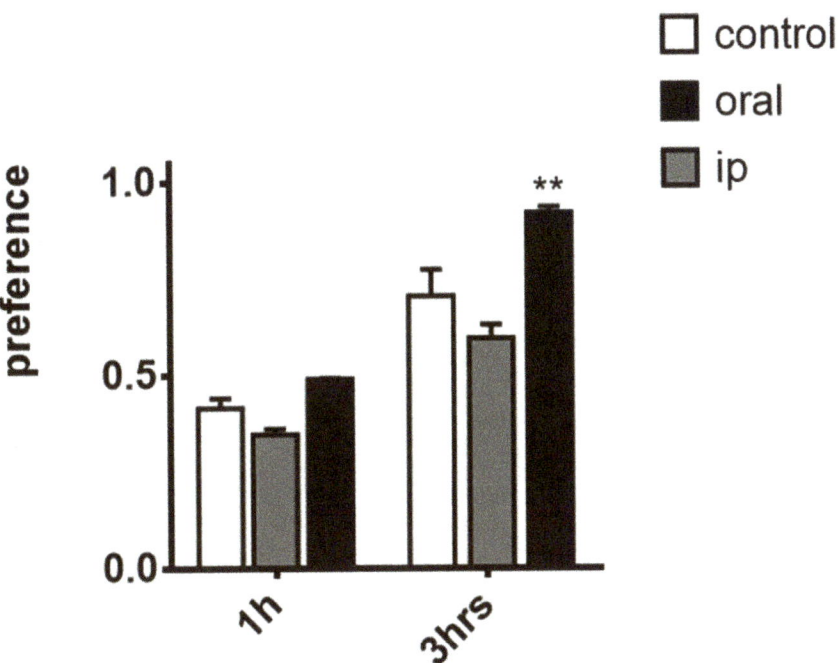

Figure 3. Sucrose preference test. Sucrose preference was calculated as the quantity of sucrose solution drunk/total fluid intake and is considered an index of the motivational state of the animal, ($n = 10$ per group) represented as mean ± SEM. Repeated-measures two-way ANOVA with Bonferroni post-hoc test: ** $p < 0.001$; differences between the oral group and the control group. The tests were administered on day one of treatment and on day 21 for the chronic group, 50 min after drug administration.

The results showed that the oral administration of affron® may ameliorate some depressive-like behaviors both acutely and after long-term treatment. Interestingly, no effects were observed with the intraperitoneal administration. Additionally, repeated oral administration reduced anhedonic behavior, assessed in the sucrose preference test—an effect that was not observed under ip administration. Overall, these results are congruent with reports describing the beneficial effects of saffron extract consumption in patients suffering from anxiety or depression [41,42].

Considering the fact that drugs used to treat mental disorders are best studied in models of the disease, we used a rat model of depression, based on isolation [60]. Thus, individual housing has been shown to induce depressive-like behavior [61]. For that, animals were individually housed from arrival at the facilities until the end of the experiments, which allowed us to monitor any possible improvement or amelioration in behaviors related to anxiety, depression or anhedonia after affron® supplementation.

Regarding the anxiolytic effects in the elevated plus maze, no significant differences were found between any of the groups in our study. In other studies, higher doses of saffron ip (56 and 80 mg/kg) showed anxiolytic effects in the EPM with a single dose, and a dose-dependent effect that decreased with doses up to 300 mg/kg [62]. It is possible that the lower dose used in our study limited the expression of the anxiolytic potential of affron®. It is also possible that differences in the source of plant material could explain the different findings in our study.

Data on the forced-swimming test assessing depressive-like behavior were clearer. On the one hand, affron® did not affect immobility time or latency to the immobility period. However, a clear effect in the escape behavior (swimming and climbing) with the oral administration of affron® can be observed. Our data are interpreted in line with the presence of antidepressant effect, since the animals clearly show more motivation to fight against the adverse conditions of being exposed to the water environment. These data appear relevant as they highlight the ability of saffron extracts to acutely improve depressive-like behavior.

To our knowledge, the antianhedonic effects of affron® in the sucrose preference test have not been previously reported in animal studies. This is the clearest effect found with affron® in the study. Oral dose was able to increase the preference for the sweet drink, which is indicative of a positive motivational state. Again, in this situation, oral administration was effective instead of intraperitoneal injection. Interestingly, intraperitoneal administration may even induce the opposite effect (i.e., anhedonia, indicative of desensitization of the brain reward system). It is worth mentioning that the antianhedonic response, measured by sucrose preference, differs in response to antidepressants with different mechanisms of action, such as SSRI and TCA [63].

The fact that the oral administration of affron® was the effective route to observe the positive effects of this compound, and not ip administration, may be related to the fact that the active form of crocin isomers from saffron extract is crocetin, which is formed in the intestinal tract by glycosidases of enterocytes [64–66]. Thus, the saffron extract must, apparently, be taken orally to induce its antidepressant effect. In any case, oral administration is the preferred route for any potential nutraceutical since the majority of nutraceuticals are intended for this route of administration.

The neurobiological mechanisms that explain affron's antianhedonic effect and possible antidepressant effect have not been directly assessed yet. Regulation of mood was initially attributed to downregulations in monoamines, such as dopamine, serotonin or noradrenaline [67–69]. Whereas anhedonia is associated with low levels of dopamine, anxiety and depression appear to be more associated with the decreased activity of both serotonin and dopamine. The clear actions of affron® in the amelioration of anhedonia suggest a more potent action in the regulation of dopamine than serotonin or other monoamines. Indeed, regarding dopamine modulation, it has been proven that saffron affected monoamine oxidases MAO-A and MAO-B in the brain [68], and the administration of *C. sativus* and its constituents increased brain dopamine levels in a dose-dependent manner [68]. These effects of *C. Sativus* in dopamine, together with the modulation of the excitatory amino acid, glutamate, and interactions with the opioid system have been reported to reduce withdrawal syndrome and may contribute to the amelioration of behavioral symptoms observed here [68].

However, the regulation of mood has been more recently associated with other factors, such as the alteration of neurotrophic factors, dysregulation in the hypothalamus–hypophysis–adrenal axis (HPA), low-grade inflammation or increased oxidative stress [70–72]. Certain evidence suggests that saffron regulates some of these mechanisms [73]. Indeed, saffron and its constituents, crocin and safranal, as well as crocetin, are potent antioxidants that can reduce oxidative stress, as demonstrated in animal models [74–76]. Its anti-inflammatory properties [77,78] and the modulation of the activity HPA in animal models of stress (i.e., by reducing levels of plasma corticosterone [79,80]) have also been proven. Future studies are needed to explore the specific actions of different doses of affron® in these processes.

3. Material and Methods

3.1. Materials

Affron® is a patented compound (ES2573542A1) and has been previously characterized [33]. Samples of saffron stigma extracts marketed under the brand name affron® were provided by Pharmactive Biotech Products SL, standardized to ≥3.5% Lepticrosalides®, a term which characterizes the sum of the bioactive compounds safranal and crocin isomers, analyzed by HPLC [33]. The compound was presented in powder form and stored in darkness until the experiment was performed.

3.2. Animals

A total of 30 adult male Wistar rats (ENVIGO, Barcelona, Spain) weighting 300–350 g at the beginning of the experiments were kept under a 12-h light/dark cycle (lights off at 12:00 p.m.) in conditions of constant temperature (23 ± 1 °C). Standard food and tap water were available ad libitum at the home-cage outside the schedules assigned to experimental manipulation.

All experimental protocols adhered to the guidelines of the Animal Welfare Committee of the Universidad Complutense of Madrid, following European legislation (European Directive 2010/63/UE).

3.3. Experimental Design

Animals had an acclimation period of one week, after which they were habituated to manipulation for several days before the experiment started. Upon arrival at the facilities, animals were housed in isolation for the duration of the study, according to a social isolation model of anxious/depressive-like behavior [81]. Animals' weights were recorded every two days during the experiment. Rats were randomly assigned to one of the three of the following experimental groups: Oral affron® (Oral), Intraperiotoneally administered affron® (ip) and Vehicle (10 rats per group). In the Oral group, affron® was dissolved in their tap water and the rats were monitored to ensure they consumed an adequate dose during the first hours of the morning (See Figure 4 for a schematic representation of the experimental schedule used).

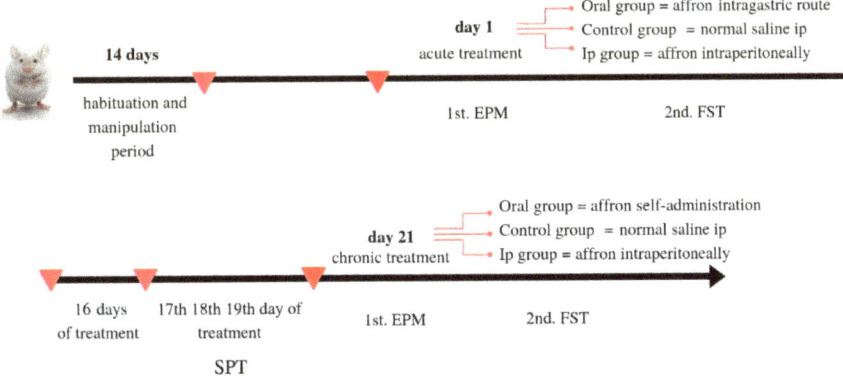

Figure 4. Schematic representation of the treatment schedule.

Behavioral tests were performed on the first day of the experiment in order to assess the acute effects of the treatment, and also after the chronic treatment. The tests used were the elevated plus maze (EPM), the Forced swim test (FST) and the sucrose preference test (SPT).

3.3.1. Treatment

The animals received a single dose of affron®, dissolved in distilled water at the beginning of the experiment. Rats in the oral group received 200 mg/kg affron®, which was delivered via the use of an intra-gastric cannula in a volume of 2 mL/kg. The control group was treated with 0.9% saline solution via intraperitoneal injection (ip) in a volume of 2 mL/kg. The ip group received 50 mg/kg affron® dissolved in saline. Thirty minutes after each administration, the animals were tested on the elevated plus maze (EPM) and 30 min later they were assessed in the forced swim test (FST). For the next 20 days, rats in the oral group had free access to 200 mg/kg affron dissolved in their drinking water until they consumed the whole daily dose, which took place in less than 4 h, after which tap water was reintroduced. The rest of the animals received their daily dose via ip. The animals underwent the sucrose preference test on the 17th day of the experiment 30 min after affron® administration. Likewise, on the 21st day of the experiment, the animals were assessed at the elevated plus maze, and 30 min later, at the forced swimming test. All treatments were prepared and administered daily, and all tests took place between 9:00 and 14:00.

3.3.2. Anxiety and Depression-Like Behavior

Several different models were used for the assessment of anxiety- and depression-related behaviors in rodents [82]. The Forced Swim Test and the Sucrose Preference Test were employed to assess any depressive-like behavioral responses, being some of the most commonly used tests to assess this kind of behavior in animal models [83,84]. The elevated plus maze test was chosen to assess anxiety-related behavior. In addition, in the chronic study, sucrose preference was used as a complementary test for anhedonia [63,85]. Anhedonia is defined as the inability to experience pleasure from rewarding or enjoyable activities and constitutes a core symptom of depression in humans [86]. The order of the tests was chosen to minimize any possible interference. Considering the relative distance and difference in environments between the animal facilities and the testing room, 10 min of acclimation were granted prior to the behavioral tests.

3.3.3. Elevated Plus Maze Test

The elevated plus maze (EPM) is based upon the conflict between an innate aversion to open spaces and a tendency to explore new environments (Suo et al., 2013). The apparatus consisted of two open arms (50 × 10 cm), two closed arms (50 × 10 × 20 cm) and a central platform (10 × 10 cm), which raised to a height of 50 cm. The maze was placed in the center of a quiet room and testing was performed under dim light. Each animal was gently placed on the central platform facing one of the closed arms and allowed to explore the maze for 5 min. The light of the test room was adjusted at 350 lux at the center of the maze. Then, the animals were removed and the EPM was cleaned with 30% ethanol between each test to prevent interference resulting from any residual odors of the previous rat. Data were registered automatically using the Mazesoft software. The analysis of exploratory activity in rats included four parameters: number of entries into open arms; number of entries into closed arms; time spent in open arms; time spent in closed arms.

3.3.4. Forced Swim Test (Porsolt Test)

The forced swimming test (FST) was originally introduced in 1977 by Porsolt and has since become a standard for the evaluation of antidepressant drugs [87]. In preparation, 24 h prior to the test, animals were placed in the testing apparatus for 10 min in order to become familiar with the testing environment and to minimize novelty effects [82,88]. Briefly, the rats were individually placed in a transparent methacrylate cylinder (height 50 cm, diameter 30 cm) filled with water (23 ± 1 °C) to a height of 40 cm (a modified version of the FST was used to increase water depth to 40 cm, so the rats were unable to touch the bottom of the tank). Water was replaced for each test. Following each test session, rats were dried using cotton towels and returned to their home cages. All sessions were recorded with a video camera (SONY HDR-CX115, New York, NY, USA). Afterwards, four behavioral categories were quantified using the freeware for behavioral quantification, Raton Time 1.0 (Fixma SL, Valencia, Spain), including immobility latency (latency to immobility), immobility (rat floating in the water with only movements necessary to keep the nose above water), swimming (active horizontal movements around the cylinder) and climbing (upward-directed movement of the forepaws, usually directed against the walls). Animals underwent the test 30 min after the elevated plus maze.

3.3.5. Sucrose Preference Test

The sucrose preference test (SPT) is a reward-related test commonly used as an indicator of anhedonia [89]. No previous food or water deprivation was applied before the test. During the adaptation period, the animals were presented in their home cages with two bottles of the type used for the test, in order to habituate them to testing conditions. The rats were allowed simultaneous access to two identical drinking bottles that contained a 1% sucrose solution for 3 h. The sucrose solution was prepared daily before the experiment and kept at 4 °C for no longer than 24 h. The position of the drinking bottles was changed after each measurement to exclude the effect of place preference [89,90]. The consumption of water and sucrose solution was calculated by weighing each bottle before, during and after the test. Sucrose preference was calculated as the quantity of sucrose solution drunk/total fluid intake [2]. The sucrose preference test was performed on the 17th day of treatment in order to avoid interferences with the other tests.

3.4. Statistical Analyses

The data are expressed as mean ± standard error of mean (SEM). Normality data were assessed by D'Agostino and Pearson test. Data were analyzed using GraphPad Prism version 6.0. In order to detect significant differences among the experimental groups, depending on the behavioral test, either one-way analysis of variance with one factor (treatment) or two-way ANOVA comparing two factors—treatment (oral, intraperitoneal, control) and time—was used. Data of the behavioral tests were analyzed as dependent variables, and the Bonferroni post-hoc test for multiple comparisons was used when appropriate. Values of $p \leq 0.05$ were considered statistically significant.

4. Conclusions

In conclusion, this study provides evidence of the antianhedonic, and mild antidepressant actions of a 50 mg/kg acute ip dose and a 200 mg/kg oral dose of affron®, a standardized saffron extract, when administered acutely or repeatedly, orally. Future studies are required to ascertain the specific mechanisms of this action. Anyhow, these results open new fields for the possible application of affron® to prevent negative emotional states or as a co-adjuvant therapy in the treatment of depression.

Author Contributions: L.O., R.G.d.H. and F.A.: Experimental design, supervision and writing. A.B. and R.M.: experimental procedures and data analyses. All authors have read and agree to the published version of the manuscript.

Funding: This research received no external funding.

Acknowledgments: The authors gratefully acknowledge the Pharmactive Biotech Products, SL Company, for funding the project and supplying affron®. We also thank Alberto Espinel, Paula Almodóvar and Daniel González Hedström for their help and support.

Conflicts of Interest: Other than the funding of this work by Pharmactive Biotech Products SL, the authors declare no conflict of interest.

References

1. Fajemiroye, J.O.; Galdino, P.M.; Florentino, I.F.; Da Rocha, F.F.; Ghedini, P.C.; Polepally, P.R.; Zjawiony, J.K.; Costa, E.A. Plurality of anxiety and depression alteration mechanism by oleanolic acid. *J. Psychopharmacol.* **2014**, *28*, 923–934. [CrossRef] [PubMed]
2. Kessler, R.C.; Berglund, P.; Demler, O.; Jin, R.; Merikangas, K.R.; Walters, E.E. Lifetime prevalence and age-of-onset distributions of DSM-IV disorders in the National Comorbidity Survey Replication. *Arch. Gen. Psychiatry* **2005**, *62*, 593–602. [CrossRef] [PubMed]
3. McManus, S.; Meltzer, H.; Brugha, T.; Bebbington, P.; Jenkins, R. *Adult Psychiatric Morbidity in England, 2007. Results of a Household Survey*; The Health and Social Care Information Centre; National Centre for Social Research: Leeds, UK, 2009; p. 12.
4. World Health Organization. International Classification of Diseases for Mortality and Morbidity Statistics (11th Revision). 2018. Available online: https://icd.who.int/browse11/l-m/en (accessed on 1 July 2020).
5. Newby, J.M.; McKinnon, A.; Kuyken, W.; Gilbody, S.; Dalgleish, T. Systematic review and meta-analysis of transdiagnostic psychological treatments for anxiety and depressive disorders in adulthood. *Clin. Psychol. Rev.* **2015**, *40*, 91–110. [CrossRef] [PubMed]
6. Keller, M.C.; Nesse, R.M. Is low mood an adaptation? Evidence for subtypes with symptoms that match precipitants. *J. Affect. Disord.* **2005**, *86*, 27–35. [CrossRef] [PubMed]

7. Nettle, D. Understanding of evolution may be improved by thinking about people. *Evol. Psychol.* **2010**, *8*, 205–228. [CrossRef]
8. Gelenberg, A.J.; Freeman, M.P.; Markowitz, J.C.; Rosenbaum, J.F.; Thase, M.E.; Trivedi, M.H.; Van Rhoads, R.S.; Reus, V.I.; DePaulo, J.R., Jr.; Fawcett, J.A. Practice guideline for the treatment of patients with major depressive disorder third edition. *Am. J. Psychiatry* **2010**, *167*.
9. Bolmont, B.; Abraini, J.H. State-anxiety and low moods: Evidence for a single concept. *Physiol. Behav.* **2001**, *74*, 421–424. [CrossRef]
10. Baumeister, H.; Knecht, A.; Hutter, N. Direct and indirect costs in persons with chronic back pain and comorbid mental disorders–a systematic review. *J. Psychosom. Res.* **2012**, *73*, 79–85. [CrossRef]
11. Salum, G.A.; Isolan, L.R.; Bosa, V.L.; Tocchetto, A.G.; Teche, S.P.; Schuch, I.; Costa, J.R.; Costa Mde, A.; Jarros, R.B.; Mansur, M.A.; et al. The multidimensional evaluation and treatment of anxiety in children and adolescents: Rationale, design, methods and preliminary findings. *Rev. Bra. Psiquiatria.* **2011**, *33*, 181–195. [CrossRef]
12. National Institute for Health and Clinical Excellence. *National Collaborating Centre for Mental Health. The Treatment and Management of Depression in Adults (Updated Edition)*; National Clinical Practice Guideline 90; National Institute for Health and Care Excellence: London, UK, 2010; pp. 466–536.
13. Fajemiroye, J.O.; da Silva, D.M.; de Oliveira, D.R.; Costa, E.A. Treatment of anxiety and depression: Medicinal plants in retrospect. *Fund. Clin. Pharmacol.* **2016**, *30*, 198–215. [CrossRef]
14. Sarris, J. Herbal medicines in the treatment of psychiatric disorders: 10-year updated review. *Phytother. Res.* **2018**, *32*, 1147–1162. [CrossRef] [PubMed]
15. Dome, P.; Tombor, L.; Lazary, J.; Gonda, X.; Rihmer, Z.J.B.R.B. Natural health products, dietary minerals and over-the-counter medications as add-on therapies to antidepressants in the treatment of major depressive disorder: A review. *Brain Res. Bull.* **2019**, *146*, 51–78. [CrossRef]
16. Mischoulon, D.; Rapaport, M.H.A. Current Role of Herbal and Natural Preparations. *Antidepressants* **2019**, *250*, 225–252.
17. Bathaie, S.Z.; Mousavi, S.Z. Historical uses of saffron: Identifying potential new avenues for modern Research. *Avicenna, J. Phytomed.* **2011**, *1*, 57–66.
18. Fernández, J. Biology, biotechnology and biomedicine of saffron. *Recent Res. Dev. Plant. Sci.* **2004**, *2*, 127–159.
19. Grigg, D.B. *The Agricultural Systems of the World: An. Evolutionary Approach*; Cambridge University Press: Cambridge, UK, 1974.
20. Leone, S.; Recinella, L.; Chiavaroli, A.; Orlando, G.; Ferrante, C.; Leporini, L.; Brunetti, L.; Menghini, L. Phytotherapic use of the Crocus sativus L. (Saffron) and its potential applications: A brief overview. *Phytother. Res.* **2018**, *32*, 2364–2375. [CrossRef]
21. Srivastava, R.; Ahmed, H.; Dixit, R.K.; Dharamveer, P.; Saraf, S.A. Crocus sativus L.: A comprehensive review. *Pharmacogn. Rev.* **2010**, *4*, 200–208. [CrossRef]
22. Sampathu, S.; Shivashankar, S.; Lewis, Y.; Wood, A. Saffron (Crocus sativus Linn.)—Cultivation, processing, chemistry and standardization. *Crit. Rev. Food Sci. Nutr.* **1984**, *20*, 123–157. [CrossRef]
23. Kyriakoudi, A.; Ordoudi, S.; Roldan-Medina, M.; Tsimidou, M. Saffron, a Functional Spice. *Austin J. Nutr. Food Sci.* **2015**, *3*, 1051–1059.
24. Farahmand, S.K.; Samini, F.; Samini, M.; Samarghandian, S. Safranal ameliorates antioxidant enzymes and suppresses lipid peroxidation and nitric oxide formation in aged male rat liver. *Biogerontology* **2013**, *14*, 63–71. [CrossRef]
25. Asdaq, S.M.B.; Inamdar, M.N. Potential of Crocus sativus (saffron) and its constituent, crocin, as hypolipidemic and antioxidant in rats. *Appl. Biochem. Biotechnol.* **2010**, *162*, 358–372. [CrossRef] [PubMed]
26. Ardebili, D.; Hosseinzadeh, H.; Abnous, K.; Hasani, F.V.; Robati, R.Y.; Razavi, B.M. Involvement of brain-derived neurotrophic factor (BDNF) on malathion induced depressive-like behavior in subacute exposure and protective effects of crocin. *Iran. J. Basic Med. Sci.* **2015**, *18*, 958.
27. Pitsikas, N.; Boultadakis, A.; Georgiadou, G.; Tarantilis, P.A.; Sakellaridis, N. Effects of the active constituents of Crocus sativus L., crocins, in an animal model of anxiety. *Phytomedicine* **2008**, *15*, 1135–1139. [CrossRef] [PubMed]
28. Ghasemi, R.; Moosavi, M.; Zarifkar, A.; Rastegar, K. The interplay of Akt and ERK in Aβ toxicity and insulin-mediated protection in primary hippocampal cell culture. *J. Mol. Neurosci.* **2015**, *57*, 325–334. [CrossRef]

29. Nam, K.N.; Park, Y.M.; Jung, H.J.; Lee, J.Y.; Min, B.D.; Park, S.U.; Jung, W.S.; Cho, K.H.; Park, J.H.; Kang, I.; et al. Anti-inflammatory effects of crocin and crocetin in rat brain microglial cells. *Eur. J. Pharmacol.* **2010**, *648*, 110–116. [CrossRef]
30. Rathore, B.; Jaggi, K.; Thakur, S.K.; Mathur, A.; Mahdi, F. Anti-inflammatory activity of *Crocus sativus* extract in experimental arthritis. *Int. J. Pharm. Sci. Res.* **2015**, *6*, 1473.
31. Hosseinzadeh, H.; Younesi, H.M. Antinociceptive and anti-inflammatory effects of *Crocus sativus* L. stigma and petal extracts in mice. *BMC Pharmacol.* **2002**, *2*, 7. [CrossRef]
32. Hosseinzadeh, H.; Parvardeh, S. Anticonvulsant effects of thymoquinone, the major constituent of *Nigella sativa* seeds, in mice. *Phytomedicine* **2004**, *11*, 56–64. [CrossRef]
33. Kell, G.; Rao, A.; Beccaria, G.; Clayton, P.; Inarejos-Garcia, A.; Prodanov, M. affron((R)) a novel saffron extract (Crocus sativus L.) improves mood in healthy adults over 4 weeks in a double-blind, parallel, randomized, placebo-controlled clinical trial. *Complement. Ther. Med.* **2017**, *33*, 58–64. [CrossRef]
34. Abe, K.; Sugiura, M.; Shoyama, Y.; Saito, H. Crocin antagonizes ethanol inhibition of NMDA receptor-mediated responses in rat hippocampal neurons. *Brain Res.* **1998**, *787*, 132–138. [CrossRef]
35. Hosseini, A.; Razavi, B.M.; Hosseinzadeh, H. Pharmacokinetic Properties of Saffron and its Active Components. *Eur. J. Drug Metab. Pharmacokinet.* **2018**, *43*, 383–390. [CrossRef] [PubMed]
36. Chen, M.C.; Gotlib, I.H. 13 Molecular Foundations of the Symptoms of Major Depressive Disorder. *Oxf. Handb. Mol. Psychol.* **2015**, 258.
37. Roy, A.; Roy, R.N. Stress and Major Depression: Neuroendocrine and Biopsychosocial Mechanisms. In *Stress Neuroendocrinology Neurobiology: Handbook of Stress Series 2*; Elsevier: San Diego, CA, USA, 2017; pp. 173–184.
38. Palta, P.; Samuel, L.J.; Miller, E.R.; Szanton, S.L. Depression and oxidative stress: Results from a meta-analysis of observational studies. *Psychosom. Med.* **2014**, *76*, 12–19. [CrossRef] [PubMed]
39. Leonard, B.; Maes, M. Mechanistic explanations how cell-mediated immune activation, inflammation and oxidative and nitrosative stress pathways and their sequels and concomitants play a role in the pathophysiology of unipolar depression. *Neurosci. Biobehav. R.* **2012**, *36*, 764–785. [CrossRef] [PubMed]
40. Jones, K. Review of neuroplasticity and depression: Evidence for the neurotrophic or neuroplasticity theory of depression pathophysiology and systematic review of the neurophysiological implications of long-term antidepressant treatment. 2016. [CrossRef]
41. Marx, W.; Lane, M.; Rocks, T.; Ruusunen, A.; Loughman, A.; Lopresti, A.; Marshall, S.; Berk, M.; Jacka, F.; Dean, O.M. Effect of saffron supplementation on symptoms of depression and anxiety: A systematic review and meta-analysis. *Nutr. Rev.* **2019**. [CrossRef]
42. Tóth, B.; Hegyi, P.; Lantos, T.; Szakács, Z.; Kerémi, B.; Varga, G.; Tenk, J.; Pétervári, E.; Balaskó, M.; Rumbus, Z. The efficacy of saffron in the treatment of mild to moderate depression: A meta-analysis. *Planta Med.* **2019**, *85*, 24–31. [CrossRef]
43. Lopresti, A.L.; Smith, S.J.; Hood, S.D.; Drummond, P.D. Efficacy of a standardised saffron extract (affron(R)) as an add-on to antidepressant medication for the treatment of persistent depressive symptoms in adults: A randomised, double-blind, placebo-controlled study. *J. Psychopharmacol.* **2019**, *33*, 1415–1427. [CrossRef]
44. Hosseinzadeh, H.; Karimi, G.; Niapoor, M. Antidepressant effects of Crocus sativus stigma extracts and its constituents, crocin and safranal, in mice. *J. Med. Plants* **2004**, *3*, 48–58.
45. Hassani, F.V.; Naseri, V.; Razavi, B.M.; Mehri, S.; Abnous, K.; Hosseinzadeh, H. Antidepressant effects of crocin and its effects on transcript and protein levels of CREB, BDNF, and VGF in rat hippocampus. *DARU* **2014**, *22*, 16. [CrossRef]
46. Razavi, B.M.; Sadeghi, M.; Abnous, K.; Hasani, F.V.; Hosseinzadeh, H. Study of the role of CREB, BDNF, and VGF neuropeptide in long term antidepressant activity of crocin in the rat cerebellum. *DARU* **2017**, *16*, 1452.
47. Bostan, H.B.; Mehri, S.; Hosseinzadeh, H. Toxicology effects of saffron and its constituents: A review. *Irn. J. Basic Med. Sci.* **2017**, *20*, 110–121. [CrossRef]
48. Lymperopoulou, C.; Lamari, F.J.M.A.P. Saffron safety in humans: Lessons from the animal and clinical studies. *Med. Aromat Plants* **2015**, *4*, e164.
49. Agha-Hosseini, M.; Kashani, L.; Aleyaseen, A.; Ghoreishi, A.; Rahmanpour, H.; Zarrinara, A.R.; Akhondzadeh, S. Crocus sativus L.(saffron) in the treatment of premenstrual syndrome: A double-blind, randomised and placebo-controlled trial. *BJOG: Int. J. Obstet. Gy.* **2008**, *115*, 515–519. [CrossRef] [PubMed]

50. Ahmadpanah, M.; Ramezanshams, F.; Ghaleiha, A.; Akhondzadeh, S.; Bahmani, D.S.; Brand, S. Crocus Sativus, L.(saffron) versus sertraline on symptoms of depression among older people with major depressive disorders–a double-blind, randomized intervention study. *Psychiat. Res.* **2019**, *282*, 112–613. [CrossRef] [PubMed]
51. Akhondzadeh, S.; Fallah-Pour, H.; Afkham, K.; Jamshidi, A.-H.; Khalighi-Cigaroudi, F. Comparison of Crocus sativus L. and imipramine in the treatment of mild to moderate depression: A pilot double-blind randomized trial [ISRCTN45683816]. *BMC Complem. Altern. M.* **2004**, *4*, 12. [CrossRef]
52. Basti, A.A.; Moshiri, E.; Noorbala, A.-A.; Jamshidi, A.-H.; Abbasi, S.H.; Akhondzadeh, S. Comparison of petal of Crocus sativus L. and fluoxetine in the treatment of depressed outpatients: A pilot double-blind randomized trial. *Prog. Neuro-Psychoph.* **2007**, *31*, 439–442. [CrossRef]
53. Ghajar, A.; Neishabouri, S.M.; Velayati, N.; Jahangard, L.; Matinnia, N.; Haghighi, M.; Ghaleiha, A.; Afarideh, M.; Salimi, S.; Meysamie, A. Crocus sativus L. versus citalopram in the treatment of major depressive disorder with anxious distress: A double-blind, controlled clinical trial. *Pharmacopsychiatry* **2017**, *50*, 152–160. [CrossRef]
54. Jelodar, G.; Javid, Z.; Sahraian, A.; Jelodar, S. Saffron improved depression and reduced homocysteine level in patients with major depression: A Randomized, double-blind study. *Avicenna, J. Phytomed.* **2018**, *8*, 43.
55. Kashani, L.; Eslatmanesh, S.; Saedi, N.; Niroomand, N.; Ebrahimi, M.; Hosseinian, M.; Foroughifar, T.; Salimi, S.; Akhondzadeh, S. Comparison of saffron versus fluoxetine in treatment of mild to moderate postpartum depression: A double-blind, randomized clinical trial. *Pharmacopsychiatry* **2017**, *50*, 64–68. [CrossRef]
56. Noorbala, A.A.; Akhondzadeh, S.H.; Tahmacebi-Pour, N.; Jamshidi, A.H. Hydro-alcoholic extract of Crocus sativus L. versus fluoxetine in the treatment of mild to moderate depression: A double-blind, randomized pilot trial. *J. Ethnopharmacol.* **2005**, *97*, 281–284. [CrossRef]
57. Sahraian, A.; Jelodar, S.; Javid, Z.; Mowla, A.; Ahmadzadeh, L. Study the effects of saffron on depression and lipid profiles: A double blind comparative study. *Asian J. Psychiatr.* **2016**, *22*, 174–176. [CrossRef] [PubMed]
58. Shahmansouri, N.; Farokhnia, M.; Abbasi, S.-H.; Kassaian, S.E.; Tafti, A.-A.N.; Gougol, A.; Yekehtaz, H.; Forghani, S.; Mahmoodian, M.; Saroukhani, S. A randomized, double-blind, clinical trial comparing the efficacy and safety of Crocus sativus L. with fluoxetine for improving mild to moderate depression in post percutaneous coronary intervention patients. *J. Affect. Dis.* **2014**, *155*, 216–222. [CrossRef] [PubMed]
59. Shakiba, M.; Moazen-Zadeh, E.; Noorbala, A.A.; Jafarinia, M.; Divsalar, P.; Kashani, L.; Shahmansouri, N.; Tafakhori, A.; Bayat, H.; Akhondzadeh, S. Saffron (Crocus sativus) versus duloxetine for treatment of patients with fibromyalgia: A randomized double-blind clinical trial. *Avicenna J. Phytomed.* **2018**, *8*, 513.
60. Russell, V.A.; Sagvolden, T.; Johansen, E.B. PMC1180819; Animal models of attention-deficit hyperactivity disorder. *Behav. Brain. Funct.* **2005**, *1*, 9. [CrossRef] [PubMed]
61. Djordjevic, J.; Djordjevic, A.; Adzic, M.; Radojcic, M.B. Effects of chronic social isolation on Wistar rat behavior and brain plasticity markers. *Neuropsychobiology* **2012**, *66*, 112–119. [CrossRef]
62. Hosseinzadeh, H.; Noraei, N.B. Anxiolytic and hypnotic effect of Crocus sativus aqueous extract and its constituents, crocin and safranal, in mice. *Phytother. Res. PTR* **2009**, *23*, 768–774. [CrossRef] [PubMed]
63. Scheggi, S.; De Montis, M.G.; Gambarana, C. PMC6209858; Making Sense of Rodent Models of Anhedonia. *Int. J. Neuropsychopharmacol.* **2018**, *21*, 1049–1065. [CrossRef]
64. Asai, A.; Nakano, T.; Takahashi, M.; Nagao, A. Orally administered crocetin and crocins are absorbed into blood plasma as crocetin and its glucuronide conjugates in mice. *J. Agric. Food. Chem.* **2005**, *53*, 7302–7306. [CrossRef]
65. Xi, L.; Qian, Z.; Du, P.; Fu, J. Pharmacokinetic properties of crocin (crocetin digentiobiose ester) following oral administration in rats. *Phytomedicine* **2007**, *14*, 633–636. [CrossRef]
66. Lautenschlager, M.; Sendker, J.; Huwel, S.; Galla, H.J.; Brandt, S.; Dufer, M.; Riehemann, K.; Hensel, A. Intestinal formation of trans-crocetin from saffron extract (*Crocus sativus* L.) and in vitro permeation through intestinal and blood brain barrier. *Phytomedicine* **2015**, *22*, 36–44. [CrossRef]
67. Delgado, P.L. Depression: The case for a monoamine deficiency. *J. Clin. Psychiatry* **2000**.
68. Khazdair, M.R.; Boskabady, M.H.; Hosseini, M.; Rezaee, R.; Tsatsakis, A. The effects of *Crocus sativus* (saffron) and its constituents on nervous system: A review. *Avicenna, J. Phytomed.* **2015**, *5*, 376.

69. Hosseinzadeh, H.; Sadeghnia, H.R.; Rahimi, A.J.P.m. Effect of safranal on extracellular hippocampal levels of glutamate and aspartate during kainic acid treatment in anesthetized rats. *Planta Med.* **2008**, *74*, 1441–1445. [CrossRef]
70. Maes, M.; Mihaylova, I.; Kubera, M.; Leunis, J.C.; Geffard, M. IgM-mediated autoimmune responses directed against multiple neoepitopes in depression: New pathways that underpin the inflammatory and neuroprogressive pathophysiology. *J. Affect. Dis.* **2011**, *135*, 414–418. [CrossRef]
71. Miller, A.H.; Raison, C.L. Are Anti-inflammatory Therapies Viable Treatments for Psychiatric Disorders?: Where the Rubber Meets the Road. *JAMA Psychiatry* **2015**, *72*, 527–528. [CrossRef]
72. Moylan, S.; Eyre, H.A.; Maes, M.; Baune, B.T.; Jacka, F.N.; Berk, M. Exercising the worry away: How inflammation, oxidative and nitrogen stress mediates the beneficial effect of physical activity on anxiety disorder symptoms and behaviours. *Neurosci. Biobehav. R.* **2013**, *37*, 573–584. [CrossRef]
73. Lopresti, A.L.; Drummond, P.D. Saffron (Crocus sativus) for depression: A systematic review of clinical studies and examination of underlying antidepressant mechanisms of action. *Human Psychopharmacol.* **2014**, *29*, 517–527. [CrossRef]
74. Boskabady, M.H.; Farkhondeh, T. Antiinflammatory, Antioxidant, and Immunomodulatory Effects of *Crocus sativus* L. and its Main Constituents. *Phytother. Res. PTR* **2016**, *30*, 1072–1094. [CrossRef]
75. Broadhead, G.K.; Chang, A.; Grigg, J.; McCluskey, P. Efficacy and Safety of Saffron Supplementation: Current Clinical Findings. *Crit. Rev. Food Sci. Nutr.* **2016**, *56*, 2767–2776. [CrossRef]
76. Samarghandian, S.; Samini, F.; Azimi-Nezhad, M.; Farkhondeh, T. Anti-oxidative effects of safranal on immobilization-induced oxidative damage in rat brain. *Neurosci. Lett.* **2017**, *659*, 26–32. [CrossRef]
77. Poma, A.; Fontecchio, G.; Carlucci, G.; Chichiricco, G. Anti-inflammatory properties of drugs from saffron crocus. *Anti-Inflamm. Anti-Allergy Agents Med. Chem.* **2012**, *11*, 37–51. [CrossRef] [PubMed]
78. Wiedlocha, M.; Marcinowicz, P.; Krupa, R.; Janoska-Jazdzik, M.; Janus, M.; Debowska, W.; Mosiolek, A.; Waszkiewicz, N.; Szulc, A. Effect of antidepressant treatment on peripheral inflammation markers—A meta-analysis. *Prog. Neuro-Psychoph* **2018**, *80*, 217–226. [CrossRef] [PubMed]
79. Halataei, B.A.; Khosravi, M.; Arbabian, S.; Sahraei, H.; Golmanesh, L.; Zardooz, H.; Jalili, C.; Ghoshooni, H. Saffron (*Crocus sativus*) aqueous extract and its constituent crocin reduces stress-induced anorexia in mice. *Phytother. Res. PTR* **2011**, *25*, 1833–1838. [CrossRef] [PubMed]
80. Hooshmandi, Z.; Rohani, A.H.; Eidi, A.; Fatahi, Z.; Golmanesh, L.; Sahraei, H. Reduction of metabolic and behavioral signs of acute stress in male Wistar rats by saffron water extract and its constituent safranal. *Pharm. Biol.* **2011**, *49*, 947–954. [CrossRef]
81. Ieraci, A.; Mallei, A.; Popoli, M. Social isolation stress induces anxious-depressive-like behavior and alterations of neuroplasticity-related genes in adult male mice. *Neural Plast.* **2016**, *33*, 58–64. [CrossRef]
82. Cryan, J.F.; Markou, A.; Lucki, I. Assessing antidepressant activity in rodents: Recent developments and future needs. *Trends Pharmacol. Sci.* **2002**, *23*, 238–245. [CrossRef]
83. Bogdanova, O.V.; Kanekar, S.; D'Anci, K.E.; Renshaw, P.F. Factors influencing behavior in the forced swim test. *Physiol. Behav.* **2013**, *118*, 227–239. [CrossRef]
84. Zhang, J.C.; Wu, J.; Fujita, Y.; Yao, W.; Ren, Q.; Yang, C.; Li, S.X.; Shirayama, Y.; Hashimoto, K. Antidepressant effects of TrkB ligands on depression-like behavior and dendritic changes in mice after inflammation. *Int. J. Neuropsychopharmacol.* **2014**, *18*. [CrossRef]
85. Eagle, A.L.; Mazei-Robison, M.; Robison, A.J. Sucrose preference test to measure stress-induced anhedonia. *Bio. Protoc.* **2016**, *6*, 1822. [CrossRef]
86. Malhi, G.S.; Mann, J.J. Depression. *Lancet* **2018**, *392*, 2299–2312. [CrossRef]
87. Porsolt, R.D.; Le Pichon, M.; Jalfre, M. Depression: A new animal model sensitive to antidepressant treatments. *Nature* **1977**, *266*, 730–732. [CrossRef]
88. Lucki, I. The forced swimming test as a model for core and component behavioral effects of antidepressant drugs. *Behav. Pharmacol.* **1997**, *8*, 523–532. [CrossRef]
89. Warner-Schmidt, J.L.; Duman, R.S. VEGF as a potential target for therapeutic intervention in depression. *Curr. Opin. Pharmacol.* **2008**, *8*, 14–19. [CrossRef]

90. Pothion, S.; Bizot, J.C.; Trovero, F.; Belzung, C. Strain differences in sucrose preference and in the consequences of unpredictable chronic mild stress. *Behav. Brain Res.* **2004**, *155*, 135–146. [CrossRef] [PubMed]

Sample Availability: Samples of the compound affron® are available from Pharmactive Biotech Products SL.

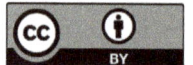

© 2020 by the authors. Licensee MDPI, Basel, Switzerland. This article is an open access article distributed under the terms and conditions of the Creative Commons Attribution (CC BY) license (http://creativecommons.org/licenses/by/4.0/).

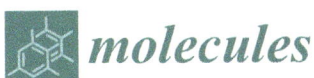

Article

Crocetin Mitigates Irradiation Injury in an In Vitro Model of the Pubertal Testis: Focus on Biological Effects and Molecular Mechanisms

Giulia Rossi [1,†], Martina Placidi [1,†], Chiara Castellini [2], Francesco Rea [1], Settimio D'Andrea [2], Gonzalo Luis Alonso [3], Giovanni Luca Gravina [4], Carla Tatone [1], Giovanna Di Emidio [1,*] and Anna Maria D'Alessandro [5]

1. Lab of Reproductive Technologies, Department of Life, Health and Environmental Sciences, University of L'Aquila, 67100 L'Aquila, Italy; giulia.rossi1@guest.univaq.it (G.R.); martina.placidi@graduate.univaq.it (M.P.); frea@unite.it (F.R.); carla.tatone@univaq.it (C.T.)
2. Andrology Unit, Department of Life, Health and Environmental Sciences, University of L'Aquila, 67100 L'Aquila, Italy; chiara.castellini@univaq.it (C.C.); settimio.dandrea@alice.it (S.D.)
3. Química Agrícola, E.T.S.I. Agrónomos y Montes, Departamento de Ciencia y Tecnología Agroforestal y Genética, Universidad de Castilla-La Mancha, Avda. de España s/n, 02071 Albacete, Spain; gonzalo.alonso@uclm.es
4. Laboratory of Radiobiology, Division of Radiotherapy, Department of Biotechnological and Applied Clinical Sciences, University of L'Aquila, 67100 L'Aquila, Italy; giovanniluca.gravina@univaq.it
5. Lab of Nutritional Biochemistry, Department of Life, Health and Environmental Sciences, University of L'Aquila, 67100 L'Aquila, Italy; annamaria.dalessandro@univaq.it
* Correspondence: giovanna.diemidio@univaq.it
† These authors contributed equally to this work.

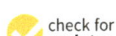

Citation: Rossi, G.; Placidi, M.; Castellini, C.; Rea, F.; D'Andrea, S.; Alonso, G.L.; Gravina, G.L.; Tatone, C.; Di Emidio, G.; D'Alessandro, A.M. Crocetin Mitigates Irradiation Injury in an In Vitro Model of the Pubertal Testis: Focus on Biological Effects and Molecular Mechanisms. *Molecules* 2021, 26, 1676. https://doi.org/10.3390/molecules26061676

Academic Editors: Nikolaos Pitsikas and Konstantinos Dimas

Received: 22 February 2021
Accepted: 14 March 2021
Published: 17 March 2021

Publisher's Note: MDPI stays neutral with regard to jurisdictional claims in published maps and institutional affiliations.

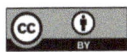

Copyright: © 2021 by the authors. Licensee MDPI, Basel, Switzerland. This article is an open access article distributed under the terms and conditions of the Creative Commons Attribution (CC BY) license (https://creativecommons.org/licenses/by/4.0/).

Abstract: Infertility is a potential side effect of radiotherapy and significantly affects the quality of life for adolescent cancer survivors. Very few studies have addressed in pubertal models the mechanistic events that could be targeted to provide protection from gonadotoxicity and data on potential radioprotective treatments in this peculiar period of life are elusive. In this study, we utilized an in vitro model of the mouse pubertal testis to investigate the efficacy of crocetin to counteract ionizing radiation (IR)-induced injury and potential underlying mechanisms. Present experiments provide evidence that exposure of testis fragments from pubertal mice to 2 Gy X-rays induced extensive structural and cellular damage associated with overexpression of PARP1, PCNA, SOD2 and HuR and decreased levels of SIRT1 and catalase. A twenty-four hr exposure to 50 µM crocetin pre- and post-IR significantly reduced testis injury and modulated the response to DNA damage and oxidative stress. Nevertheless, crocetin treatment did not counteract the radiation-induced changes in the expression of SIRT1, p62 and LC3II. These results increase the knowledge of mechanisms underlying radiation damage in pubertal testis and establish the use of crocetin as a fertoprotective agent against IR deleterious effects in pubertal period.

Keywords: saffron; crocetin; pubertal testis; X-rays; radiotherapy; fertility preservation; SIRT1; HuR; oxidative stress; autophagy

1. Introduction

Infertility is a potential side effect of cancer therapies and significantly affects the quality of life for survivors during their pre-reproductive and reproductive years [1,2]. Although modern radiotherapy techniques have evolved to ensure a reduction of the potential risk of infertility, radiotherapy can still result in permanent or temporary gonadal toxicity in male patients [3]. The formation of sperm by the testes through the process of spermatogenesis is highly radiosensitive. Rapidly dividing testicular germ cells are highly affected by ionizing radiation (IR) and their loss is proportional to the radiation dose. Low radiation doses can cause a profound reduction or even transient complete loss of sperms [4].

A critical period for development of reproductive organs and function and establishment of fertility potential is puberty. Spermatogenesis is known to start at very early stages of pubertal development [5–7] and may occur before the ability to produce an ejaculate [8]. This makes it difficult to apply fertility preservation strategies in pubertal cancer patients. Cryopreservation of ejaculated spermatozoa prior to anticancer therapy, routinely used to preserve fertility in men, represents the first line treatment in adolescents, as well [9,10]. However, for some patients it may not be possible to recover sperm prior to the onset of ablative therapies. Although semen samples can be obtained from boys from the age of 12 years onwards, the onset of sperm production (spermarche) can be very difficult to predict [11]. Since there is no reliable sensitive estimate for the presence of spermatozoa in the testes, sperm extraction from testicular tissue biopsy is not reliable [12]. Therefore, new strategies to protect male fertility against IR deleterious effects in pubertal period need to be considered. One of the possible reasons for limited progress in the field is the partial understanding of the mechanistic events that could be targeted to provide protection or repair from gonadotoxicity in this peculiar period of life. Very few studies have addressed this issue in pubertal models. Proteomics results from pubertal mice testes revealed that carbon ion radiations exert acute and chronic injury by activating early and long-term mechanisms. Most proteins that are differentially expressed in early and long-term response are involved in energy supply, endoplasmic reticulum, cell proliferation, cell cycle, antioxidant capacity and mitochondrial respiration categories. Importantly, a significant increase in ROS levels was observed clearly demonstrating that high doses of carbon ion radiations disrupt the antioxidant system in testicular tissue [13,14].

The data obtained using various models including cells, animals, and recently humans suggest that radioprotective agents working through a variety of mechanisms have the potential to decrease free radical damage produced by IR [15]. Therefore, recently, much interest has been ignited to discover antioxidants which would counteract or minimize radiation-induced testicular toxicity [16–22].

In this context, recent research has reported that intake of saffron, or its constituents crocin and safranal, exerts protective effects against genotoxicity associated to 1–2 Gy total body irradiation in testis of adult mice [23,24]. Crocin is the glycosylated form of crocetin, a symmetric di-carboxylic acid diterpene: about 94% of the total amount of crocetin in saffron is glycosylated to crocin and 6% is present in the free form [23,24]. Similarly to flavonoids [25], crocin shows a poor bioavailability after oral administration [26]. In the intestine, crocins are hydrolyzed to the deglycosylated trans-crocetin, which is rapidly absorbed [27–29]. On this basis, most of the saffron therapeutic activities have been attributed to this carotenoid, known for its elevated anti-inflammatory and free radical scavenger activity [30].

In the present study, we investigated the hypothesis that crocetin may exert a radioprotective effect by preventing IR-induced damage in testis of pubertal mice. This hypothesis is based on the knowledge of the potent anti-tumor effects of this molecule, a feature essential for a potential fertoprotective agent, and on its ability to prevent ovarian toxicity induced by cyclophosphamide, an anticancer drug with strong pro-oxidant power [31]. In this study, we utilized an in vitro culture system of prepubertal mouse testes as an experimental model of spermatogenesis to investigate the efficacy of crocetin to counteract X-ray-induced testicular injury and the mechanisms underlying IR insult and potential crocetin effects. Exposure to IR initiates a cascade of events that are based on direct DNA damage and generation of free radicals. It is well documented that oxidative stress adversely affects spermatogenesis, whereas anti-oxidative enzymes like superoxide dismutase (SOD) and catalase (CAT) protect the testicular germ cells against the oxidative stress-induced apoptosis [32]. A crucial player in sensing and modulating the testis redox status is sirtuin 1 (SIRT1), a NAD+-dependent deacetylates targeting key proteins involved in the cellular stress response [33,34]. An actor of the antioxidant and radioprotective adaptive response is HuR (human antigen R), a RNA-binding protein known to stabilize mRNAs containing AU-rich elements [35–37]. One of the primary repair mechanisms to resolve DNA lesions caused by IR is poly (ADP-ribose) polymerase 1 (PARP1) over-activation and intracellular NAD+ level depletion [18,38]. Pathways that mitigate the effects of DNA damage during replication include translesion synthesis and template switching under the regulation of proliferating cell nuclear antigen (PCNA) [39]. A further process that deserves investigation in this context is the autophagic pathway. Autophagy is crucial for the formation and degradation of specific structures that guarantee successful spermatogenesis, and can be induced or enhanced by various external gonadotoxic stimuli [40].

Based on the knowledge and hypotheses reported above, in this study, testes obtained from pubertal mice were exposed to 2 Gy IR in the presence or absence of crocetin and subjected to the analysis of morphological parameters associated with the integrity of germinative epithelium and to the evaluation of the molecular signaling related to IR damage response including antioxidant defenses, DNA damage response and autophagy.

2. Results

2.1. Effect of Crocetin on Tubule Diameter, Cross-Sectional Area, Seminiferous Epithelium Height and Presence of Sperm in the Lumen in Pubertal Testis Exposed to IR

Histomorphometrical examination of testes exposed to 2 Gy X-rays showed a significant increase in diameter (195.06 ± 2.84 µm) and cross-sectional area (30.55 × 10^3 ± 0.90 µm^2) of seminiferous tubules associated with a decrease of seminiferous epithelium height (50.52 ± 1.21 µm) when compared with the control (CTRL) group (183.76 ± 2.39 µm; 27.04 × 10^3 ± 0.2 µm^2; 56.75 ± 1.04 µm, respectively, Table 1). In addition, the percentage of tubules with active spermatogenesis (29.18% ± 2.68) appeared significantly reduced in comparison to the control group (39.57% ± 2.77). Treatment with crocetin was able to counteract X-rays deleterious effects on testis when compared to the IR group. Values of mean diameter of seminiferous tubules and cross-sectional area (184.15 ± 2.73 µm; 27.51 × 10^3 ± 0.86 µm^2, respectively) in testes exposed to crocetin were not significantly different from the control group. Moreover, the lumen of seminiferous tubules presented a germinal epithelium with a thickness (56.14 ± 1.39 µm) similar to control. A higher percentage of tubules with active spermatogenesis (58.58% ± 3.99) was observed in comparison to control group (Table 1, Figure 1).

Table 1. Morphometric parameters in pubertal testis exposed to IR in the presence/absence of crocetin.

Group of Treatment	n	Mean Tubule Diameter [1] (µm)	n	Cross-Sectional Area [1] (×10^3 µm^2)	n	Seminiferous Epithelium [1] Height (µm)	n	Spermatogenesis [1] (%)
CTRL	120	183.76 ± 2.39 [a]	120	27.04 ± 0.72 [a]	57	56.75 ± 1.04 [a]	359	39.57 ± 2.77 [a]
IR	108	195.06 ± 2.84 [b]	108	30.55 ± 0.90 [b]	52	50.52 ± 1.20 [b]	240	29.18 ± 2.68 [b]
CRO + IR	153	184.15 ± 2.73 [a]	153	27.51 ± 0.86 [a]	76	56.14 ± 1.39 [a]	324	58.58 ± 3.99 [c]
p value *		p = 0.006		p = 0.01		p = 0.002		p < 0.001

[1] Data as presented mean ± SEM. * Statistical analysis by one-way ANOVA. [a,b,c] Post hoc multiple comparison by Holm–Sidak. Different letters indicate $p < 0.05$.

2.2. Effect of Crocetin on Protein Expression of PARP1 and PCNA in Pubertal Testis Exposed to IR

To investigate the IR effects on DNA, we evaluated the expression of markers involved in DNA strand breaks repair such as PCNA and PARP1. As shown in Figure 2, we detected an upregulation of PCNA and PARP1 to the control group, confirming the activation of the DNA repair response. The group treated with crocetin showed a lower amount of PCNA than the irradiated group and similar levels than control. The ability of crocetin to restore the basal levels of PARP1 and PCNA levels highlighted the establishment of a protective mechanism against radiation-induced DNA damage.

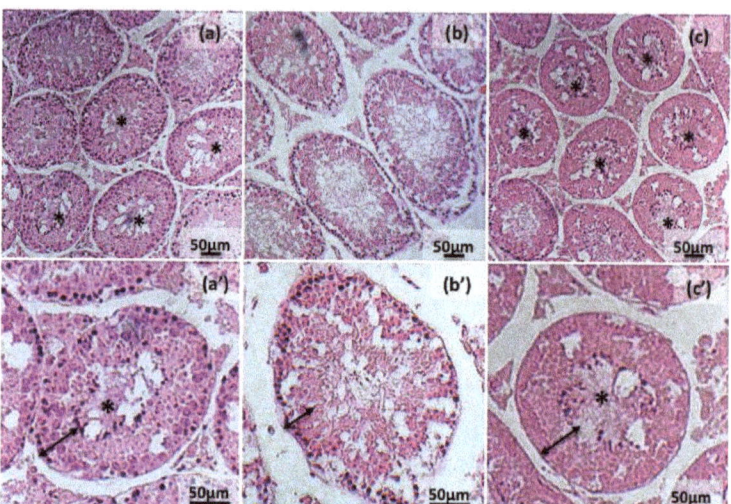

Figure 1. Representative images showing H&E stained testis sections from control (**a,a'**), irradiated (**b,b'**) and crocetin + irradiated group (**c,c'**). Histological features of irradiated testes show a significant increase in diameter and cross-sectional area of seminiferous tubules, a decrease of seminiferous epithelium height compared with the control group. Crocetin pretreatment significantly protects irradiated testes from X-rays injury. Seminiferous epithelium height is delimited by black double arrow. Mature spermatozoa located into the lumen of tubules are indicated with asterisk.

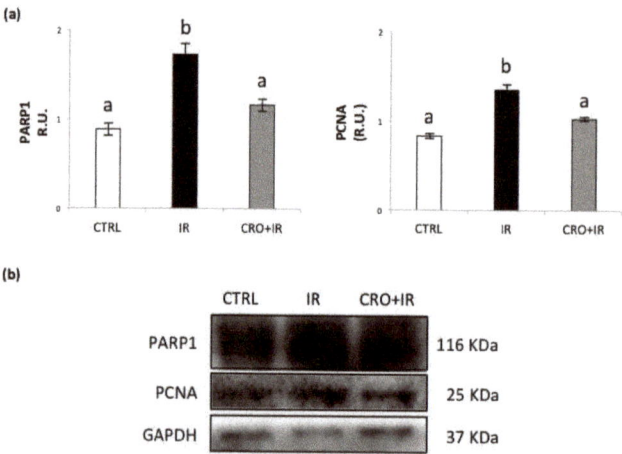

Figure 2. (**a**) Western blot analysis of PARP1 and PCNA protein levels. (**b**) Representative images of immunoreactive bands. Data are presented as means ± SEM of densitometric analysis of immunoreactive bands normalized to internal reference protein (GAPDH). One-way ANOVA $p < 0.05$; ^{a,b} $p < 0.05$, Holm–Sidak post hoc multiple comparison.

2.3. Effect of Crocetin on Protein Expression of SIRT1, Hur, SOD2 and CAT in Pubertal Testis Exposed to IR

To investigate the involvement of oxidative stress in the response to IR, we analysed the levels of SIRT1, HuR, SOD2 and CAT. The group exposed to IR showed lower levels of SIRT1 and CAT and higher levels of SOD2 and HuR. The crocetin supplementation was able to restore the basal levels of SOD2, CAT and HuR but had no effects on SIRT1 expression following IR (Figure 3). The establishment of a condition of oxidative stress in IR testes was confirmed by evaluating lipid peroxidation [41,42]. As shown in Supplementary Figure S1, IR insult induced a significant increase in 4-HNE immunostaining, which was prevented by medium supplementation with crocetin.

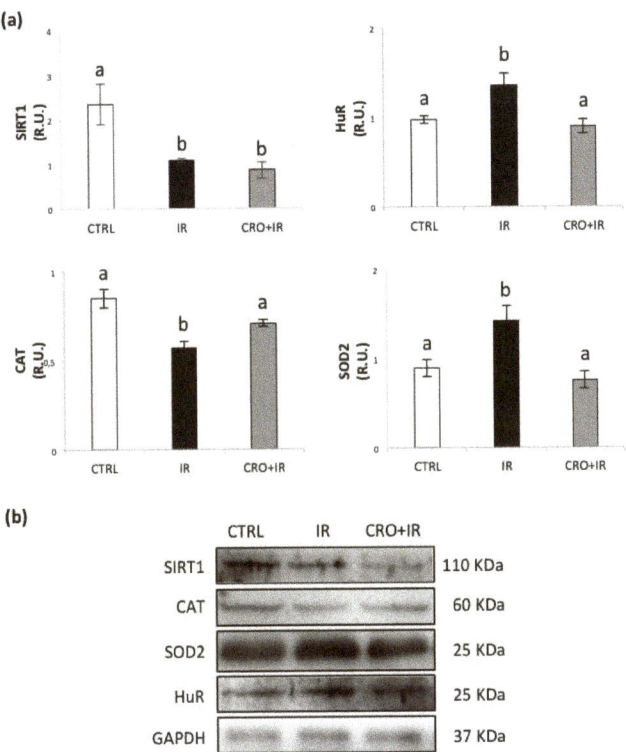

Figure 3. (a) Western blot analysis of SIRT1, HuR, CAT, and SOD2 protein levels. (b) Representative images of immunoreactive bands. Data are presented as means ± SEM of densitometric analysis of immunoreactive bands normalized to internal reference protein (GAPDH). One-way ANOVA $p < 0.05$; [a,b] $p < 0.05$, Holm–Sidak post hoc multiple comparison.

2.4. Effect of Crocetin on Autophagy Markers on Pubertal Testis Exposed to IR

To evaluate the role of autophagy, we analysed the proteins implicated in this process. Our data showed that IR significantly decreased the content of p62 and raised LC3-II in mice testes compared with control as an evidence of increased autophagy. Crocetin pretreatment was not capable to restore the basal levels of p62 and LC3-II and so to prevent the autophagic activation (Figure 4).

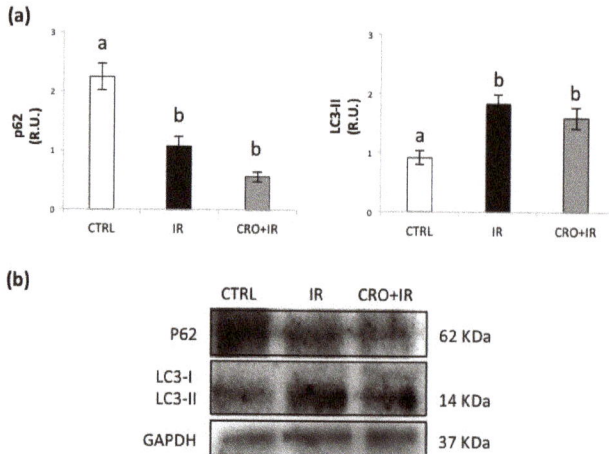

Figure 4. (a) Western blot analysis of p62 and LC3-II. (b) Representative images of immunoreactive bands. Data are presented as means ± SEM of densitometric analysis of immunoreactive bands normalized to internal reference protein (GAPDH). One-way ANOVA $p < 0.05$; [a,b] $p < 0.05$, Holm–Sidak post hoc multiple comparison.

3. Discussion

In this study, we utilized an in vitro model of the pubertal testis as an experimental model to investigate the efficacy of crocetin to counteract IR-induced injury and potential underlying mechanisms in the pubertal male gonad. Results from our experiments provide evidence that exposure of pubertal testicular tissue to 2 Gy irradiation induced extensive structural and cellular damage associated with activation of DNA damage and antioxidant responses and induction of autophagy. A twenty-four hour exposure to 50 μM crocetin pre- and post-IR significantly reduced testis injury and modulated the response signalling pathways to cell damage.

Radioprotectors targeting oxidative damage and inflammatory reaction have been studied for decades with limited success, because of the limited effect, toxicity or risk of tumorigenesis [15]. In this context, we have hypothesized the potential of crocetin as a protective agent in relation to its antioxidant, anti-inflammatory and antitumor activities which would facilitate clinical application [43]. According to [32], the in vitro culture system selected to test IR and crocetin effects was able to sustain in vitro spermatogenesis. We observed that about 40% of tubules from pubertal testicular fragments were characterized by the presence of sperm in the lumen after 48 hr in vitro culture. In this system, the gonadotoxic effects of IR were evidenced by the appearance of enlarged seminiferous tubules in association with reduced germinal epithelium thickness and percentage of tubules with complete spermatogenesis (sperm in the lumen). By focusing on these parameters, we established that crocetin supplementation was able to counteract IR insult and sustain spermatogenesis as evidenced by an increased percentage of tubules showing sperm in the lumen. This conclusion, which represents the first evidence for crocetin radioprotective effects in the male gonad, is consistent with previous findings in adult mice receiving saffron extracts or crocin after IR [23,24] and provides evidence that the effects of saffron carotenoids intake described in these studies may be mediated by the direct action of crocetin obtained from hydrolyzation of ingested crocin [27,44].

Exposure to IR initiates a cascade of events that are based on direct DNA damage and generation of free radicals. PARP1 is involved in primary repair mechanisms to resolve DNA lesions caused by toxicants and plays an important role in safeguarding DNA integrity in spermatogenesis [45]. Gamma-irradiation-dependent increase of PARP1 activity has been recently reported in testis of adult rat [18]. For these reasons, PARP1 overexpression in irradiated pubertal testes here described is considered an evidence of the activation of a DNA damage response and/or excessive amount of ROS [46,47]. Cell response to DNA damage may involve functional association between PARP1 and PCNA [48]. Accordingly, in our experimental model, increased PARP1 protein was associated with overexpression of PCNA. The finding that PARP1 and PCNA levels did not change in irradiated testes exposed to crocetin strongly suggests that crocetin exposure is able to mitigate the IR gonadotoxic insult in this experimental model.

Radioprotective effects of crocetin observed in somatic tissues have been ascribed to elevated activities of endogenous antioxidant enzymes [49]. Here we have found that response to irradiation of pubertal testis fragments is characterized by overexpression of SOD2 and downregulation of CAT. SOD2, also known as manganese-dependent superoxide dismutase (MnSOD), is a mitochondrial protein that converts superoxide ion into oxygen and hydrogen peroxide. This, in turn, is transformed into water and oxygen by CAT. In contrast to SOD2, CAT levels were reduced in the irradiated sample, revealing an altered process of mitochondrial detoxification of the superoxide anion, resulting in a condition of oxidative stress. The observation that crocetin exposure was effective in maintaining basal protein levels of SOD2 and CAT during IR supports the hypothesis that radioprotective activity of crocetin is mediated by its ROS scavenging activity or modulation of antioxidants genes [31,48,50–52]. A further evidence is the observation in testes cultured in the presence of crocetin prior and after irradiation of a reduction of oxidative damage measured by levels of 4-HNE, a well-known marker of lipid peroxidation [42].

Total body exposure to IR results in reduced gene expression and activity of SIRT1, a member of the family of sirtuin, histone NAD+-dependent deacetylases, in testes of adult rats. SIRT1 plays a crucial role as a sensor of cellular energy status and oxidative stress in the male gonad [33,34]. Here we show that the pubertal testes exposed to irradiation undergo a decrease in SIRT1 protein level, a condition known to be associated with severe oxidative stress [18,33]. However, exposure to crocetin did not counteract this effect, suggesting that the radioprotective effects of crocetin are partial and not mediated by a SIRT1-dependent response. A possible explanation for decrease of SIRT1 protein level may be the dissociation of SIRT1 mRNA from the RNA-binding protein HuR, which occurs under severe oxidative stress [52–54]. HuR overexpression has been associated with increased resistance to damage induced by irradiation and promotion of cell survival [37]. In the testis, this protein has a fine-tuned regulation that influences post-meiotic cell formation, spermatid maturation and sperm production [35,36]. In the present study, HuR expression is increased upon IR and maintained at basal levels by exposure to crocetin, revealing HuR involvement in the adaptive response to IR in the male gonad. Therefore, the low level of SIRT1 in the crocetin group may be explained by hypothesizing additional mechanisms which are out of crocetin control.

Cellular autophagy is a cellular mechanism for selective removal of damaged cytoplasmic components. Selective autophagy has been documented to play a pro-survival role in spermatogenic cells under physiological and adverse conditions. It has been reported to minimize cell damage and promote clearance of damaged proteins and mitochondria under oxidative insult [55]. According to [56], the increase in the autophagic marker LC3-II we found in this study represents an evidence that IR-exposed testis is characterized by augmented autophagic flux. This was further confirmed by the data related to p62, which decreases when autophagy is induced [57,58]. In the testis fragments subjected to IR, there was an increase in LC3II and a decrease of p62 irrespective of the crocetin treatment. Nevertheless, our observations about the status of health of the seminiferous epithelium and the pathways related to response to DNA damage and oxidative insult may suggest that activation of autophagy in the presence of crocetin reflects a cellular effort leading to repair and maintenance of spermatogenesis. Under this condition, tissue integrity is associated with that of DNA and redox modulation. However, the lack of recovery of normal SIRT1 levels is an evidence of a sublethal damage which deserves further investigation. However, the study of the molecular pathways involved in the response to IR shows that this protective effect is partial. While protecting the germinative epithelium and modulating the response to DNA damage and oxidative stress, it does not counteract the radiation-induced decrease in SIRT1 and autophagy. These results underline the need to investigate the long-term effects of crocetin, a condition that requires in vitro experimental models capable to sustain spermatogenesis in the long term.

Overall, this study provides new insights into the short-term cellular and molecular damage caused by ionizing radiation in pubertal mouse testes and reveals crocetin ability to decrease IR injury in the pubertal mouse testis. This provides the basis for establishing new strategies to protect male fertility against IR deleterious effects in adolescent patients who are unable or unwilling to produce a semen sample.

4. Materials and Methods

4.1. Animal Care

Male pubertal CD-1 mice (28–31 days, n = 12, Charles River Italia s.r.l., Calco, Italy) were maintained in a temperature-controlled environment under a 12 h light/dark cycle (7.00–19.00) with free access to feed and water ad libitum. All the experiments were carried out in conformity with national and international laws and policies (EECC 86/609, OJ 358, 1 Dec 12, 1987; Italian Legislative Decree 116/92, GU n. 40, Feb 18, 1992; National Institutes of Health Guide for the Care and Use of Laboratory Animals, NIH publication No. 85-23, 1985). The project was approved by the Italian Ministry of Health and the internal committee of the University of L'Aquila. Animals were euthanized by cervical dislocation after an inhalant overdose of carbon dioxide (CO_2, 10–30%), followed by cervical dislocation. All efforts were made to minimize animal suffering.

4.2. Crocetin Preparation

Crocetin isolation was performed by crocetin esters and purified by an internal method of the Verdù Cantò Saffron Spain Company (Novelda, Alicante, Spain) [59]. Crocetin quantification was estimated using the method based on the extinction coefficient and the related area calculated according to [60,61]. Crocetin in its free-acid form is insoluble in water and most organic solvents, except for dimethyl sulfoxide (DMSO) [62]. Crocetin was dissolved in DMSO 0.3 M and diluted in the Minimum Essential Medium-alpha (MEM-α, Euroclone, Pero, Milan, Italy) to achieve concentrations of 50 µM, prepared daily and protected from light. The final concentration of DMSO was 0.02%.

4.3. Mouse Testis Culture

After collection, tunica albuginea was removed and testes were cut in four pieces. Testis fragments were cultured in 12-well culture plates with polycarbonate nucleopore membrane (Whatman, Camlab Ltd., Cambridge, UK) in Minimum Essential Medium-alpha (MEMα) (Invitrogen, Thermo Fisher Scientific Inc., Merelbeke, Belgium) supplemented with 3 mg/mL bovine serum albumin (MEMα-BSA) (Sigma Aldrich, St. Louis, MO, USA) [32,63]. Cultures were conducted at 37 °C in a CO_2 incubator with a controlled humidified atmosphere composed of 95% air and 5% CO_2. Mouse testis fragments were randomly assigned to three experimental groups: (1) CTRL group: control testes were cultured for 24 h in MEMα-BSA, then transferred to a new plate and cultured for another 24 h in the presence of fresh culture medium; (2) IR group: testes were cultured for 24 h in MEMα-BSA, then irradiated using an X-rays linear accelerator (an Elekta 6-MV photon linear accelerator) at a dose rate of 2 Gy (200 cGy/min) at room temperature [64,65] and cultured for another 24 h in the presence of fresh culture medium; (3) CRO+IR: testes were cultured for 24 h in MEMα-BSA supplemented with 50 µM crocetin [66]. Testes were then irradiated and cultured for another 24 h in fresh culture medium containing crocetin. At the end of treatments, testes were processed to perform histological and molecular analysis.

4.4. Histological Staining and Morphometric Analysis

Testes were fixed in Bouin's solution (Sigma Aldrich, St. Louis, MO, USA), embedded in paraffin blocks, cut with a Leica sliding microtome (RM 2045, Nussloch, Germany) into section of 5 µm thick, which were mounted on microscope slides. Testicular sections were dewaxed in xylene, re-hydrated in descending ethanol concentration, 100% (v/v), 90% (v/v) and 70% (v/v), stained with Haematoxylin and Eosin (H&E) according to the manufacturer's instructions (Bio Optica, Milan, Italy) and observed by light microscopy (Zeiss Axiostar Plus, Oberkochen, Germany).

Digital images were analysed using ImageJ 1.44 p to obtain measurements of morphometric parameters as mean diameter, the cross-sectional area of round or nearly round seminiferous tubules [67,68], seminiferous epithelium height [69] and the spermatogenesis [20]. The presence of active spermatogenesis was assessed by the observation of spermatozoa in the lumen of at least 150 seminiferous tubules in each experimental group.

4.5. Western Blot Analysis

Pubertal testis fragments were lysed in RIPA Lysis buffer, containing 25 mM Tris-HCL pH 7.5, 150 mM NaCl, 1% Nonidet P-40, 1 mM EDTA pH 8.0, H2O, 1 mM PMSF, 1 mM sodium ortovanadate and 1% protease inhibitor cocktail, by repeated freeze/thaw cycles in liquid nitrogen. After centrifugation at 12,000 g for 20 min at 4 °C, supernatants were collected for protein analysis. The concentration of proteins was determined by a BCA protein assay kit (Pierce, Rockford, IL, USA).

Thirty micrograms of testicular proteins were resolved by 10% SDS-PAGE electrophoresis, transferred to a polyvinylidene difluoride membrane (PVDF, Sigma Aldrich, St. Louis, MO, USA) and blocked with 5% BSA (Sigma Aldrich, St. Louis, MO, USA) in Tris-buffered saline containing 0.05% Tween 20 (TBS-T) for 1 h at room temperature. After the blocking of non-specific binding site, membranes were incubated with polyclonal rabbit anti-SIRT1 antibody (Ab12193, Abcam, Cambridge, UK; 1:750), anti-SOD2 antibody (Ab86087, Abcam; 1:1000), anti-LC3A/B antibody (AB-83557, Immunological Sciences, 1:500), anti-P62/SQSTM1 antibody (AB-83779, Immunological Sciences, 1:500) or mouse monoclonal anti-HuR (SC-71290, Santa Cruz Biotechnology Inc., Dallas, TX, USA, 1:250), anti-PARP-1 (sc-74479, Santa Cruz Biotechnology, Inc., Dallas, TX, USA, 1:300), anti-PCNA (NB500-106, Novus Biologicals, Bio-Techne srl, Milan, Italy, 1:700) anti-GAPDH (TA802519, OriGene Technologies Inc., Rockville, MD, USA, 1:750), anti-CAT (200-4151, Rockland Inc., Gilbertsville, PA, USA, 1:10,000), overnight at 4 °C, followed by incubation with peroxidase (HRP)-conjugated goat anti-rabbit IgG (BA1054, Boster Biological Technology Co., Ltd., Pleasanton, CA, USA, 1:3000) or anti-mouse secondary antibody (Ab6728, Abcam, 1:2000) for 1 h and 30 min at room temperature. The specific immune complexes were detected by ECL kit (Life Technologies-Thermo Scientific, Waltham, MA, USA) using Uvitec Cambridge system (Alliance series, Cambridge, UK). Signal normalization was carried out by using GAPDH, as the loading control protein, using ImageJ 1.44 p software. Values were given as relative units (RU). All experiments were repeated three time.

4.6. Immunohistochemical Analysis

Paraffin-embedded sections of testes were deparaffinized and hydrated through xylenes and graded alcohol series. To increase the immunoreactivity, the sections were boiled in 10 mM citrate buffer (pH, 6.1 Bio-Optica, Milan, Italy) in a microwave at 720 W (3 cycles/3 min each). The sections were then subjected to treatment for blocking endogenous peroxidase activity (Dako). After thorough washing, sections were incubated with MOM mouse IgG blocking reagent overnight at 4 °C (Vector Laboratories) according to the manufacturer's protocol. Then, sections were incubated with rabbit polyclonal to 4-HNE (4 Hydroxynonenal, ab46545, Abcam, 1:100) diluted in MOM diluent for 30 min, according to the Vector Laboratories instructions. 4-HNE was revealed by biotinylated anti-rabbit IgG followed by streptavidin-HRP, DAB substrate buffer and DAB (Dako kit), according to manufacturer's instructions. Counterstaining was performed with hematoxylin (Bio-Optica, Milan, Italy). Negative controls were performed by omitting primary antibody and substituting it with MOM diluent alone. Finally, sections were dehydrated and mounted with Neomount (Merck, Darmstadt, Germany). They were observed and photographed under a Leitz Laborlux S microscope (Leica, Wetzler, Germany) equipped with an Olympus digital compact camera.

4.7. Statistical Analysis

Results are expressed as mean ± standard error of the mean (S.E.M.). All data were processed using the Sigma Plot 11.0 (Systat Software Inc., San Jose, CA, USA). One-way ANOVA and Holm–Sidak post hoc analyses were performed to analyse significant differences between groups. A p value < 0.05 was considered statistically significant.

Supplementary Materials: Supplementary Figure S1 is available online.

Author Contributions: Conceptualization, C.T., A.M.D., G.D.E.; methodology, G.R., M.P., C.C., F.R., S.D., G.L.A., G.L.G.; software, G.R., M.P., G.D.E.; validation, C.T., A.M.D.; formal analysis, G.R., M.P., G.D.E.; investigation, G.R., M.P., G.D.E.; resources, C.T., A.M.D.; data curation, C.T., A.M.D., G.D.E., G.R.; writing—original draft preparation, G.R., M.P., G.D.E., C.T., A.M.D.; writing—review and editing, G.D.E., C.T., A.M.D.; visualization, G.D.E., C.T., A.M.D.; supervision, C.T., A.M.D., G.D.E.; project administration, C.T., A.M.D.; funding acquisition, C.T., A.M.D. All authors have read and agreed to the published version of the manuscript.

Funding: The funds for this work were provided by the Department of Life, Health and Environmental Sciences, University of L'Aquila.

Institutional Review Board Statement: Not applicant.

Informed Consent Statement: Not applicant.

Data Availability Statement: The data presented in this study are available on request from the corresponding author.

Conflicts of Interest: The authors declare no conflict of interest.

Sample Availability: Samples of the compounds are available from the authors.

References

1. Valli, H.; Phillips, B.T.; Shetty, G.; Byrne, J.A.; Clark, A.T.; Meistrich, M.L.; Orwig, K.E. Germline stem cells: Toward the regeneration of spermatogenesis. *Fertil. Steril.* **2014**, *101*, 3–13. [CrossRef]
2. Ward, E.; DeSantis, C.; Robbins, A.; Kohler, B.; Jemal, A. Childhood and adolescent cancer statistics, 2014. *CA Cancer J. Clin.* **2014**, *64*, 83–103. [CrossRef] [PubMed]
3. Jeruss, J.S.; Woodruff, T.K. Preservation of fertility in patients with cancer. *N. Engl. J. Med.* **2009**, *360*, 902–911. [CrossRef] [PubMed]
4. Osterberg, E.C.; Ramasamy, R.; Masson, P.; Brannigan, R.E. Current practices in fertility preservation in male cancer patients. *Urol. Ann.* **2014**, *6*, 13–20. [CrossRef]
5. Müller, J.; Skakkebaek, N.E. Quantification of germ cells and seminiferous tubules by stereological examination of testicles from 50 boys who suffered from sudden death. *Int. J. Androl.* **1983**, *6*, 143–156. [CrossRef] [PubMed]
6. Müller, J.; Skakkebaek, N.E. The prenatal and postnatal development of the testis. *Baillieres Clin. Endocrinol. Metab.* **1992**, *6*, 251–271. [CrossRef]
7. Hovatta, O. Cryopreservation of testicular tissue in young cancer patients. *Hum. Reprod. Update* **2001**, *7*, 378–383. [CrossRef] [PubMed]
8. Nielsen, C.T.; Skakkebaek, N.E.; Richardson, D.W.; Darling, J.A.; Hunter, W.M.; Jørgensen, M.; Nielsen, A.; Ingerslev, O.; Keiding, N.; Müller, J. Onset of the release of spermatozoa (spermarche) in boys in relation to age, testicular growth, pubic hair, and height. *J. Clin. Endocrinol. Metab.* **1986**, *62*, 532–535. [CrossRef]
9. Sharma, V. Sperm storage for cancer patients in the UK: A review of current practice. *Hum. Reprod.* **2011**, *26*, 2935–2943. [CrossRef]
10. Daudin, M.; Rives, N.; Walschaerts, M.; Drouineaud, V.; Szerman, E.; Koscinski, I.; Eustache, F.; Saïas-Magnan, J.; Papaxanthos-Roche, A.; Cabry-Goubet, R.; et al. Sperm cryopreservation in adolescents and young adults with cancer: Results of the French national sperm banking network (CECOS). *Fertil. Steril.* **2015**, *103*, 478–486. [CrossRef]
11. Bahadur, G.; Ozturk, O.; Wafa, R.; Muneer, A.; Ralph, D.; Minhas, S. Posttreatment azoospermia in cancer patients is subgroup dependent. *Fertil. Steril.* **2006**, *85*, 531–533. [CrossRef]
12. Wyns, C.; Curaba, M.; Petit, S.; Vanabelle, B.; Laurent, P.; Wese, J.F.; Donnez, J. Management of fertility preservation in prepubertal patients: 5 years' experience at the Catholic University of Louvain. *Hum. Reprod.* **2011**, *26*, 737–747. [CrossRef] [PubMed]
13. Li, H.; He, Y.; Zhang, H.; Miao, G. Differential proteome and gene expression reveal response to carbon ion irradiation in pubertal mice testes. *Toxicol. Lett.* **2014**, *225*, 433–444. [CrossRef] [PubMed]

14. Li, H.; Zhang, H.; Di, C.; Xie, Y.; Zhou, X.; Yan, J.; Zhao, Q. Comparative proteomic profiling and possible toxicological mechanism of acute injury induced by carbon ion radiation in pubertal mice testes. *Reprod. Toxicol.* **2015**, *58*, 45–53. [CrossRef]
15. Smith, T.A.; Kirkpatrick, D.R.; Smith, S.; Smith, T.K.; Pearson, T.; Kailasam, A.; Herrmann, K.Z.; Schubert, J.; Agrawal, D.K. Radioprotective agents to prevent cellular damage due to ionizing radiation. *J. Transl. Med.* **2017**, *15*, 232. [CrossRef]
16. Naeimi, R.A.; Talebpour Amiri, F.; Khalatbary, A.R.; Ghasemi, A.; Zargari, M.; Ghesemi, M.; Hosseinimehr, S.J. Atorvastatin mitigates testicular injuries induced by ionizing radiation in mice. *Reprod. Toxicol.* **2017**, *72*, 115–121. [CrossRef] [PubMed]
17. Li, X.; Luo, L.; Karthi, S.; Zhang, K.; Luo, J.; Hu, Q.; Weng, Q. Effects of 200 Gy 60Co-γ Radiation on the Regulation of Antioxidant Enzymes, Hsp70 Genes, and Serum Molecules of Plutella xylostella (Linnaeus). *Molecules* **2018**, *23*, 1011. [CrossRef] [PubMed]
18. El-Mesallamy, H.O.; Gawish, R.A.; Sallam, A.M.; Fahmy, H.A.; Nada, A.S. Ferulic acid protects against radiation-induced testicular damage in male rats: Impact on SIRT1 and PARP1. *Environ. Sci. Pollut. Res. Int.* **2018**, *25*, 6218–6227. [CrossRef]
19. Fatehi, D.; Mohammadi, M.; Shekarchi, B.; Shabani, A.; Seify, M.; Rostamzadeh, A. Radioprotective effects of Silymarin on the sperm parameters of NMRI mice irradiated with γ-rays. *J. Photochem. Photobiol. B* **2018**, *178*, 489–495. [CrossRef]
20. Najafi, M.; Cheki, M.; Amini, P.; Javadi, A.; Shabeeb, D.; Eleojo Musa, A. Evaluating the protective effect of resveratrol, Q10, and alpha-lipoic acid on radiation-induced mice spermatogenesis injury: A histopathological study. *Int. J. Reprod. Biomed.* **2019**, *17*, 907–914. [CrossRef]
21. Ibrahim, A.A.; Karam, H.M.; Shaaban, E.A.; Safar, M.M.; El-Yamany, M.F. MitoQ ameliorates testicular damage induced by gamma irradiation in rats: Modulation of mitochondrial apoptosis and steroidogenesis. *Life Sci.* **2019**, *232*, 116655. [CrossRef]
22. Gawish, R.A.; Fahmy, H.A.; Abd El Fattah, A.I.; Nada, A.S. The potential effect of methylseleninic acid (MSA) against γ-irradiation induced testicular damage in rats: Impact on JAK/STAT pathway. *Arch. Biochem. Biophys.* **2020**, *679*, 108205. [CrossRef]
23. Koul, A.; Abraham, S.K. Intake of saffron reduces γ-radiation-induced genotoxicity and oxidative stress in mice. *Toxicol. Mech. Methods* **2017**, *27*, 428–434. [CrossRef] [PubMed]
24. Koul, A.; Abraham, S.K. Efficacy of crocin and safranal as protective agents against genotoxic stress induced by gamma radiation, urethane and procarbazine in mice. *Hum. Exp. Toxicol.* **2018**, *37*, 13–20. [CrossRef]
25. Shahidi, F.; Vasudevan Ramakrishnan, V.; Oh, W.Y. Bioavailability and metabolism of food bioactives and their health effects: A review. *J. Food Bioact.* **2019**, *8*, 6–41. [CrossRef]
26. Lautenschläger, M.; Sendker, J.; Hüwel, S.; Galla, H.J.; Brandt, S.; Düfer, M.; Riehemann, K.; Hensel, A. Intestinal formation of trans-crocetin from saffron extract (*Crocus sativus* L.) and in vitro permeation through intestinal and blood brain barrier. *Phytomedicine* **2015**, *22*, 36–44. [CrossRef]
27. Asai, A.; Nakano, T.; Takahashi, M.; Nagao, A. Orally administered crocetin and crocins are absorbed into blood plasma as crocetin and its glucuronide conjugates in mice. *J. Agric. Food Chem.* **2005**, *53*, 7302–7306. [CrossRef] [PubMed]
28. Zhang, Y.; Fei, F.; Zhen, L.; Zhu, X.; Wang, J.; Li, S.; Geng, J.; Sun, R.; Yu, X.; Chen, T.; et al. Sensitive analysis and simultaneous assessment of pharmacokinetic properties of crocin and crocetin after oral administration in rats. *J. Chromatogr. B Anal. Technol. Biomed. Life Sci.* **2017**, *1044*, 1–7. [CrossRef] [PubMed]
29. Umigai, N.; Murakami, K.; Ulit, M.V.; Antonio, L.S.; Shirotori, M.; Morikawa, H.; Nakano, T. The pharmacokinetic profile of crocetin in healthy adult human volunteers after a single oral administration. *Phytomedicine* **2011**, *18*, 575–578. [CrossRef]
30. Hashemi, M.; Hosseinzadeh, H. A comprehensive review on biological activities and toxicology of crocetin. *Food Chem. Toxicol.* **2019**, *130*, 44–60. [CrossRef]
31. Di Emidio, G.; Rossi, G.; Bonomo, I.; Alonso, G.L.; Sferra, R.; Vetuschi, A.; Artini, P.G.; Provenzani, A.; Falone, S.; Carta, G.; et al. The Natural Carotenoid Crocetin and the Synthetic Tellurium Compound AS101 Protect the Ovary against Cyclophosphamide by Modulating SIRT1 and Mitochondrial Markers. *Oxidative Med. Cell. Longev.* **2017**, *2017*, 8928604. [CrossRef]
32. Ranjan, A.; Choubey, M.; Yada, T.; Krishna, A. Direct effects of neuropeptide nesfatin-1 on testicular spermatogenesis and steroidogenesis of the adult mice. *Gen. Comp. Endocrinol.* **2019**, *271*, 49–60. [CrossRef]
33. Tatone, C.; Di Emidio, G.; Barbonetti, A.; Carta, G.; Luciano, A.M.; Falone, S.; Amicarelli, F. Sirtuins in gamete biology and reproductive physiology: Emerging roles and therapeutic potential in female and male infertility. *Hum. Reprod. Update* **2018**, *24*, 267–289. [CrossRef] [PubMed]
34. Rato, L.; Duarte, A.I.; Tomás, G.D.; Santos, M.S.; Moreira, P.I.; Socorro, S.; Cavaco, J.E.; Alves, M.G.; Oliveira, P.F. Pre-diabetes alters testicular PGC1-α/SIRT3 axis modulating mitochondrial bioenergetics and oxidative stress. *Biochim. Biophys. Acta* **2014**, *1837*, 335–344. [CrossRef]
35. Levadoux-Martin, M.; Gouble, A.; Jégou, B.; Vallet-Erdtmann, V.; Auriol, J.; Mercier, P.; Morello, D. Impaired gametogenesis in mice that overexpress the RNA-binding protein HuR. *EMBO Rep.* **2003**, *4*, 394–399. [CrossRef]
36. Nguyen Chi, M.; Chalmel, F.; Agius, E.; Vanzo, N.; Khabar, K.S.; Jégou, B.; Morello, D. Temporally regulated traffic of HuR and its associated ARE-containing mRNAs from the chromatoid body to polysomes during mouse spermatogenesis. *PLoS ONE* **2009**, *4*, e4900. [CrossRef] [PubMed]
37. Masuda, K.; Abdelmohsen, K.; Kim, M.M.; Srikantan, S.; Lee, E.K.; Tominaga, K.; Selimyan, R.; Martindale, J.L.; Yang, X.; Lehrmann, E.; et al. Global dissociation of HuR-mRNA complexes promotes cell survival after ionizing radiation. *EMBO J.* **2011**, *30*, 1040–1053. [CrossRef] [PubMed]
38. Reed, A.M.; Fishel, M.L.; Kelley, M.R. Small-molecule inhibitors of proteins involved in base excision repair potentiate the anti-tumorigenic effect of existing chemotherapeutics and irradiation. *Future Oncol.* **2009**, *5*, 713–726. [CrossRef]

39. Ripley, B.M.; Gildenberg, M.S.; Washington, M.T. Control of DNA Damage Bypass by Ubiquitylation of PCNA. *Genes* **2020**, *11*, 138. [CrossRef] [PubMed]
40. Zhu, Y.; Yin, Q.; Wei, D.; Yang, Z.; Du, Y.; Ma, Y. Autophagy in male reproduction. *Syst. Biol. Reprod. Med.* **2019**, *65*, 265–272. [CrossRef]
41. Liou, G.Y.; Storz, P. Detecting reactive oxygen species by immunohistochemistry. *Methods Mol. Biol.* **2015**, *1292*, 97–104.
42. Di Emidio, G.; Rea, F.; Placidi, M.; Rossi, G.; Cocciolone, D.; Virmani, A.; Macchiarelli, G.; Palmerini, M.G.; D'Alessandro, A.M.; Artini, P.G.; et al. Regulatory Functions of L-Carnitine, Acetyl, and Propionyl L-Carnitine in a PCOS Mouse Model: Focus on Antioxidant/Antiglycative Molecular Pathways in the Ovarian Microenvironment. *Antioxidants* **2020**, *9*, 867. [CrossRef] [PubMed]
43. Colapietro, A.; Mancini, A.; Vitale, F.; Martellucci, S.; Angelucci, A.; Llorens, S.; Mattei, V.; Gravina, G.L.; Alonso, G.L.; Festuccia, C. Crocetin Extracted from Saffron Shows Antitumor Effects in Models of Human Glioblastoma. *Int. J. Mol. Sci.* **2020**, *21*, 423. [CrossRef]
44. Xi, L.; Qian, Z.; Du, P.; Fu, J. Pharmacokinetic properties of crocin (crocetin digentiobiose ester) following oral administration in rats. *Phytomedicine* **2007**, *14*, 633–636. [CrossRef] [PubMed]
45. Celik-Ozenci, C.; Tasatargil, A. Role of poly(ADP-ribose) polymerases in male reproduction. *Spermatogenesis* **2013**, *3*, e24194. [CrossRef] [PubMed]
46. Virág, L. Structure and function of poly(ADP-ribose) polymerase-1: Role in oxidative stress-related pathologies. *Curr. Vasc. Pharmacol.* **2005**, *3*, 209–214. [CrossRef]
47. Du, Y.; Yamaguchi, H.; Wei, Y.; Hsu, J.L.; Wang, H.L.; Hsu, Y.H.; Lin, W.C.; Yu, W.H.; Leonard, P.G.; Lee, G.R., IV; et al. Blocking c-Met-mediated PARP1 phosphorylation enhances anti-tumor effects of PARP inhibitors. *Nat. Med.* **2016**, *22*, 194–201. [CrossRef]
48. Prosperi, E.; Scovassi, A.I. Dynamic Interaction between PARP-1, PCNA and p21waf1/cip1. In *Poly(ADP-Ribosyl)ation*; Springer: Boston, MA, USA, 2006; pp. 67–74.
49. Zhang, C.; Chen, K.; Wang, J.; Zheng, Z.; Luo, Y.; Zhou, W.; Zhuo, Z.; Liang, J.; Sha, W.; Chen, H. Protective Effects of Crocetin against Radiation-Induced Injury in Intestinal Epithelial Cells. *Biomed. Res. Int.* **2020**, *2020*, 2906053.
50. Milani, A.; Basirnejad, M.; Shahbazi, S.; Bolhassani, A. Carotenoids: Biochemistry, pharmacology and treatment. *Br. J. Pharmacol.* **2017**, *174*, 1290–1324. [CrossRef]
51. Cerdá-Bernad, D.; Valero-Cases, E.; Pastor, J.J.; Frutos, M.J. Saffron bioactives crocin, crocetin and safranal: Effect on oxidative stress and mechanisms of action. *Crit. Rev. Food Sci. Nutr.* **2020**, 1–18. [CrossRef]
52. López de Silanes, I.; Zhan, M.; Lal, A.; Yang, X.; Gorospe, M. Identification of a target RNA motif for RNA-binding protein HuR. *Proc. Natl. Acad. Sci. USA* **2004**, *101*, 2987–2992. [CrossRef] [PubMed]
53. Abdelmohsen, K.; Pullmann, R., Jr.; Lal, A.; Kim, H.H.; Galban, S.; Yang, X.; Blethrow, J.D.; Walker, M.; Shubert, J.; Gillespie, D.A.; et al. Phosphorylation of HuR by Chk2 regulates SIRT1 expression. *Mol. Cell.* **2007**, *25*, 543–557. [CrossRef] [PubMed]
54. Kim, H.S.; Patel, K.; Muldoon-Jacobs, K.; Bisht, K.S.; Aykin-Burns, N.; Pennington, J.D.; van der Meer, R.; Nguyen, P.; Savage, J.; Owens, K.M.; et al. SIRT3 is a mitochondria-localized tumor suppressor required for maintenance of mitochondrial integrity and metabolism during stress. *Cancer Cell* **2010**, *17*, 41–52. [CrossRef]
55. Lv, C.; Wang, X.; Guo, Y.; Yuan, S. Role of Selective Autophagy in Spermatogenesis and Male Fertility. *Cells* **2020**, *9*, 2523. [CrossRef] [PubMed]
56. Yoshii, S.R.; Mizushima, N. Monitoring and Measuring Autophagy. *Int. J. Mol. Sci.* **2017**, *18*, 1865. [CrossRef]
57. Jiang, T.; Harder, B.; de la Vega, M.R.; Wong, P.K.; Chapman, E.; Zhang, D.D. p62 links autophagy and Nrf2 signaling. *Free Radic. Biol. Med.* **2015**, *88*, 199–204. [CrossRef]
58. Katsuragi, Y.; Ichimura, Y.; Komatsu, M. p62/SQSTM1 functions as a signaling hub and an autophagy adaptor. *FEBS J.* **2015**, *282*, 4672–4678. [CrossRef]
59. Festuccia, C.; Mancini, A.; Gravina, G.L.; Scarsella, L.; Llorens, L.; Alonso, G.L.; Tatone, C.; Di Cesare, E.; Jannini, E.A.; Lenzi, A.; et al. Antitumor Effects of Saffron-Derived Carotenoids in Prostate Cancer Cell Models. *BioMed Res. Int.* **2014**, *2014*, 135048. [CrossRef]
60. Sánchez, A.M.; Carmona, M.; Zalacain, A.; Carot, J.M.; Jabaloyes, J.M.; Alonso, G.L. Rapid determination of crocetin esters and picrocrocin from saffron spice (*Crocus sativus* L.) using UV-visible spectrophotometry for quality control. *J. Agric. Food Chem.* **2008**, *56*, 3167–3175. [CrossRef]
61. Sánchez, A.M.; Carmona, M.; Ordoudi, S.A.; Tsimidou, M.Z.; Alonso, G.L. Kinetics of individual crocetin ester degradation in aqueous extracts of saffron (*Crocus sativus* L.) upon thermal treatment in the dark. *J. Agric. Food Chem.* **2008**, *56*, 1627–1637. [CrossRef]
62. Bathaie, S.Z.; Farajzade, A.; Hoshyar, R. A review of the chemistry and uses of crocins and crocetin, the carotenoid natural dyes in saffron, with particular emphasis on applications as colorants including their use as biological stains. *Biotech. Histochem.* **2014**, *89*, 401–411. [CrossRef]
63. Lopes, F.; Smith, R.; Nash, S.; Mitchell, R.T.; Spears, N. Irinotecan metabolite SN38 results in germ cell loss in the testis but not in the ovary of prepubertal mice. *Mol. Hum. Reprod.* **2016**, *22*, 745–755. [CrossRef]
64. Gravina, G.L.; Mancini, A.; Mattei, C.; Vitale, F.; Marampon, F.; Colapietro, A.; Rossi, G.; Ventura, L.; Vetuschi, A.; Di Cesare, E.; et al. Enhancement of radiosensitivity by the novel anticancer quinolone derivative vosaroxin in preclinical glioblastoma models. *Oncotarget* **2017**, *8*, 29865–29886. [CrossRef]

65. Ciccarelli, C.; Di Rocco, A.; Gravina, G.L.; Mauro, A.; Festuccia, C.; Del Fattore, A.; Berardinelli, P.; De Felice, F.; Musio, D.; Bouché, M.; et al. Disruption of MEK/ERK/c-Myc signaling radiosensitizes prostate cancer cells in vitro and in vivo. *J. Cancer Res. Clin. Oncol.* **2018**, *144*, 1685–1699. [CrossRef]
66. Nasirzadeh, M.; Rasmi, Y.; Rahbarghazi, R.; Kheradmand, F.; Karimipour, M.; Aramwit, P.; Astinfeshan, M.; Gholinejad, Z.; Daeihasani, B.; Saboory, E.; et al. Crocetin promotes angiogenesis in human endothelial cells through PI3K-Akt-eNOS signaling pathway. *EXCLI J.* **2019**, *18*, 936–949. [PubMed]
67. Nyengaard, J.R. Stereologic methods and their application in kidney research. *J. Am. Soc. Nephrol.* **1999**, *10*, 1100–1123. [PubMed]
68. Osinubi, A.A.; Noronha, C.C.; Okanlawon, A.O. Morphometric and stereological assessment of the effects of long-term administration of quinine on the morphology of rat testis. *West. Afr. J. Med.* **2005**, *24*, 200–205. [CrossRef] [PubMed]
69. Montoto, L.G.; Arregui, L.; Sánchez, N.M.; Gomendio, M.; Roldan, E.R.S. Postnatal testicular development in mouse species with different levels of sperm competition. *Reproduction* **2012**, *143*, 333–346. [CrossRef]

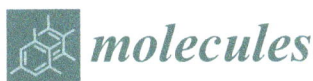

Article

Saffron Pre-Treatment Promotes Reduction in Tissue Inflammatory Profiles and Alters Microbiome Composition in Experimental Colitis Mice

Suhrid Banskota [1,2], Hassan Brim [3], Yun Han Kwon [1,2], Gulshan Singh [4], Sidhartha R. Sinha [4], Huaqing Wang [1,2], Waliul I. Khan [1,2,*] and Hassan Ashktorab [5,*]

1. Farncombe Family Digestive Health Research Institute, McMaster University, 1280 Main St. W, Hamilton, ON L8S 4K1, Canada; banskots@mcmaster.ca (S.B.); yyoon90@gmail.com (Y.H.K.); wanghu@mcmaster.ca (H.W.)
2. Department of Pathology and Molecular Medicine, McMaster University, Hamilton, ON L8S 4K1, Canada
3. Department of Pathology, Cancer Center, Howard University College of Medicine, Washington, DC 20059, USA; hbrim@howard.edu
4. Division of Gastroenterology and Hepatology, Stanford University, Stanford, CA 94305, USA; gsingh10@stanford.edu (G.S.); sidsinha@stanford.edu (S.R.S.)
5. Department of Medicine, Gastroenterology Division, Cancer Center, Howard University College of Medicine, Washington, DC 20059, USA
* Correspondence: khanwal@mcmaster.ca (W.I.K.); hashktorab@howard.edu (H.A.)

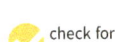

Citation: Banskota, S.; Brim, H.; Kwon, Y.H.; Singh, G.; Sinha, S.R.; Wang, H.; Khan, W.I.; Ashktorab, H. Saffron Pre-Treatment Promotes Reduction in Tissue Inflammatory Profiles and Alters Microbiome Composition in Experimental Colitis Mice. *Molecules* **2021**, *26*, 3351. https://doi.org/10.3390/molecules26113351

Academic Editors: Konstantinos Dimas and Nikolaos Pitsikas

Received: 30 April 2021
Accepted: 27 May 2021
Published: 2 June 2021

Publisher's Note: MDPI stays neutral with regard to jurisdictional claims in published maps and institutional affiliations.

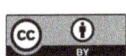

Copyright: © 2021 by the authors. Licensee MDPI, Basel, Switzerland. This article is an open access article distributed under the terms and conditions of the Creative Commons Attribution (CC BY) license (https://creativecommons.org/licenses/by/4.0/).

Abstract: Inflammatory bowel disease (IBD) is a chronic inflammatory condition of the gastrointestinal tract with an incompletely understood pathogenesis. Long-standing colitis is associated with increased risk of colon cancer. Despite the availability of various anti-inflammatory and immunomodulatory drugs, many patients fail to respond to pharmacologic therapy and some experience drug-induced adverse events. Dietary supplements, particularly saffron (*Crocus sativus*), have recently gained an appreciable attention in alleviating some symptoms of digestive diseases. In our study, we investigated whether saffron may have a prophylactic effect in a murine colitis model. Saffron pre-treatment improved the gross and histopathological characteristics of the colonic mucosa in murine experimental colitis. Treatment with saffron showed a significant amelioration of colitis when compared to the vehicle-treated mice group. Saffron treatment significantly decreased secretion of serotonin and pro-inflammatory cytokines, such as TNF-α, IL-1β, and IL-6, in the colon tissues by suppressing the nuclear translocation of NF-κB. The gut microbiome analysis revealed distinct clusters in the saffron-treated and untreated mice in dextran sulfate sodium (DSS)-induced colitis by visualization of the Bray–Curtis diversity by principal coordinates analysis (PCoA). Furthermore, we observed that, at the operational taxonomic unit (OTU) level, Cyanobacteria were depleted, while short-chain fatty acids (SCFAs), such as isobutyric acid, acetic acid, and propionic acid, were increased in saffron-treated mice. Our data suggest that pre-treatment with saffron inhibits DSS-induced pro-inflammatory cytokine secretion, modulates gut microbiota composition, prevents the depletion of SCFAs, and reduces the susceptibility to colitis.

Keywords: inflammatory bowel disease; saffron; gut microbiota; colitis; cytokines

1. Introduction

Inflammatory bowel disease (IBD) is a chronic relapsing immune-inflammatory condition of the gastrointestinal (GI) tract with increasing prevalence worldwide [1]. IBD is broadly classified into Crohn's disease (CD) and ulcerative colitis (UC) on the basis of their clinical presentation, but the risk factors implicated on the pathogenesis of both CD and UC are similar [2]. The etiology of IBD is complex and various studies suggest that its pathogenesis is associated with a dysregulated immune response, genetic factors, gut microbiota, and environmental factors [2]. Various immunosuppressive synthetic drugs and biologics, such as salicylates, corticosteroids, tumor necrosis factor (TNF) blockers, and vedolizumab, are available as therapies for IBD, and many additional options are in the pipeline [3–5]. Clinical data suggest that these therapies are limited in managing the disease in some patients, while some fail to respond over time. Moreover, failure in managing IBD over the long run deteriorates the inflammatory conditions and increases the risk of developing colon cancer [6–10]. Therefore, alternative approaches in preventing the induction or perpetuation of intestinal inflammation are important in decreasing the incidence of IBD.

Natural products, such as berberine, baicalein, curcumin, bromelain, and their chemical constituents, are reported to be effective in treating IBD, and the mechanism of action involved in ameliorating inflammation has been widely studied [11]. Saffron (*Crocus sativus*) has been used as a spice and for health management since ancient times and is reported to play a key role in treatment of different digestive system disorders [12–15]. Saffron, by virtue of its potent antioxidant property, showed a significant decrease in lipoprotein oxidation susceptibility (LOS) in human subjects and was evaluated as a promising anti-obesity drug [16]. Crocin, a biologically active carotenoid constituent of saffron, was demonstrated to protect against DSS-induced colitis in C57BL/6 J mice and suppressed tumor growth in ApcMinC/Gpt mice by suppressing NF-κB-mediated inflammation [17]. NF-κB, an oxidative stress sensitive transcription factor, is associated with tissue induction of pro-inflammatory cytokines, such as tumor necrosis factor (TNF)-α, interleukin (IL)-6, and IL-1β [18,19].

Alteration in the enterochromaffin (EC) cell numbers and intestinal 5-HT content has been observed in experimental colitis and in both UC and CD patients [20,21]. The altered 5-HT plays a key role in the activation and transportation of immune cells to produce proinflammatory cytokines by increasing angiogenesis [22–24]. Previous studies, including ours, demonstrated that excessive serotonin (5-HT) secreted from EC cells during DSS-induced inflammation in the gut plays an important role in the modulation of gut microbial composition as well as gut function [25,26]. The human GI tract is colonized with 1×10^{14} colony-forming units of bacteria and the colonization occurs soon after birth [27]. Accumulating evidence suggest that the gut microbiota has an important role on the pathogenesis of IBD. We previously demonstrated that 5-HT regulates the growth of bacteria in a species-dependent manner and selects for a more colitogenic microbiota [26]. The effect of saffron on the altered 5-HT and composition of gut microbiota in DSS-treated mice has not been evaluated so far.

The current study was conducted to investigate whether saffron has prophylactic effects on an experimental colitis mice model by evaluating the secretion of pro-inflammatory cytokines such as TNF-α, IL-6, and IL-1β in colon tissue, the colonic 5-HT level, assessing the cecal microbiota composition, and analyzing the changes in short-chain fatty acids in feces. The findings from this study will shed light on the translational perspective of the protective effect of saffron in human IBD.

2. Results

2.1. Saffron Alleviated DSS-Induced Colitis in Mice

To investigate the prophylactic effect of saffron in mice, C57BL/6 mice were orally gavaged with saffron (10 mg/kg and 20 mg/kg body weight of mice) based on a previous study [28], for four days prior to the administration of 2.5% dextran sodium sulfate solution, and continued for another seven days along with DSS (Figure 1A). The severity of the DSS-induced colitis, disease activity index (DAI), colon length, macroscopic score, and histological score was significantly improved by saffron at a 20 mg/Kg dose while saffron at the dose of 10 mg/Kg showed improvement in the DAI, macroscopic score, and histological score (Figure 1B–F). The results indicate that saffron reduces the severity of DSS-induced colitis in mice by improving the gross and histopathological characteristics of the colonic mucosa.

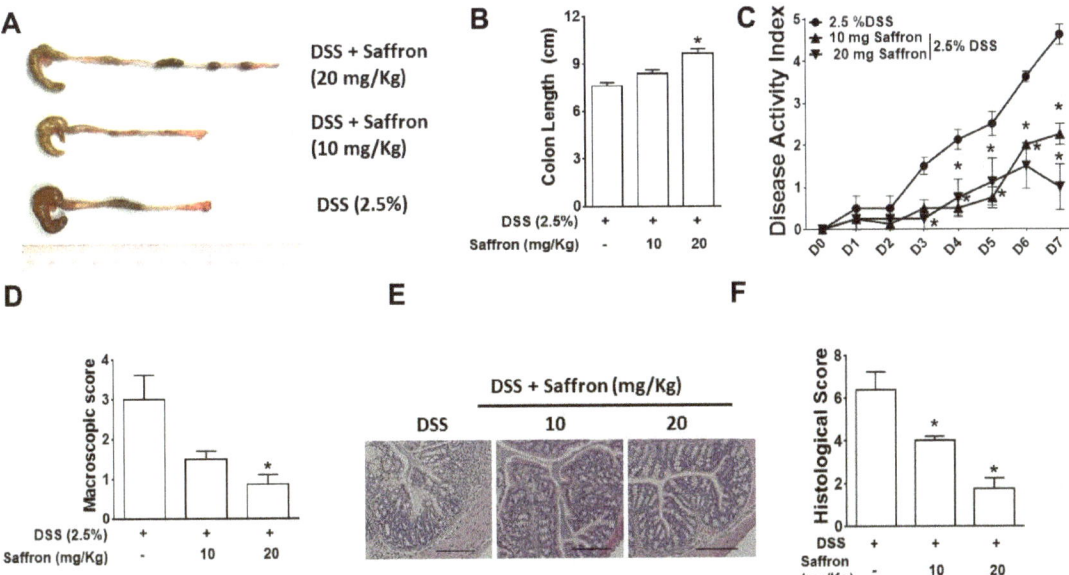

Figure 1. Saffron reduced the severity of DSS-induced colitis in mice. Mice were orally gavaged with saffron (10 mg/Kg and 20 mg/Kg) or the vehicle for 4 days before the administration of 2.5% DSS in their drinking water and continued for 7 days along with the DSS. Inflammation was assessed by (**A**) macroscopic appearance of the colon tissue; (**B**) colon length; (**C**) the disease activity index; (**D**) the macroscopic score; (**E**) representative micrographs of H&E-stained colon cross-sections on day 7 post-DSS, bar = 100 µM; and (**F**) the histological score. Data represent the mean ± SEM (n = 4/group). * $p < 0.05$, compared to the vehicle-treated mice.

2.2. Saffron Prevented Increase in DSS-Induced Pro-Inflammatory Cytokines and 5-HT Level in Mice Colonic Tissue

A number of different immune cells, such as macrophages and dendritic cells, promote the recruitment of additional immune cells to inflamed tissue. [29,30]. The increase in the pro-inflammatory cytokines such as IL-6, IL-1β, and TNF-α in tissue indicates an aggravated immune response at the site of inflammation. Therefore, we analyzed the secreted pro-inflammatory cytokines in colonic tissue of mice and found that the DSS-induced increased secretion of IL-6, IL-1β, and TNF-α was significantly reduced by saffron (20 mg/kg), reducing the severity of the DSS-induced colitis. (Figure 2A–C). Additionally, we found that the DSS-induced increased 5-HT level in the colon tissue was significantly inhibited by the saffron at a higher dose (Figure 2E), further supporting the beneficial effect of saffron in preventing colitis. To investigate the mechanism by which saffron suppressed the DSS-induced pro-inflammatory cytokines, we analyzed NF-κB in the cytoplasmic and nuclear protein of the colon tissues. The nuclear translocation of NF-κB by DSS was significantly decreased by a higher dose of saffron in mice (Figure 2E). These data indicate that saffron inhibits DSS-induced secretion of pro-inflammatory cytokines in mice colons by decreasing the nuclear translocation of NF-κB.

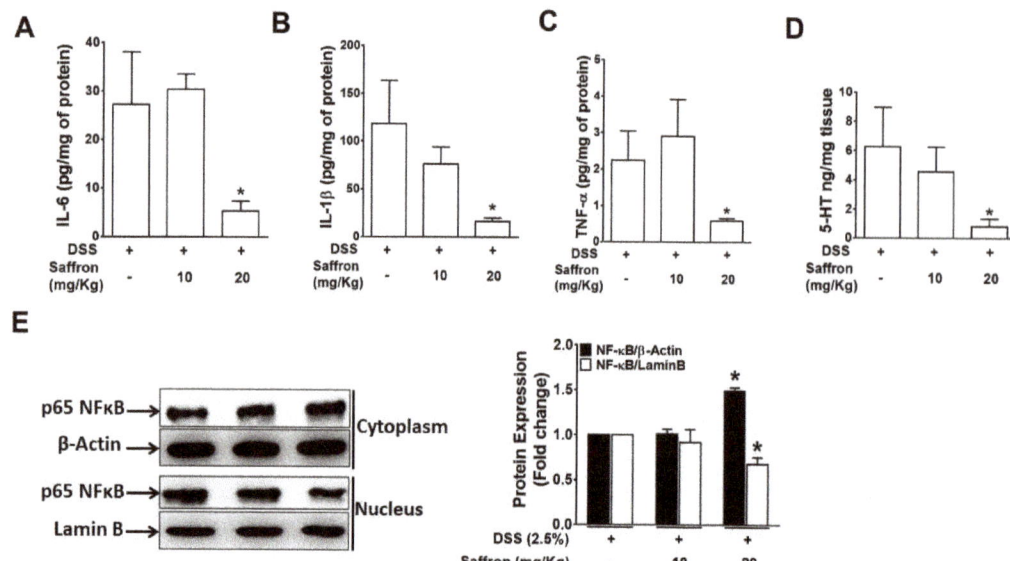

Figure 2. Pre-treatment with saffron inhibited the DSS-induced secretion of pro-inflammatory cytokines and the serotonin level in colon tissue. The supernatants from the homogenized colon tissue were analyzed for (**A**) IL-6, (**B**) IL-1β, (**C**) TNF-α, and (**D**) Serotonin (5-HT). Data represent the mean ± SEM ($n = 4$/group). * $p < 0.05$, compared to the vehicle-treated mice. (**E**) Cytoplasmic and nuclear protein extracted from colon tissues were analyzed for NF-κB. Representative blots of the cytoplasmic and nuclear NF-κB from the colon tissue of three random mice from each group. The bar graph represents the mean ± SEM. * $p < 0.05$, compared to the vehicle-treated mice.

2.3. Saffron Alters the Mouse Gut Microbiota Composition in DSS-Treated Mice

To determine whether saffron alters the mouse gut microbiota composition, we analyzed the cecal microbial composition in three different groups of mice which received DSS, DSS plus 10 mg/kg of saffron, and DSS plus 20 mg/kg of saffron. As shown in Figure 3A, the alpha diversity of the three groups was not different. However, the three groups of mice were separated into distinct clusters, as shown by visualization of the Bray–Curtis diversity by principal coordinate analysis (PCoA) (Figure 3B; $p < 0.05$). The two groups of saffron-treated mice appeared more similar in composition while largely differed when compared to the DSS-treated group. In addition, the taxonomic summaries (average of each group) at the phylum level revealed greater similarity between the saffron-treated mice. Moreover, saffron administration depleted the Proteobacteria phylum, in which the effect seems to be much greater at 20 mg/kg compared to 10 mg/kg of saffron (Figure 3C; $p < 0.05$); in turn, this phylum is absent in naïve SPF mice [31]. Similarly, we observed that, at the operational taxonomic unit (OTU) level, Cyanobacteria were depleted in the saffron-treated mice and the effect was greater at the dose of 20 mg/kg (Figure 3D, $p < 0.05$).

2.4. Saffron Increased Beneficial Short-Chain Fatty Acids (SCFAs) in DSS-Treated Mice

SCFAs are vital for regulation of intestinal epithelial cell (IEC) functioning, to modulate their proliferation, differentiation, and promoting gut barrier function. SCFAs are known to be altered by a change in the microbiota composition [32]. To confirm the functional effect of the altered microbiota by saffron administration during DSS-induced colitis, we analyzed the SCFA levels in the feces by using gas chromatography–mass spectrometry (GC/MS). We found that saffron at both doses significantly increased isobutyric acid and acetic acid, while at higher dose it also increased propionic acid in feces (Figure 4).

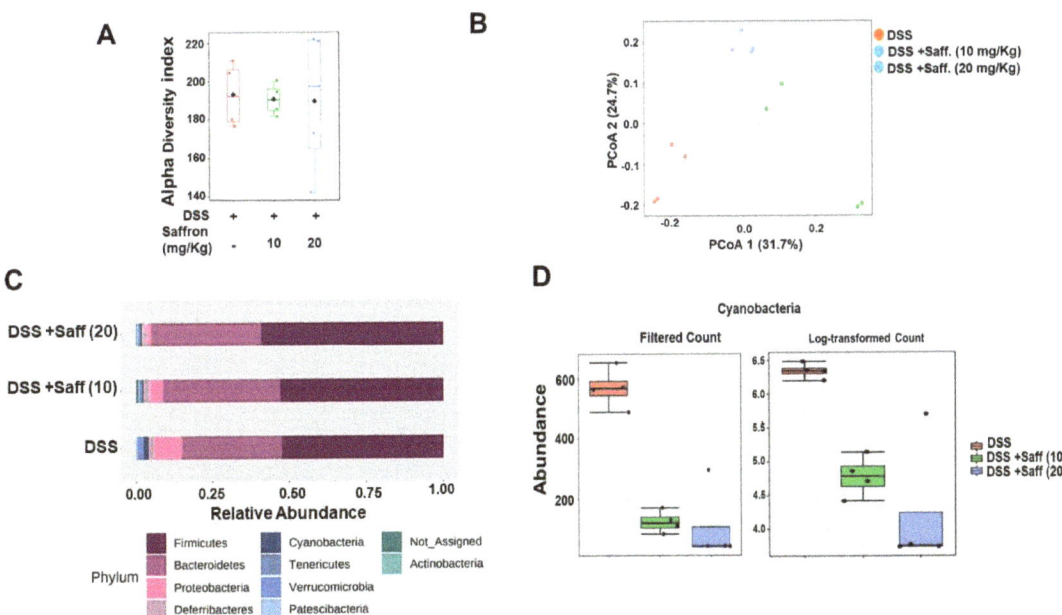

Figure 3. Microbial composition analysis in the cecal samples of saffron pre-treated and untreated mice challenged with DSS. The cecal content of mice were subjected to 16S rRNA partial sequencing profiling analysis and the figure represents (**A**) the alpha diversity of the three group of mice using the Chao1 index. (**B**) PCoA of the Bray–Curtis dissimilarity, showing distinct microbiota in each group of mice. (**C**) Taxonomic summaries at the phylum level. (**D**) Abundance of Cyanobacteria in the saffron-treated and untreated groups ($n = 4$/group).

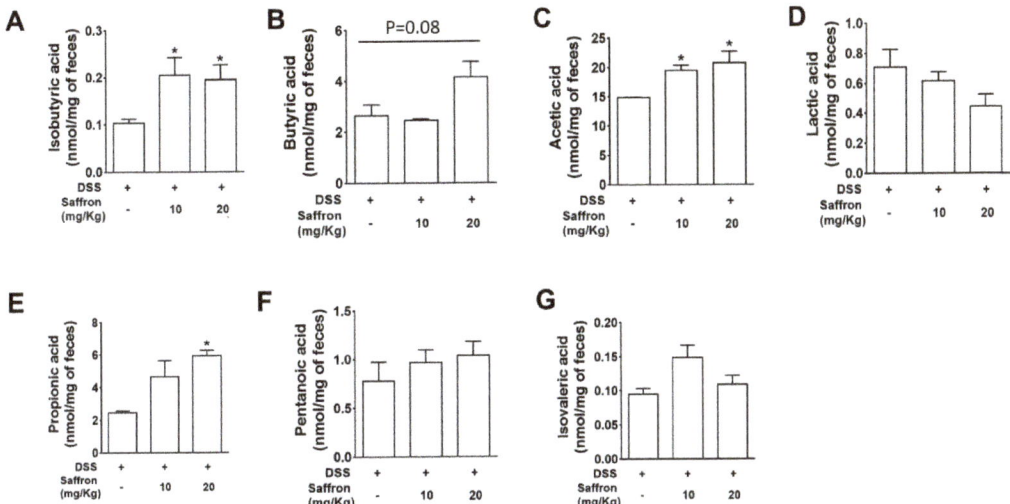

Figure 4. Saffron prevented depletion of the SCFA concentrations in fecal samples of DSS-treated mice. Fecal samples of mice were analyzed for determining the concentration of (**A**) isobutyric acid, (**B**) butyric acid, (**C**) acetic acid, (**D**) lactic acid, (**E**) propionic acid, (**F**) pentanoic acid, and (**G**) isovaleric acid. Data represent the mean ± SEM ($n = 4$/group). * $p < 0.05$, compared to the vehicle-treated mice fecal sample.

3. Discussion

The application of natural and traditionally trusted medicinal product provides a safe alternative to manage inflammatory conditions in the gut. Saffron has been used since ancient days in diets, and its various components, such as crocin, crocetin, picrocrocin, and safranal, are reported to have significant efficacy in peptic ulcer, stomach cancer, ulcerative colitis, colorectal cancer, and pancreatic disorder [15,33,34]. A randomized, double blind, placebo control trial conducted on mild to moderate ulcerative colitis patient suggested that dietary saffron may be effective in reducing the severity of disease in UC patients by improving the antioxidant factors [33]. Some other studies illustrated the protective effects of the active constituents of saffron, such as crocin and safranal, against experimental colitis [35,36]. In the present study, we investigated the effect of unfractionated saffron in preventing DSS-induced colitis in mice by evaluating its effect on the serotonin level, microbiota, and short-chain fatty acids. We found that supplementation of saffron along with diet reduced the severe effect of DSS. A previous study reported slight, although not significant restoration of colon length and percentage of weight loss in the safranal (200 mg/kg, 500 mg/kg)-treated groups of mice, with a significant decrease in the DAI score [37]. We found that the unfractionated saffron (20 mg/kg) treatment significantly increased the colon length, decreased the DAI, and improved the histopathological characteristics of the colonic mucosa, exhibiting its protective effects during experimental colitis. The tissue levels of pro-inflammatory cytokines, such as IL-6, IL-1β, and TNF-α, were significantly reduced in mice treated with saffron at the dose of 20 mg/Kg (Figure 2A–C). This effect of saffron may be achieved by the virtue of its antioxidant property. NF-κB, being a redox-sensitive transcription factor, is activated by various inflammatory insults and translocate to the nucleus to induce proinflammatory cytokines during inflammation [16,17]. Saffron pre-treatment inhibited the nuclear translocation of p65 NF-κB in mice colonic tissue samples, which corresponds to inhibition of the secretion of IL-6, IL-1β, and TNF-α. Saffron at the same dose significantly inhibited the serotonin level in colon tissue (Figure 2D). Serotonin was previously demonstrated to play a key role in the pathogenesis of experimental colitis by priming colon epithelial cells to inflammation. It has been previously revealed that serotonin modulates the gut function and gut microbiota composition by selecting colitogenic microbiota [38]. The amount of serotonin was significantly decreased in the saffron-pretreated mice, and it can be speculated that saffron may inhibit the oxidative stress probably by activating an antioxidant mechanism [33]. Additionally, disturbance in gut microbiota composition is largely associated with various diseases, as gut microbiota perform various important functions, such as digestion of polysaccharides, vitamin synthesis, and boosting of the immune system [39,40]. There were no significant changes in the alpha diversity of the gut microbiome, but each group showed distinct clusters while analyzing beta diversity (Figure 3B). The group that only received DSS was different compared to the mice that received saffron. An increased abundance of Proteobacteria has been implicated in a Crohn's disease and its load has been suggested as a potential criterion in the diagnosis of dysbiosis in gut microbiota [41]. Saffron-treated mice showed depletion in the Proteobacteria phylum. Furthermore, unlike in human IBD, Cyanobacteria, which are reported to increase in DSS-induced colitis [42,43], which is in agreement with our study, were depleted by saffron as observed at the OTU-level analysis (Figure 3C,D). This reduction in colitogenic bacteria (Proteobacteria and Cyanobacteria) is likely to be sensed directly by the immune system, leading to a reduction in pro-inflammatory signals and markers. However, further in-depth studies are warranted to validate these findings. SCFAs, such as butyric acid, acetic acid, and propionic acid, are reported to participate in controlling inflammation and repair the colon epithelium [32]. SCFA levels are known to be reduced in fecal samples of IBD patients and in experimental colitis [44–46]. Saffron preserved the essential SCFAs in mice feces, indicating its beneficial attributes in maintaining colonic microbial populations during colitis. The cumulative effects of saffron treatment, leading to the positive changes in observed macroscopic, histological, and immune markers, have potential translational implications for patients with intestinal inflammation. In fact, based on our previous and the present findings [28], we calculated the human equivalent dose (20 mg/Kg) of saffron that showed the best outcome in DSS-induced colitis mice and started a clinical trial in patients with mild to moderate ulcerative colitis. We have already registered our clinical trial for this application at clinicaltrials.gov (https://www.clinicaltrials.gov/ct2/results?cond=saffron&term=&cntry=&state=&city=&dist= accessed on 1 June 2021) (NCT04749576).

4. Materials and Methods

4.1. Mice

Age-matched C57BL/6N mice were purchased from Taconic Biosciences (Rensselaer, NY, USA). All experimental animal procedures were in accordance with the guidelines and principles of the Canadian Council of Animal Care and were approved by the Animal Care Committee McMaster University (AUP # 19-02-09).

4.2. Pre-Treatment with Saffron and Evaluation of DSS-Induced Colitis

Saffron aqueous extract at two different doses (10 mg and 20 mg per kg body weight) were given to the mice (N = 4 mice/group) by oral gavage for four days prior to the administration of DSS (mol wt. 36–54 kilo daltons; ICN Biomedicals Inc., Soho, OH, USA) in their drinking water at 2.5% weight/volume (w/v) along with saffron for 7 more days. The average DSS consumption per cage was recorded every day for the duration of the experiment. Mice were sacrificed on the 7th day after the beginning of DSS administration to examine the severity of colitis using previously published scoring systems. The disease activity index (DAI) was calculated using the scores of body weight loss, bloody feces, and consistency of stool. Macroscopic scoring was done after the mice were sacrificed by careful observation of rectal bleeding, rectal prolapse, colonic bleeding, and diarrhea. Colonic histological damage score was based on goblet cell depletion, the loss of crypt architectures, inflammatory cell infiltration, and crypt abscess.

4.3. Enzyme Linked Immunosorbent Assay (ELISA)

Colon tissues from mice in each group were homogenized in tissue lysis buffer and the supernatant were used to analyze the level of IL-1β, IL-6, and TNF-α using commercially available ELISA kits from R&D System Inc. (Minneapolis, MN, USA) and expressed in units/mg of protein.

The serotonin level in tissue were measured as previously described [26], using commercially available enzyme-linked immunosorbent assay (ELISA) kits (Cat. # IM1749; Beckman Coulter, Fullerton, CA, USA). The serotonin level was expressed as a function of tissue weight (ng/mg).

4.4. Western Blot

Cytoplasmic and nuclear proteins were extracted by using the NE-PER nuclear and cytoplasmic extraction reagent kit (no. 78833, Thermo Scientific, Waltham, MA, USA) as described earlier [5]. Briefly, the protein concentration in the extract was determined by the DC Protein Assay Kit (Bio-Rad Laboratories, Mississauga, ON, Canada). Protein samples were separated using sodium dodecyl sulfate-polyacrylamide gel electrophoresis and were electrophoretically transferred onto nitrocellulose or polyvinylidene difluoride membranes. The membranes were incubated with 5% bovine serum albumin (BSA) in s 1× Tris-buffered saline Tween 20 at room temperature for 1 h and then probed with primary antibodies overnight at 4 °C. The membranes were then washed 3 times with Tris-buffered saline containing 0.1% Tween 20 followed by incubation with corresponding secondary antibodies for 1 h at room temperature. Immunodetection was performed by visualization of the membrane using a chemiluminescent reagent (Thermo Scientific) and by exposure to a luminescent image analyzer, the ChemiDoc Touch Imaging System (Bio-Rad Laboratories, Hercules, CA, USA). NF-κB p65 (1:1000; catalog no. ab16502) and lamin B1 (1:1000; catalog no. ab65986) were purchased from Abcam (Cambridge, MA, USA). β-actin (1:1000; catalog no. 4970) was purchased from Cell Signaling Technology, Inc. (Boston, MA, USA). The rabbit polyclonal antibody was obtained from Abbiotec (San Diego, CA, USA).

4.5. Bacterial Diversity and Profiling Analysis of the Cecal Microbiota

Bacterial profiling of cecal samples was carried out by amplification of the V3–V4 regions of the 16S rRNA gene, as described previously [47,48]. Amplification products were sequenced on an Illumina MiSeq with 2 × 250 nt paired end reads. The OTU abundance table obtained were given as input to Microbiome Analyst using default parameters and rarefying the data to the minimum library size with total sum normalization. The low variance filter was set at 10% using the inter-quartile range, and 20% prevalence was kept with four minimum counts [49]. The Microbiome Analyst platform was used to analyze alpha and beta diversities, and to compare the relative abundance of taxa at the phylum level [49].

4.6. Analysis of Fecal Short-Chain Fatty Acid Using Gas Chromatography—Mass Spectrometry

The concentrations of SCFAs in feces of mice were determined by gas chromatography–mass spectrometry, as described previously [26]. Briefly, e-tubes in which fecal samples were acidified with a weight equivalent amount of 3.7% hydrochloric acid were sonicated in methanol for 20 min before use. To the acidified samples, internal standards (14.72 mmol/L butyric acid-d_7) were added, followed by the addition of diethyl ether to obtain a diethyl ether–fecal extract. The acidified samples were extracted three times with propyl formate containing butyric acid-d_7 as the internal standard, and a 60 µL extract aliquot was derivatized with 25 µL MTBSTFA at 40 °C for 1 h and then analyzed by GCMS Then the derivatized samples were run through the 6890N Network GC system (Agilent Technologies, Mississauga, ON, Canada) equipped with DB-17HT (30 m × 0.25 mm ID, 0.15 mm film) and 5973N Mass Selective Detector (Agilent Technologies). Acetic acid, propionic acid, isobutyric acid, butyric acid, isovaleric acid, pentanoic acid, and lactic acid were quantified and reported as nmol/mg of fecal sample. The calibration curves were obtained for all seven targets by injecting all the standards as a mixture.

4.7. Statistical Analysis

Student's *t*-test or one-way ANOVA in GraphPad Prism ver. 9.0 (San Diego, CA, USA) was used to determine the significance of the intergroup differences. Data are expressed as the mean ± SEM. *p* values of less than 0.05 were considered statistically significant.

5. Conclusions

Our data suggest that saffron exhibits its prophylactic effect on DSS-induced colitis in mice by reducing the serotonin levels, inhibiting pro-inflammatory cytokine secretion, and maintaining the diversity of the gut microbiota and the SCFA level. Our pre-clinical study provides an alternative and safe approach to reduce the susceptibility to GI disorders, including IBD, by incorporating saffron, a natural and edible product, into diets. However, a well-designed clinical trial may shed some light on the efficacy of saffron in different GI disorders, such as IBD.

Author Contributions: S.B., H.A. and W.I.K. conceived and designed the research; S.B., Y.H.K. and H.W. performed the experiments; S.B., Y.H.K. and W.I.K. analyzed and interpreted the results of the experiments; S.B. and W.I.K. drafted the manuscript; S.B., H.B., H.A., G.S., S.R.S. and W.I.K. edited and revised the manuscript. All authors have read and agreed to the published version of the manuscript.

Funding: This work was supported by grants from the Canadian Institutes of Health Research (PJT156262). S.B. is supported by Post-Doctoral Fellowship Award from Canadian Institutes of Health Research.

Institutional Review Board Statement: Not applicable. Animal experiment approval number has been added above in method section.

Informed Consent Statement: Not applicable.

Data Availability Statement: The data presented in this study are available on request from the corresponding author.

Acknowledgments: We would like to thank Michael Surette and his laboratory for the support in the microbiota work. We also thank all saffron growers and gp-food.com (http://www.gp-food.com/index.php/about-us.html) (accessed on 1 June 2021) for providing saffron.

Conflicts of Interest: The authors declare no conflict of interest.

Sample Availability: Samples are available from the authors.

References

1. Jairath, V.; Feagan, B.G. Global burden of inflammatory bowel disease. *Lancet Gastroenterol. Hepatol.* **2020**, *5*, 2–3. [CrossRef]
2. Ananthakrishnan, A.N. Epidemiology and risk factors for IBD. *Nat. Rev. Gastroenterol. Hepatol.* **2015**, *12*, 205–217. [CrossRef]
3. Li, P.; Zheng, Y.; Chen, X. Drugs for autoimmune inflammatory diseases: From small molecule compounds to anti-TNF biologics. *Front. Pharmacol.* **2017**, *8*, 460. [CrossRef] [PubMed]
4. Manuc, T.E.; Manuc, M.M.; Diculescu, M.M. Recent insights into the molecular pathogenesis of Crohn's disease: A review of emerging therapeutic targets. *Clin. Exp. Gastroenterol.* **2016**, *9*, 59. [PubMed]
5. Banskota, S.; Wang, H.; Kwon, Y.H.; Gautam, J.; Gurung, P.; Haq, S.; Hassan, F.N.; Bowdish, D.M.; Kim, J.A.; Carling, D.; et al. Salicylates Ameliorate Intestinal Inflammation by Activating Macrophage AMPK. *Inflamm. Bowel Dis.* **2021**, *27*, 914–926. [CrossRef]
6. Yanai, H.; Hanauer, S.B. Assessing response and loss of response to biological therapies in IBD. *Am. J. Gastroenterol.* **2011**, *106*, 685–698. [CrossRef]
7. Biancone, L.; Armuzzi, A.; Scribano, M.L.; Castiglione, F.; D'incà, R.; Orlando, A.; Papi, C.; Daperno, M.; Vecchi, M.; Riegler, G.; et al. Cancer Risk in Inflammatory Bowel Disease: A 6-Year Prospective Multicenter Nested Case–Control. IG-IBD Study. *Inflamm. Bowel Dis.* **2020**, *26*, 450–459. [CrossRef]
8. Jawad, N.; Direkze, N.; Leedham, S.J. Inflammatory bowel disease and colon cancer. In *Inflammation and Gastrointestinal Cancers*; Springer: Berlin, Germany, 2011; pp. 99–115.
9. Munkholm, P. The incidence and prevalence of colorectal cancer in inflammatory bowel disease. *Aliment. Pharmacol. Ther.* **2003**, *18*, 1–5. [CrossRef] [PubMed]
10. Isbell, G.; Levin, B. Ulcerative colitis and colon cancer. *Gastroenterol. Clin. N. Am.* **1988**, *17*, 773–791. [CrossRef]
11. Guo, B.J.; Bian, Z.X.; Qiu, H.C.; Wang, Y.T.; Wang, Y. Biological and clinical implications of herbal medicine and natural products for the treatment of inflammatory bowel disease. *Ann. N. Y. Acad. Sci.* **2017**, *1401*, 37–48. [CrossRef]
12. Serrano-Díaz, J.; Sánchez, A.M.; Martínez-Tomé, M.; Winterhalter, P.; Alonso, G.L. A contribution to nutritional studies on Crocus sativus flowers and their value as food. *J. Food Compos. Anal.* **2013**, *31*, 101–108. [CrossRef]
13. Alavizadeh, S.H.; Hosseinzadeh, H. Bioactivity assessment and toxicity of crocin: A comprehensive review. *Food Chem. Toxicol.* **2014**, *64*, 65–80. [CrossRef] [PubMed]
14. Khorasany, A.R.; Hosseinzadeh, H. Therapeutic effects of saffron (*Crocus sativus* L.) in digestive disorders: A review. *Iran. J. Basic Med. Sci.* **2016**, *19*, 455.
15. Ashktorab, H.; Soleimani, A.; Singh, G.; Amin, A.; Tabtabaei, S.; Latella, G.; Stein, U.; Akhondzadeh, S.; Solanki, N.; Gondré-Lewis, M.C.; et al. Saffron: The golden spice with therapeutic properties on digestive diseases. *Nutrients* **2019**, *11*, 943. [CrossRef] [PubMed]
16. Verma, S.; Bordia, A. Antioxidant property of saffron in man. *Indian J. Med. Sci.* **1998**, *52*, 205–207.
17. Teng, S.; Hao, J.; Bi, H.; Li, C.; Zhang, Y.; Zhang, Y.; Han, W.; Wang, D. The protection of crocin against ulcerative colitis and colorectal cancer via suppression of NF-κB-mediated inflammation. *Front. Pharmacol.* **2021**, *12*, 639458. [CrossRef] [PubMed]
18. Banskota, S.; Regmi, S.C.; Kim, J.-A. NOX1 to NOX2 switch deactivates AMPK and induces invasive phenotype in colon cancer cells through overexpression of MMP-7. *Mol. Cancer* **2015**, *14*, 123. [CrossRef]
19. Tak, P.P.; Firestein, G.S. NF-κB: A key role in inflammatory diseases. *J. Clin. Investig.* **2001**, *107*, 7–11. [CrossRef]
20. Khan, W.I.; Motomura, Y.; Wang, H.; El-Sharkawy, R.T.; Verdu, E.F.; Verma-Gandhu, M.; Rollins, B.J.; Collins, S.M. Critical role of MCP-1 in the pathogenesis of experimental colitis in the context of immune and enterochromaffin cells. *Am. J. Physiol. Gastrointest. Liver Physiol.* **2006**, *291*, G803–G811. [CrossRef]
21. Manocha, M.; Khan, W.I. Serotonin and GI disorders: An update on clinical and experimental studies. *Clin. Transl. Gastroenterol.* **2012**, *3*, e13. [CrossRef]
22. Ghia, J.E.; Li, N.; Wang, H.; Collins, M.; Deng, Y.; El–Sharkawy, R.T.; Côté, F.; Mallet, J.; Khan, W.I. Serotonin has a key role in pathogenesis of experimental colitis. *Gastroenterology* **2009**, *137*, 1649–1660. [CrossRef]
23. Regmi, S.C.; Park, S.Y.; Ku, S.K.; Kim, J.A. Serotonin regulates innate immune responses of colon epithelial cells through Nox2-derived reactive oxygen species. *Free Radic. Biol. Med.* **2014**, *69*, 377–389. [CrossRef]
24. Banskota, S.; Gautam, J.; Regmi, S.C.; Gurung, P.; Park, M.H.; Kim, S.J.; Nam, T.G.; Jeong, B.S.; Kim, J.A. BJ-1108, a 6-Amino-2, 4, 5-Trimethylpyridin-3-ol analog, inhibits serotonin-induced angiogenesis and tumor growth through PI3K/NOX Pathway. *PLoS ONE* **2016**, *11*, e0148133. [CrossRef]

25. Banskota, S.; Ghia, J.E.; Khan, W.I. Serotonin in the gut: Blessing or a curse. *Biochimie* **2019**, *161*, 56–64. [CrossRef]
26. Kwon, Y.H.; Wang, H.; Denou, E.; Ghia, J.E.; Rossi, L.; Fontes, M.E.; Bernier, S.P.; Shajib, M.S.; Banskota, S.; Collins, S.M.; et al. Modulation of gut microbiota composition by serotonin signaling influences intestinal immune response and susceptibility to colitis. *Cell. Mol. Gastroenterol. Hepatol.* **2019**, *7*, 709–728. [CrossRef] [PubMed]
27. Hill, D.A.; Artis, D. Intestinal bacteria and the regulation of immune cell homeostasis. *Annu. Rev. Immunol.* **2009**, *28*, 623–667. [CrossRef] [PubMed]
28. Singh, G.; Haileselassie, Y.; Brim, H.; Ashktorab, H.; Habtezion, A. Tu1284 Protective Effect of Saffron in Mouse Colitis Models through Immune Modulation. *Gastroenterology* **2020**, *158*, S-1043. [CrossRef]
29. Striz, I.; Brabcova, E.; Kolesar, L.; Sekerkova, A. Cytokine networking of innate immunity cells: A potential target of therapy. *Clin. Sci.* **2014**, *126*, 593–612. [CrossRef]
30. Coombes, J.; Powrie, F. Dendritic cells in intestinal immune regulation. *Nat. Rev. Immunol.* **2008**, *8*, 435–446. [CrossRef] [PubMed]
31. Osbelt, L.; Thiemann, S.; Smit, N.; Lesker, T.R.; Schröter, M.; Gálvez, E.J.; Schmidt-Hohagen, K.; Pils, M.C.; Mühlen, S.; Dersch, P.; et al. Variations in microbiota composition of laboratory mice influence Citrobacter rodentium infection via variable short-chain fatty acid production. *PLoS Pathog.* **2020**, *16*, e1008448. [CrossRef]
32. Parada Venegas, D.; De la Fuente, M.K.; Landskron, G.; González, M.J.; Quera, R.; Dijkstra, G.; Harmsen, H.J.; Faber, K.N.; Hermoso, M.A. Short chain fatty acids (SCFAs)-mediated gut epithelial and immune regulation and its relevance for inflammatory bowel diseases. *Front. Immunol.* **2019**, *10*, 277. [CrossRef]
33. Tahvilian, N.; Masoodi, M.; Faghihi Kashani, A.; Vafa, M.; Aryaeian, N.; Heydarian, A.; Hosseini, A.; Moradi, N.; Farsi, F. Effects of saffron supplementation on oxidative/antioxidant status and severity of disease in ulcerative colitis patients: A randomized, double-blind, placebo-controlled study. *Phytother. Res.* **2021**, *35*, 946–953. [CrossRef] [PubMed]
34. Cerdá-Bernad, D.; Valero-Cases, E.; Pastor, J.J.; Frutos, M.J. Saffron bioactives crocin, crocetin and safranal: Effect on oxidative stress and mechanisms of action. *Crit. Rev. Food Sci. Nutr.* **2020**, 1–18. [CrossRef] [PubMed]
35. Kawabata, K.; Tung, N.H.; Shoyama, Y.; Sugie, S.; Mori, T.; Tanaka, T. Dietary crocin inhibits colitis and colitis-associated colorectal carcinogenesis in male ICR mice. *Evid. Based Complement. Altern. Med.* **2012**, *2012*, 820415. [CrossRef]
36. Khodir, A.E.; Said, E.; Atif, H.; ElKashef, H.A.; Salem, H.A. Targeting Nrf2/HO-1 signaling by crocin: Role in attenuation of AA-induced ulcerative colitis in rats. *Biomed. Pharmacother.* **2019**, *110*, 389–399. [CrossRef]
37. Lertnimitphun, P.; Jiang, Y.; Kim, N.; Fu, W.; Zheng, C.; Tan, H.; Zhou, H.; Zhang, X.; Pei, W.; Lu, Y.; et al. Safranal alleviates dextran sulfate sodium-induced colitis and suppresses macrophage-mediated inflammation. *Front. Pharmacol.* **2019**, *10*, 1281. [CrossRef]
38. Banskota, S.; Regmi, S.C.; Gautam, J.; Gurung, P.; Lee, Y.J.; Ku, S.K.; Lee, J.H.; Lee, J.; Chang, H.W.; Park, S.J.; et al. Serotonin disturbs colon epithelial tolerance of commensal E. coli by increasing NOX2-derived superoxide. *Free Radic. Biol. Med.* **2017**, *106*, 196–207. [CrossRef]
39. Campieri, M.; Gionchetti, P. Bacteria as the cause of ulcerative colitis. *Gut* **2001**, *48*, 132–135. [CrossRef]
40. Sekirov, I.; Russell, S.L.; Antunes, L.C. Finlay BB Gut microbiota in health and disease. *Physiol. Rev.* **2010**, *90*, 859–904. [CrossRef]
41. Vester-Andersen, M.K.; Mirsepasi-Lauridsen, H.C.; Prosberg, M.V.; Mortensen, C.O.; Träger, C.; Skovsen, K.; Thorkilgaard, T.; Nøjgaard, C.; Vind, I.; Krogfelt, K.A.; et al. Increased abundance of proteobacteria in aggressive Crohn's disease seven years after diagnosis. *Sci. Rep.* **2019**, *9*, 1–10. [CrossRef] [PubMed]
42. Wang, J.; Zhu, G.; Sun, C.; Xiong, K.; Yao, T.; Su, Y.; Fang, H. TAK-242 ameliorates DSS-induced colitis by regulating the gut microbiota and the JAK2/STAT3 signaling pathway. *Microb. Cell Factories* **2020**, *19*, 1–17. [CrossRef] [PubMed]
43. Santoru, M.L.; Piras, C.; Murgia, A.; Palmas, V.; Camboni, T.; Liggi, S.; Ibba, I.; Lai, M.A.; Orrù, S.; Blois, S.; et al. Cross sectional evaluation of the gut-microbiome metabolome axis in an Italian cohort of IBD patients. *Sci. Rep.* **2017**, *7*, 1–14. [CrossRef] [PubMed]
44. Huda-Faujan, N.; Abdulamir, A.S.; Fatimah, A.B.; Anas, O.M.; Shuhaimi, M.; Yazid, A.M.; Loong, Y.Y. The impact of the level of the intestinal short chain fatty acids in inflammatory bowel disease patients versus healthy subjects. *Open Biochem. J.* **2010**, *4*, 53. [CrossRef] [PubMed]
45. Machiels, K.; Joossens, M.; Sabino, J.; De Preter, V.; Arijs, I.; Eeckhaut, V.; Ballet, V.; Claes, K.; Van Immerseel, F.; Verbeke, K.; et al. A decrease of the butyrate-producing species Roseburia hominis and Faecalibacterium prausnitzii defines dysbiosis in patients with ulcerative colitis. *Gut* **2014**, *63*, 1275–1283. [CrossRef] [PubMed]
46. Zhou, Y.; Xu, H.; Xu, J.; Guo, X.; Zhao, H.; Chen, Y.; Zhou, Y.; Nie, Y. F. prausnitzii and its supernatant increase SCFAs-producing bacteria to restore gut dysbiosis in TNBS-induced colitis. *AMB Express* **2021**, *11*, 1–10. [CrossRef]
47. Bartram, A.K.; Lynch, M.D.; Stearns, J.C.; Moreno-Hagelsieb, G.; Neufeld, J.D. Generation of multimillion-sequence 16S rRNA gene libraries from complex microbial communities by assembling paired-end Illumina reads. *Appl. Environ. Microbiol.* **2011**, *77*, 3846–3852. [CrossRef]
48. Stearns, J.C.; Davidson, C.J.; McKeon, S.; Whelan, F.J.; Fontes, M.E.; Schryvers, A.B.; Bowdish, D.M.; Kellner, J.D.; Surette, M.G. Culture and molecular-based profiles show shifts in bacterial communities of the upper respiratory tract that occur with age. *ISME J.* **2015**, *9*, 1246–1259. [CrossRef]
49. Chong, J.; Liu, P.; Zhou, G.; Xia, J. Using MicrobiomeAnalyst for comprehensive statistical, functional, and meta-analysis of microbiome data. *Nat. Protoc.* **2020**, *15*, 799–821. [CrossRef]

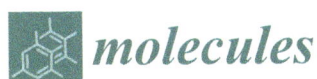

Article

Crocins from *Crocus sativus* L. in the Management of Hyperglycemia. In Vivo Evidence from Zebrafish

Eleni Kakouri [1,†], **Adamantia Agalou** [2,†], **Charalabos Kanakis** [1], **Dimitris Beis** [2,*] and **Petros A. Tarantilis** [1,*]

[1] Laboratory of Chemistry, Department of Food Science & Human Nutrition, School of Food and Nutritional Sciences, Agricultural University of Athens, 111855 Athens, Greece; elenikakouri@aua.gr (E.K.); chkanakis@aua.gr (C.K.)

[2] Developmental Biology, Biomedical Research Foundation Academy of Athens, 11527 Athens, Greece; agalou@bioacademy.gr

* Correspondence: dbeis@bioacademy.gr (D.B.); ptara@aua.gr (P.A.T.)

† These authors contributed equally to this work.

Academic Editors: Nikolaos Pitsikas and Konstantinos Dimas

Received: 7 October 2020; Accepted: 7 November 2020; Published: 10 November 2020

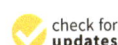

Abstract: Diabetes mellitus is a disease characterized by persistent high blood glucose levels and accompanied by impaired metabolic pathways. In this study, we used zebrafish to investigate the effect of crocins isolated from *Crocus sativus* L., on the control of glucose levels and pancreatic β-cells. Embryos were exposed to an aqueous solution of crocins and whole embryo glucose levels were measured at 48 h post-treatment. We showed that the application of crocins reduces zebrafish embryo glucose levels and enhances insulin expression. We also examined whether crocins are implicated in the metabolic pathway of gluconeogenesis. We showed that following a single application of crocins and glucose level reduction, the expression of *phosphoenolpyruvate carboxykinase 1* (*pck1*), a key gene involved in glucose metabolism, is increased. We propose a putative role for the crocins in glucose metabolism and insulin management.

Keywords: crocins; glucose; β-pancreatic cells; insulin; *pck1*

---

1. Introduction

Diabetes mellitus (DM) is a chronic metabolic disease characterized by persistent high blood glucose levels and accompanied by impaired metabolic pathways of carbohydrates, proteins, and lipids. Diabetes is essentially caused either by the loss of β-cells, or of their ability to produce insulin (type I). Type II diabetes refers to the inability of the organism to properly regulate and sense insulin, known as resistance to insulin. Hyperglycemia is the result of both types. Since insulin is the main transporter, responsible for removing glucose from the blood-stream, its deficiency can inescapably lead to elevated blood glucose levels. Persistent hyperglycemia can lead to severe micro and macrovascular complications causing long-term damage to nerves and blood vessels, affecting different body organs. In this regard, the management of blood glucose levels in diabetic patients is the main focus of the available antidiabetic treatment including either administration of insulin and/or synthetic drugs [1].

Numerous medicines have been developed over the past years to alleviate symptoms, increase life expectancy, and maintain the progression of the disease in remission. Medical treatments through synthetic formulations can overcome risk factors. There are several cases where synthetic formulations lead to severe side effects that are not associated with the disease itself. In order to avoid treatment related side effects, scientists are driven towards the development of new therapeutic molecules, able to replace current therapeutic strategies.

Phytochemicals are emerging as powerful alternatives towards the fight against chronic diseases, including diabetes. These plant-derived molecules used as a mixture or as a single compound, contribute to the prevention and treatment of several chronic disorders such as cancer, neurodegenerative and metabolic diseases. It has been proposed that their efficacy is mainly due to their antioxidant activity [2,3]. Treatment with natural products is yet preliminary and much information is still needed regarding their mechanism of action. These include pharmacological parameters such as pharmacokinetics and pharmacodynamics, drug tolerance, and possible side effects. Accumulating data of several in vitro, in vivo, and clinical trial studies provide evidence that these substances are of great therapeutic importance and may consist a new era of treatment against the above-mentioned long-term conditions [4–6].

Crocus sativus L. is a stemless, perennial plant belonging to the Iridaceae family and the genus Crocus. The plant is commonly known as saffron, a name which is referred to its dried red stigmas. Stigmas are considered the pharmacologically active part of the plant and their chemical composition has been widely studied [7–11]. More than 150 volatile and non-volatile compounds have been identified. Crocins (CRCs) are the predominant constituents of the stigmas and give them their characteristic deep red color [10–13]. On the contrary to other carotenoids, CRCs due to their glycosylated terminals, are water soluble molecules.

Zebrafish, *Danio rerio*, a small tropical fish, has become a popular model for studying a wide range of human diseases. These include cancer [14], cardiovascular [15], neurodegenerative [16] and metabolic diseases [17,18]. This is due to the high genetic homology with humans and the similarities in organ physiology and metabolism, offering several unique advantages. Among those, most useful for this study are the external fertilization, development, and transparency of the embryos allowing non-invasive in vivo imaging, as well as the plethora of synchronized progeny. In vivo phenotypic screens using zebrafish embryos have been particularly valuable in identifying novel bioactive natural compounds or optimizing the activity of lead compounds [19]. Chemical library screens using zebrafish embryos for the identification of melanogenesis inhibitors [20] and or transgenic-based screens for angiogenesis [21] or neoglucogenesis [18] have been very productive.

In addition, zebrafish has become a popular experimental model regarding the study of metabolic diseases, including diabetes. Similarities regarding the exocrine and endocrine pancreas between mammals and zebrafish [22], the conservation of key proteins that control glucose metabolism [18], the capability of measuring glucose levels in larvae and adult zebrafish, as well as the unique capacity of this model to recover its β-cells [23,24], make zebrafish a promising experimental model for testing compounds that alter glucose metabolism or regulate glucose levels [25,26].

We aimed to investigate the effect of CRCs isolated from *Crocus sativus* L., on the control of glucose levels using zebrafish as an animal model. We also examined whether the addition of crocins would regulate the levels of *phosphoenolpyruvate carboxykinase 1 (pck1)*, a key regulatory gene for the gluconeogenesis process that contributes to the maintenance of normoglycemia. Finally, we evaluated the effect of crocins on β-pancreatic cells.

2. Results

2.1. LC-QTOF HRMS Analysis

Although the chemical profile of CRCs is well documented in previous studies [10–13], we evaluated the quality of the fresh prepared extract used in this study. Crocins are found in the extract of *Crocus sativus* L. stigmas conjugated with different types of sugars. Identification of the types of CRCs presented was performed by the LC/Q-TOF/HRMS analysis. The quadrupole time-of-flight tandem mass spectrometer (Q-TOF/MS) is a hybrid analyzer, as it couples a TOF instrument with a quadrupole instrument. Therefore, on the contrary to conventional HPLC-MS systems, LC/Q-TOF/MS offers more accurate results since Q-TOF/MS, not only provide the chemical formula of a compound based on accurate mass measurement (mass error less than 5 ppm), but also high resolution and high detection sensitivity make this technique, a powerful tool for precise analysis of a mixture. The compounds presented in Table 1 confirm previous studies [10–13], as five types of CRCs were tentatively identified.

Table 1. Identified compounds at the negative ionization mode.

t_R	Compound Name *	Chemical Formula	m/z Theoretical	m/z Observed [M − H]$^-$	% of CRCs	Δm
10.658	Crocin 5 (trans 5GGG)	$C_{50}H_{74}O_{29}$	1137.4230	1137.4218	0.73	−1.05
13.677	Crocin 5 (cis 5GGG)	$C_{50}H_{74}O_{29}$	1137.4230	1137.4220	1.34	−0.88
14.971	Crocin 4 (trans 4GG)	$C_{44}H_{64}O_{24}$	975.37148	975.3707	46.84	−0.80
15.047	Crocin 2 (trans 2G)	$C_{32}H_{44}O_{14}$	651.26583	651.2639	29.30	−2.96
15.402	Crocin 4 (cis 4GG)	$C_{44}H_{64}O_{24}$	975.37148	975.3699	14.96	−1.62
15.783	Crocin 3 (trans 3Gg)	$C_{38}H_{54}O_{19}$	813.31865	813.317	18.29	−2.02
16.062	Crocin 3 (cis 3Gg)	$C_{38}H_{54}O_{19}$	813.31865	813.3172	78.09	−1.78
16.645	Crocin 1 (trans 1g)	$C_{26}H_{34}O_9$	489.21301	489.2117	4.84	−2.68
18.142	Crocin 2 (cis 2G)	$C_{32}H_{44}O_{14}$	651.26583	651.2639	5.61	−2.96

* Nomenclature of CRCs followed that proposed by Carmona et al. (2006) [8]. (G) is referred to gentiobiose and (g) to glucose.

2.2. Determination of LC50

We used zebrafish larvae to evaluate the effect of crocins on glucose metabolism in vivo during embryo development. In order to avoid toxic effects for the treated embryos from the CRCs application, a toxicity test was performed before proceeding with the biological experiments. LC50 was estimated according to the OECD guidelines [27] as described in the Materials and Methods Section and it was calculated at 0.681 mg/mL in an extract of crocins used in this study (Table 1).

2.3. Zebrafish Glucose Levels Are Lowered by CRCs

To investigate whether the treatment of crocins can regulate glucose levels of zebrafish embryos, larvae at 72 h post fertilization (hpf) were treated with 0.2 mg/mL CRCs for 48 h. This concentration corresponds to approximately 1/3 of the calculated LC50 and is considered safe since no effects in terms of mortality or any abnormalities were detected in the developing embryos. Three independent experiments were performed and the results showed that there was a significant decrease ($p < 0.05$) of glucose levels on treated embryos compared with the untreated embryos (Figure 1), indicating that the application of crocins can affect glucose levels.

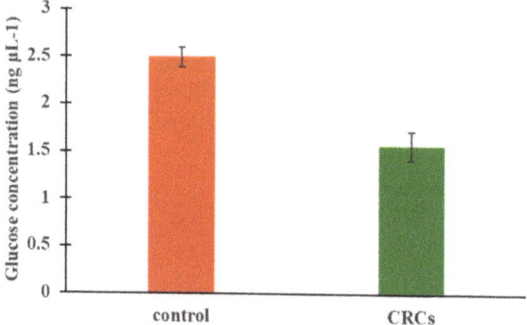

Figure 1. Glucose levels at zebrafish larvae following 48h treatment with CRCs at the concentration of 0.2 mg/mL. Data are mean +/− standard error of the mean (SEM), n = 3, $p < 0.05$.

2.4. Enhanced Fluorescence of β-Cells Indicate Insa Upregulation

Since pancreatic β-cells secrete insulin to regulate glucose metabolism, we aimed to investigate the effect of CRCs on the β-cell formation of developing zebrafish embryos. For this purpose, we used the transgenic zebrafish line *Tg(ins:DsRed)*, where the expression of the red fluorescent protein is driven by the zebrafish prepro-insulin promoter providing a convenient fluorescent marker for β-cells. Zebrafish embryos at 72 hpf were treated with CRCs and after 48 h of incubation the insulin-expressing cells of the pancreatic islets were visualized under a fluorescent microscope. A significant increase in fluorescent intensity was observed on the CRCs-treated embryos compared to the control group (Figure 2). Since the fluorescence of β-cells in this transgenic line is driven by the insulin reporter, these results indicate that the application of crocins promoted insulin expression.

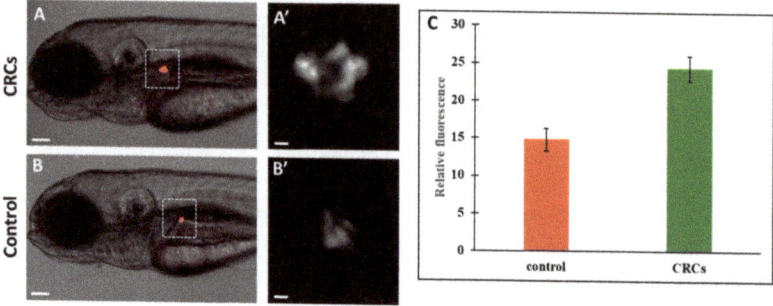

Figure 2. Zebrafish pancreas monitoring after treatment with CRCs. Transgenic zebrafish *Tg(ins:DsRed)* were treated at 72hpf with 0.2 mg/mL CRCs for 48h and visualized under fluorescent microscope. There was significant increase of fluorescence on the pancreatic islets of CRCs-treated embryos (**A**,**A′**) compared to the control group (**B**,**B′**). **A′** and **B′** are micrographs of **A** and **B**, respectively. (**C**) fluorescence intensity was quantified using Fiji software. Results shown are the mean +/− SEM. $p < 0.01$. Scale bars: A and B: 100 μm, A′ and B′:10 μm.

2.5. Insulin Expression by Quantitative Real-Time PCR

In order to confirm that the enhanced fluorescence of the zebrafish pancreatic islets is the result of increased endogenous insulin expression, rather than that of the transgene only, we determined the levels of insulin mRNA by RT-PCR. Three insulin genes have been discovered in zebrafish, namely insulin a (*insa*), insulin b (*insb*), and insulin c (*insc*). *Insa* and *insb* are expressed as early as 1 hpf indicating that both genes are maternally expressed [28,29]. However, *insa* reaches its peak at 72 hpf, a time point in which an almost mature zebrafish pancreas is established, on the contrary to *insb*, whose expression is restricted only during very early developmental stages. In addition, *insa* is expressed specifically at the pancreas, whereas *insb* is expressed also in the brain. Therefore, it has been hypothesized that *insa* is the prominent responsible gene for glucose homeostasis regulation [30]. *Insc* is quite a newly discovered gene, expressed in the gut and internal organs [29], but its exact function is still not clear. In this respect, we focused on the study of *insa*. In addition, the promoter elements of this gene were also used for the generation of the transgene. The expression of *insa* gene were evaluated using qRT-PCR on 120 hpf zebrafish larvae treated at 72 hpf for 48 h with 0.2 mg/mL of CRCs. Our data showed that after the administration of CRCs expression of *insa*, it was significantly upregulated compared to the control group ($p < 0.01$ (Figure 3), supporting the implication of crocins in glucose homeostasis.

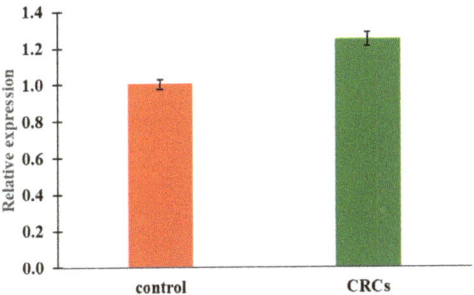

Figure 3. Expression of *insa* following 48h treatment with CRCs at the concentration of 0.2 mg/mL. *Insa* is significantly upregulated compared to the control treated embryos whose gene expression was set as 1. mRNA expression was normalized against *ef1a*. Data are mean +/− standard error of the mean (SEM), n = 3, $p < 0.01$.

2.6. Pck1 Expression Induced as a Response to Lower Glucose Levels

Pck is one of the main genes involved in glucose metabolism and is transcriptionally regulated among others by insulin. It can be found in the cytosol (*pck1*) and the mitochondria (*pck2*). However, only the cytosolic isoform, expressed in the liver, is responsible for catalyzing the formation of phosphoenolpyruvate from oxaloacetate and is predominantly implicated in the gluconeogenesis pathway [30]. In order to uncover the mechanism of implication of CRCs on glucose regulation we evaluated the expression of *pck1* gene using RT-PCR at 48 hpt. Our results showed that treatment of the zebrafish embryos with crocins lead to an induction of *pck1* following the reduced glucose levels (Figure 4). These data indicate that the reduction of glucose on CRCs-treated zebrafish larvae is not via the inhibition of the gluconeogenesis pathway (*pck1*), but rather induce a homeostatic response.

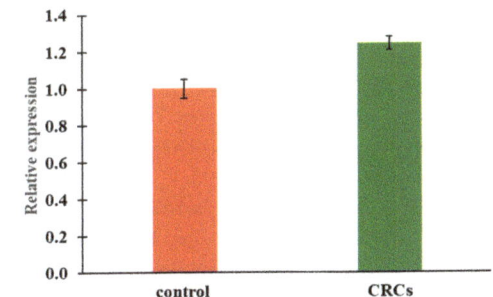

Figure 4. Expression of *pck1* following 48h treatment with CRCs at the concentration of 0.2 mg/mL. *Pck1* is significantly upregulated compared to the control treated embryos whose gene expression was set as 1. mRNA expression was normalized against *ef1a*. Data are mean +/− standard error of the mean (SEM), n = 3, $p < 0.0001$.

3. Discussion

Crocus sativus L., is a plant with rich pharmacologic activities. It has been studied in the context of several diseases such as cancer, neurodegenerative disorders, inflammation, heart related, and metabolic disorders. These properties are mainly attributed to the stigmas of the plant and specifically to its main constituents, crocins (CRCs), picrocrocin, and safranal [31–34].

However, growing, harvesting, storage, and environmental conditions, in addition to the extraction procedure, are important criteria to consider for the quality of the raw material. In herbal medicine, the quality of the material is directly linked to the efficacy of the natural product when tested in either in vivo or in vitro experiments and has a high impact on the study results. However, environmental conditions are rather uncontrolled and thus, a quality control test is always needed in order to guarantee the presence of the desired compounds. Furthermore, storage conditions including temperature, humidity, and light strongly affect the stability of the compounds presented. The above-mentioned quality criteria for the raw material used in this study are followed identically for each harvesting crop.

Saffron safety has been evaluated in clinical trials and in vivo studies [35–37]. Generally, saffron extracts as well as its constituents are relatively safe. For example, the intraperitoneal administration of stigmas ethanolic extract in rats at a range of a concentration between 1–5 g/kg bw (body weight), caused lethal effects at the highest administered dose (100% mortality), whereas the lowest dose resulted in no death at the end of 48 h. Authors estimated the LD50 value at 3.5 g kg^{-1} bw [35]. Similarly, Hosseinzadeh et al., (2010) [36] examined the safety of an extract of CRCs in mice and rats, after oral or intraperitoneal administration. No toxic effect was stated by the authors at mice treated with the extract since no mortality was observed at 2 h and after 48 h of treatment. The oral administrated dose was 3 g/kg, while the intraperitoneal injection was within the range of 0.5–3 g/kg. According to these data, stigmas of *Crocus sativus* L., and its active constituent CRCs, show a safe profile, since, an LD50 value within the range of 1–5 g/kg is attributed to low-toxic chemicals according to the toxicity classification [38].

In our experiments, the administration of CRCs is performed via immersion of the embryos in an aqueous solution of the tested compound. Even though the exact amount of crocin uptake is not known, this is a standard method for toxicity evaluation of compounds in zebrafish. Since, to our knowledge, this is the first time that a purified extract of crocins is tested in zebrafish, we investigated a range of concentrations up to 2 mg/mL in order to evaluate the toxicity. To investigate the effect of crocins on the control of glucose levels, we performed all the experiments at a concentration that corresponds to 1/3 of the LC50, and did not result in any phenotypic abnormalities. In this way, we are ensured that all measurements are not affected by any toxic response of the developing larvae.

The antidiabetic and hypoglycemic potential of *Crocus sativus* L., is supported by many studies and saffron is nowadays considered as a promising candidate in the field of metabolic diseases. For example, Kianbakht and Hajiaghaee, 2011 [39] discussed the anti-glycemic effect of crocins, safranal, and saffron extracts in diabetic rats. Their results indicated that these compounds managed to control glycemia without triggering any toxic effect in the liver or the kidney. Another study performed by Kang et al., 2012 [40] demonstrated the in vitro capacity of saffron extract to activate glucose uptake and ameliorate insulin sensitivity in skeletal muscle cells. Furthermore, Dehghan et al., 2016 [41] showed the effectiveness of saffron to improve diabetic biochemical markers, such as blood glucose and glycosylated hemoglobin, in in vivo and in vitro models. In addition, several clinical trials have confirmed the antidiabetic effect of saffron in type II diabetes patients. Milajerdi et al., 2018 [42] performed a triple-blinded randomized clinical trial in type II diabetic patients and suggested that saffron extracts, administrated twice a day and used in combination with current antidiabetic therapy, lowered blood glucose levels. In addition, the administration of saffron in overweight/obese patients diminished both sugar levels and hemoglobin A1c [43,44].

Streptozotocin-induced diabetic models have been used to evaluate the effect of CRCs on glucose levels and pancreatic function. Rajaei et al., 2013 [45] evaluated serum glucose levels of hyperglycemic rats treated intraperitoneally with crocins. Lower glucose levels observed in the study with respect to the control group were attributed to higher insulin production or to the strong antioxidant activity of the extract used. The latter antidiabetic mechanism was further investigated by Yaribeygi et al., 2019 [46], who measured SOD and catalase levels of pancreas in diabetic rats. In this study, they found that CRCs significantly increased both enzymes and thus, harmful effects caused by oxidative stress due to hyperglycemia were avoided.

In another study, the hypoglycemic and hypolipidemic effects of CRCs were evaluated in streptozotocin-induced type II diabetes rats, where advanced glycation products, glucose and HbA1c levels, and fasting insulin levels were measured. All these parameters were significantly decreased in treated animals [47].

Despite the fact that zebrafish is widely used as a model for many human disorders, including metabolic diseases, there are only few studies analyzing the effect of saffron and/or its bioactive compounds on glucose management. In our study, we used zebrafish embryos to investigate the effect of the main bioactive compounds of *Crocus sativus* L. on the regulation of the glucose levels and the insulin secretion. We found that the administration of CRCs can significantly reduce glucose levels and in parallel increase insulin expression in developing embryos, suggesting a putative hypoglycemic role of this compound. Our study used a single application of CRCs in the water of developing embryos and more studies including adult feeding with CRCs would be needed to address long-term effects in zebrafish glucose homeostasis.

In general, various mechanisms have been proposed based on histopathologic observations and on measurement of blood glucose levels in several in vitro experimental models to explain the hypoglycemic and antidiabetic activity of saffron. Among them, enhanced stimulation of insulin secretion from β-cells, increased capacity of the peripheral tissues to use it properly, restoration of the β-cells of the endocrine pancreas, and inhibition of glucose production. In addition, the antioxidant activity of the stigmas seems to drastically influence its hypoglycemic effect [45,48,49]. Here, we present elevated fluorescence levels of the pancreatic islets in the *Tg(ins:DsRed)* transgenic fish and increased transcription of the endogenous insulin gene as a result of CRCs treatment of zebrafish larvae. These observations support the hypothesis that the hypoglycemic activity of crocins is at least in part, due to the enhanced insulin production of β-cells.

Pck1 is a key gene in the process of gluconeogenesis. It is often used as an indicator of blood glucose levels since it is normally downregulated in cases of hypoglycemia and upregulated when blood glucose levels are elevated. In our study, lowering the levels of glucose were linked with a slight but significant increase in *pck1* expression. This could be explained as a homeostatic, compensatory response of the zebrafish larvae to the reduced glucose levels induced by CRCs. Nevertheless, glucose production is simultaneously related to stimulated metabolism, an issue that needs to be further investigated taking into account that diabetes patients suffer metabolism complications. The same effect of low glucose levels and overexpression of *pck1* was also in the *Tg(pck1:Luc2, cryaa:mCherry)^{s952}* bioluminescence transgenic zebrafish line [18]. Authors tested several chemical compounds for their capacity to reduce glucose levels and also studied their effect on *pck1* expression. Among the tested compounds PK1195, a translocator protein 18 kDA (TSPO) ligand, induced *pck1* expression simultaneously to a reduction in glucose levels. Authors concluded that compounds that belong to the TPSO family, regardless of their gluconeogenetic effect, can effectively interfere with levels of glucose in zebrafish larvae.

In summary, we employed zebrafish as a tool in order to explore the effect of crocins isolated from *Crocus sativus* L. on glucose metabolism. Our results suggest that the treatment of zebrafish larvae with non-toxic levels of crocins can significantly reduce the basal total glucose levels and increase insulin expression. These data provide some evidence that crocins are implicated in the glucose regulation, but further studies are needed in order to elucidate the exact mechanism of action and its potential as a putative agent on the antidiabetic field.

4. Materials and Methods

4.1. Extraction and Chemical Analysis of Crocins

Stigmas of *Crocus sativus* L. were cultivated at the Kozani prefecture and were kindly offered by the "Cooperative of Saffron producers, Kozani Greece". Stigmas were collected in 2018.

Crocus sativus L. is a male-sterile triploid lineage that ever since its origin has been propagated vegetatively. No wild population has been found so far and all the available plant material comes from cultivation. The crop is an autotriploid that evolved in Attica by combining two different genotypes of *C. cartwrightianus* (a species endemic to Attica and some Aegean islands, Greece) [50]. Triploid sterility and vegetative propagation prevented afterwards segregation of the favorable traits of saffron, resulting in worldwide cultivation of a unique clonal lineage. As a result, no infraspecific taxa have been recognized.

Five grams of dried stigmas were shattered and extracted with petroleum ether in order to remove lipid compounds, in an ultrasonic water bath (GRANT type, 300 × 140 × 150 mm internal dimensions), for 15 min at 25 °C and at the frequency of 35 kHz. The extraction was repeated 5 times and proceeded under the same conditions using diethyl ether. Extraction with petroleum ether and diethyl ether proceed prior to methanol extractions in order to eliminate the final extract from the presence of unwanted compounds such as lipids and safranal. The received powder was dried under nitrogen steam and the final extraction step took place as described above, using methanol. The organic solvent was evaporated in a rotary evaporator and a purified extract of CRCs was received. The final product that consisted of a red colored powder was kept at −4 °C for further analysis.

In order to ensure total evaporation of the organic solvent, an aqueous extract of CRCs was prepared and Raman spectroscopy was performed. No characteristic peaks that correspond to the presence of methanol were observed, indicating that the final product was methanol free.

The analysis of the extract was performed on an HPLC system (Agilent Series 1260-Agilent Technologies, Waldbronn, Germany) coupled to a 6530 Q-TOF mass spectrometer (Agilent Technologies, Singapore). The HPLC system consists of degasser, autosampler, quaternary pump, diode array detector, and a thermostatically controlled column oven. Chromatographic separation was performed at 40 °C on a Poroshell 120 EC-C18 4.6 × 50 mm, 2.7 μm reversed phase column. The following chromatographic conditions were applied: Flow rate 0.4 mL/min, injection volume 5 μL, mobile phase A (water LC/MS-0.1% formic acid), and mobile phase B (acetonitrile LC/MS-0.1% formic acid). The gradient elution program was applied as follows: 5–95% solvent B from 0 to 33 min and maintained at 95% up to 38 min. The sample was detected at 440 nm. The Q-TOF mass spectrometer was operated with a dual ESI source in the negative ionization mode and according to the following operating parameters: Capillary voltage 4000 V, gas temperature 300 °C, skimmer 65 V, octapole RF 750 V, drying gas 10 L/min, nebulizer pressure 450 psig, and fragmentor voltage 150 V. Scanning was performed from 100–1700. The Q-TOF-MS was calibrated on a daily basis using a reference mass solution (calibrant solution, Agilent Technologies) with internal reference masses at m/z 112.9856 and 1033.9881. The data acquisition and qualitative analysis were processed by MassHunter software (Agilent Technologies).

4.2. Determination of LC50

The toxicity of crocins on zebrafish embryos was evaluated according to OECD guidelines (OECD 2013 Toxicity test TG236, 2013). Briefly, fertilized embryos were collected at 3 hpf and treated with an aqueous solution of CRCs extract. A range of concentrations from 0–2 mg/mL was tested. The concentration of 0 mg/mL corresponds to the control group.

During the experiment the test media was not renewed, embryos were kept at 28 °C, and the plate was covered with aluminum foil to protect the crocins from degradation. Embryos were monitored daily up to 96 hpf and scored for lethality Three replicates were performed for each concentration tested. Results were calculated using the probit analysis (IBM SPSS Statistics v23). In order to ensure the stability of the extract, extracts of the same concentration were stored under the same conditions, and their UV-Vis spectra were recorded daily. The extracts remained stable during the experiment (data not shown).

4.3. Zebrafish Maintenance and Breeding

Zebrafish were raised under standard laboratory conditions at 28 °C on a 14/10 h day/night cycle in the animal facility of Biomedical Research Foundation of the Academy of Athens (EL25BIO003). Zebrafish are maintained according to the Recommended Guidelines for Zebrafish Husbandry Conditions [51]. The genetic backgrounds used were the wild-type Ab strain for all toxicity, glucose level quantification and RT-PCR experiments, and the transgenic line *Tg(ins:DsRed)* for visualizing pancreatic β-cells. The experimental protocols described in this study were completed by day 5 of the zebrafish embryo development and therefore, are not subject to the regulations of European animal protection guidelines, in accordance with the European Directive 2010/63 for the protection of animals used for scientific purposes.

4.4. Measurement of Glucose Levels

The measurement of glucose levels was performed on larvae zebrafish using a colorimetric/fluorimetric based enzymatic detection kit (Biovision-K606) and according to Jurczyk et al., 2011 [22]. Zebrafish larvae at 72 hpf were placed in a 12-well plate and treated with the extract of crocins at a concentration of 0.2 mg/mL. Embryos were incubated at 28 °C for 48 h. The treatment was performed in triplicate.

The measurement of glucose was performed according to the protocol provided with slight modifications. Briefly, 20 embryos were placed in eppendorf tubes and the medium was removed. The collected embryos were frozen in liquid nitrogen and were kept at −80 °C for a minimum of 30 min. Then, 80 µL of phosphate-buffered saline (PBS) were added in each tube and embryos were homogenized using a pestle. Tubes were centrifuged and collection of the supernatant took place 8 µL of each sample were added in 42 µL of PBS in a 96-well plate. After that, 50 µL of the reaction mix containing one µL of glucose probe, one µL of glucose enzyme, and 48 µL of glucose buffer were added so as to adjust the final volume at 100 µL. To calculate the results, a standard curve of glucose was constructed (0–3.5 nmol/well). Reactions were incubated at 37 °C for 30 min and absorbance was measured at 570 nm.

4.5. RNA Isolation and cDNA Synthesis

Total RNA extraction from 120 hpf zebrafish larvae was carried out using TRIzol reagent (15596026-Invitrogen) and purification was performed with Turbo DNase (2238G2-Ambion), according to the manufacturers' protocols. The RNA concentration and purity were determined by NanoDrop 2000c Spectrophotometer (Thermo Scientific, Waltham, MA, USA) and cDNA was synthesized using the PrimeScript RT reagent kit (RR037A-Takara).

4.6. Quantitative Real-Time PCR

RT-PCRs were performed with a Roche cycler system (Light Cycler 96) using the KAPA SYBR FAST qPCR kit (KK4611-KAPA Biosystems) and gene-specific primers. The sequences of primers used are the following:

pck1f: TCTCCATCCCTCCGCTCATCA, *pck1r*: GGCCCAGCTGACTGCTCCT, *insaf*: TAAGCAC TAACCCAGGCACA, *insar*: GATTTAGGAGGAAGGAAACC.

As a reference gene, the elongation factor was used with the following primers: *efa1f*: TCTCT ACCTACCCTCCTCTTGGTC and *efa1r*: TTGGTCTTGGCAGCCTTCTGTG. The relative amounts of the different mRNAs were quantified with the ΔΔCt method [52] and the fold-change ratio was calculated and expressed as mean ± SEM.

4.7. Monitoring Pancreas Development

Zebrafish larvae from the transgenic line *Tg(ins:DsRed)* were treated with 0.2 mg/mL of CRCs at 72 hpf. Embryos were incubated at 28 °C for 48 h and subsequently anesthetized using 0.4 mg/mL of Tricaine (BIA 1347-Apollo scientific) in order to proceed to imaging. To facilitate imaging, the embryos were mounted in a 1.2% low melting agarose. Fluorescent and brightfield images were captured using a Leica DMRA2 microscope (Leica, Switzerland) equipped with a HamamatsuORCA-Flash 4.0 V2 camera and analyzed using the Fiji software. Data are presented as mean ± SEM. Differences were analyzed using the two-tailed Student's *t*-test. In addition, p was considered significant when less than 0.05.

Author Contributions: Conceptualization, D.B. and P.A.T.; methodology, D.B. and P.A.T.; formal analysis, E.K. and A.A.; investigation, E.K. and A.A.; data curation, E.K., A.A., and C.K.; writing—original draft preparation, E.K.; writing—review and editing, A.A., C.K., D.B., and P.A.T.; supervision, D.B. and P.A.T. All authors have read and agreed to the published version of the manuscript.

Funding: This research received no external funding.

Conflicts of Interest: The authors declare no conflict of interest.

References

1. Choudhury, H.; Pandey, M.; Hua, C.K.; Mun, C.S.; Jing, J.K.; Kong, L.; Ern, L.Y.; Ashraf, N.A.; Kit, S.W.; Yee, T.S.; et al. An update on natural compounds in the remedy of diabetes mellitus: A systematic review. *J. Tradit. Complement. Med.* **2017**, *8*, 361–376. [CrossRef] [PubMed]
2. Sarikurkcu, C.; Kakouri, E.; Sarikurkcu, T.R.; Tarantilis, P.A. Study on the chemical composition, enzyme inhibition and antioxidant activity of Ziziphora taurica subsp. cleonioides. *Appl. Sci.* **2019**, *9*, 5515. [CrossRef]
3. Prince, P.S.M.; Kannan, N.K. Protective effect of rutin on lipids, lipoproteins, lipid metabolizing enzymes and glycoproteins in streptozotocin-induced diabetic rats. *J. Pharm. Pharmacol.* **2006**, *58*, 1373–1383. [CrossRef]
4. Al-Ishaq, R.K.; Abotaleb, M.; Kubatka, P.; Kajo, K.; Büsselberg, D. Flavonoids and Their Anti-Diabetic Effects: Cellular Mechanisms and Effects to Improve Blood Sugar Levels. *Biomolecules* **2019**, *9*, 430. [CrossRef] [PubMed]
5. Eid, H.M.; Haddad, P.S. The Antidiabetic Potential of Quercetin: Underlying Mechanisms. *Curr. Med. Chem.* **2017**, *24*, 355–364. [CrossRef] [PubMed]
6. Ghorbani, A. Mechanisms of antidiabetic effects of flavonoid rutin. *Biomed. Pharmacother.* **2017**, *96*, 305–312. [CrossRef] [PubMed]
7. Caballero-Ortega, H.; Pereda-Miranda, R.; Riveron-Negrete, L.; Hernandez, J.M.; Medécigo-Ríos, M.; Castillo-Villanueva, A.; Abdullaev, F.I. Chemical composition of saffron (*Crocus sativus* L.) from four countries. *Acta Hortic.* **2004**, *650*, 321–326. [CrossRef]
8. Carmona, M.; Zalacain, A.; Sanchez, A.M.; Novella, J.L.; Alonso, G.L. Crocetin esters, picrocrocin and its related compounds present in *Crocus sativus* stigmas and Gardenia jasminoides fruits. Tentative identification of seven new compounds by LC-ESI-MS. *J. Agric. Food Chem.* **2006**, *54*, 973–979. [CrossRef] [PubMed]
9. Ríos, J.L.; Recio, M.C.; Giner, R.M.; Máñez, S. An Update Review of Saffron and its Active Constituents. *Phytother. Res.* **1996**, *10*, 189–193. [CrossRef]
10. Tarantilis, P.A.; Tsoupras, G.; Polissiou, M. Determination of saffron (*Crocus sativus* L.) components in crude plant extract using high-performance liquid chromatography-UV-visible photodiode-array detection-mass spectrometry. *J. Chromatogr. A* **1995**, *699*, 107–118. [CrossRef]
11. Mohajeri, S.A.; Hosseinzadeh, H.; Keyhanfar, F.; Aghamohammadian, J. Extraction of crocin from saffron (*Crocus sativus*) using molecularly imprinted polymer solid-phase extraction. *J. Sep. Sci.* **2010**, *33*, 2302–2309. [CrossRef] [PubMed]
12. Karkoula, E.; Angelis Koulakiotis, N.S.; Gikas, E.; Halabalaki, M.; Tsarbopoulos, A.; Skaltsounis, A.L. Rapid isolation and characterization of crocins, picrocrocin, and crocetin from saffron using centrifugal partition chromatography and LC-MS. *J. Sep. Sci.* **2018**, *41*, 4105–4114. [CrossRef] [PubMed]

13. Kanakis, C.D.; Daferera, D.J.; Tarantilis, P.A.; Polissiou, M.G. Qualitative determination of volatile compounds and quantitative evaluation of safranal and 4-hydroxy-2,6,6-trimethyl-1-cyclohexene-1-carboxaldehyde (HTCC) in Greek saffron. *J. Agric. Food Chem.* **2004**, *52*, 4515–4521. [CrossRef] [PubMed]
14. Letrado, P.; de Miguel, I.; Lamberto, I.; Díez-Martínez, R.; Oyarzabal, J. Zebrafish: Speeding Up the Cancer Drug Discovery Process. *Cancer Res.* **2018**, *78*, 6048–6058. [CrossRef]
15. Giardoglou, P.; Beis, D. On Zebrafish Disease Models and Matters of the Heart. *Biomedicines* **2019**, *7*, 15. [CrossRef] [PubMed]
16. Bandmann, O.; Burton, A.E. Genetic zebrafish models of neurodegenerative diseases. *Neurobiol. Dis.* **2010**, *40*, 58–65. [CrossRef] [PubMed]
17. Zang, L.; Maddison, L.A.; Chen, W. Zebrafish as a Model for Obesity and Diabetes. *Front. Cell Dev. Biol.* **2018**, *6*, 91. [CrossRef]
18. Gut, P.; Baeza-Raja, B.; Andersson, O.; Hasenkamp, L.; Hsiao, J.; Hesselson, D.; Akassoglou, K.; Verdin, E.; Hirschey, M.D.; Stainier, Y.R.D. Whole-organism screening for gluconeogenesis identifies activators of fasting metabolism. *Nat. Chem. Biol.* **2012**, *9*, 97–104. [CrossRef]
19. Wiley, D.S.; Redfield, S.E.; Zon, L.I. Chemical screening in zebrafish for novel biological and therapeutic discovery. *Methods Cell Biol.* **2017**, *138*, 651–679. [CrossRef]
20. Papakyriakou, A.; Kefalos, P.; Sarantis, P.; Tsiamantas, C.; Xanthopoulos, K.P.; Vourloumis, D.; Beis, D. A zebrafish in vivo phenotypic assay to identify 3-aminothiophene-2-carboxylic acid-based angiogenesis inhibitors. *Assay Drug Dev. Technol.* **2014**, *12*, 527–535. [CrossRef]
21. Agalou, A.; Thrapsianiotis, M.; Angelis, A.; Papakyriakou, A.; Skaltsounis, A.L.; Aligiannis, N.; Beis, D. Identification of Novel Melanin Synthesis Inhibitors from Crataegus pycnoloba Using an in Vivo Zebrafish Phenotypic Assay. *Front. Pharmacol.* **2018**, *9*, 265. [CrossRef] [PubMed]
22. Jurczyk, A.; Roy, N.; Bajwa, R.; Gut, P.; Lipson, K.; Yang, C.; Covassin, L.; Racki, W.J.; Rossini, A.A.; Phillips, N.; et al. Dynamic glucoregulation and mammalian-like responses to metabolic and developmental disruption in zebrafish. *Gen. Comp. Endocrinol.* **2011**, *170*, 334–345. [CrossRef] [PubMed]
23. Curado, S.; Anderson, R.M.; Jungblut, B.; Mumm, J.; Schroeter, E.; Stainier, D.Y. Conditional targeted cell ablation in zebrafish: A new tool for regeneration studies. *Dev. Dyn.* **2007**, *236*, 1025–1035. [CrossRef] [PubMed]
24. Anderson, R.M.; Bosch, J.A.; Goll, M.G.; Hesselson, D.; Dong, P.D.; Shin, D.; Chi, N.C.; Shin, C.H.; Schlegel, A.; Halpern, M.; et al. Loss of Dnmt1 catalytic activity reveals multiple roles for DNA methylation during pancreas development and regeneration. *Dev. Biol.* **2009**, *334*, 213–223. [CrossRef]
25. Elo, B.; Villano, C.M.; Govorko, D.; White, L.A. Larval zebrafish as a model for glucose metabolism: Expression of phosphoenolpyruvate carboxykinase as a marker for exposure to anti-diabetic compounds. *J. Mol. Endocrinol.* **2007**, *38*, 433–440. [CrossRef]
26. Seth, A.; Stemple, D.L.; Barroso, I. The emerging use of zebrafish to model metabolic disease. *Dis. Model Mech.* **2013**, *6*, 1080–1088. [CrossRef]
27. OECD (2013). Test No. 236: Fish Embryo Acute Toxicity (FET) Test, OECD Guidelines for the Testing of Chemicals, Section 2. Home Page. Available online: https://www.oecd-ilibrary.org/environment/test-no-236-fish-embryo-acute-toxicity-fet-test_9789264203709-en (accessed on 14 June 2020).
28. Papasani, M.R.; Robison, B.D.; Hardy, R.W.; Hill, R.A. Early developmental expression of two insulins in zebrafish (Danio rerio). *Physiol. Genom.* **2006**, *27*, 79–85. [CrossRef]
29. Irwin, D.M. Duplication and diversification of insulin genes in ray-finned fish. *Zool. Res.* **2019**, *40*, 185–197. [CrossRef]
30. Koren, D.; Palladino, A. *Hypoglycemia, in Genetic Diagnosis of Endocrine Disorders*, 2nd ed.; Roy, E., Samuel Refetoff, W., Eds.; Academic Press: Cambridge, MA, USA, 2016; pp. 31–75.
31. Hatziagapiou, K.; Kakouri, E.; Lambrou, G.I.; Bethanis, K.; Tarantilis, P.A. Antioxidant Properties of *Crocus sativus* L. and Its Constituents and Relevance to Neurodegenerative Diseases; Focus on Alzheimer's and Parkinson's Disease. *Curr. Neuropharmacol.* **2019**, *17*, 377–402. [CrossRef]
32. Azimi, P.; Ghiasvand, R.; Feizi, A.; Hosseinzadeh, J.; Bahreynian, M.; Hariri, M.; Khosravi-Boroujeni, H. Effect of cinnamon, cardamom, saffron and ginger consumption on blood pressure and a marker of endothelial function in patients with type 2 diabetes mellitus: A randomized controlled clinical trial. *Blood Press* **2016**, *25*, 133–140. [CrossRef]

33. Pitsikas, N.; Tarantilis, P.A. Effects of the active constituents of *Crocus sativus* L. crocins and their combination with memantine on recognition memory in rats. *Behav. Pharmacol.* **2018**, *29*, 400–412. [CrossRef] [PubMed]
34. Ayatollahi, H.; Javan, A.O.; Khajedaluee, M.; Shahroodian, M.; Hosseinzadeh, H. Effect of *Crocus sativus* L. (saffron) on coagulation and anticoagulation systems in healthy volunteers. *Phytother. Res.* **2014**, *28*, 539–543. [CrossRef] [PubMed]
35. Mohajeri, D.; Mousavi, G.; Mesgari, M.; Doustar, Y.; Nouri, M.H.K. Subacute Toxicity of *Crocus sativus* L. (Saffron) Stigma Ethanolic Extract in Rats. *Am. J. Pharmacol. Toxicol.* **2007**, *2*, 189–193. [CrossRef]
36. Hosseinzadeh, H.; Sadeghi Shakib, S.; Khadem Sameni, A.; Taghiabadi, E. Acute and subacute toxicity of safranal, a constituent of saffron, in mice and rats. *Iran. J. Pharm. Res. IJPR* **2013**, *12*, 93–99. [CrossRef]
37. Mehri, S.; Razavi, B.M.; Hosseinzadeh, H. *Safety and Toxicity of Saffron, in Saffron*; Woodhead Publishing: Cambridge, UK, 2020; pp. 517–530. [CrossRef]
38. United States Environmental Protection Agency, Chemical Hazard Classification and Labeling: Comparison of OPP Requirements and the GHS: Draft. 2004. Available online: https://www.epa.gov/sites/production/files/2015-09/documents/ghscriteria-summary.pdf (accessed on 30 October 2020).
39. Kianbakht, S.; Hajiaghaee, R. Anti-hyperglycemic Effects of Saffron and its Active Constituents, Crocin and Safranal, in Alloxan-Induced Diabetic Rats. *J. Med. Plants.* **2011**, *3*, 82–89.
40. Kang, C.; Lee, H.; Jung, E.S.; Seyedian, R.; Jo, M.; Kim, J.; Kim, J.S.; Kim, E. Saffron (*Crocus sativus* L.) increases glucose uptake and insulin sensitivity in muscle cells via multipathway mechanisms. *Food Chem.* **2012**, *135*, 2350–2358. [CrossRef]
41. Dehghan, F.; Hajiaghaalipour, F.; Yusof, A.; Muniandy, S.; Hosseini, S.A.; Heydari, S.; Salim, L.Z.; Azarbayjani, M.A. Saffron with resistance exercise improves diabetic parameters through the GLUT4/AMPK pathway in-vitro and in-vivo. *Sci. Rep.* **2016**, *6*, 25139. [CrossRef]
42. Milajerdi, A.; Jazayeri, S.; Hashemzadeh, N.; Shirzadi, E.; Derakhshan, Z.; Djazayeri, A.; Akhondzadeh, S. The effect of saffron (*Crocus sativus* L.) hydroalcoholic extract on metabolic control in type 2 diabetes mellitus: A triple-blinded randomized clinical trial. *J. Res. Med. Sci.* **2018**, *20*, 23. [CrossRef]
43. Karimi-Nazari, E.; Nadjarzadeh, A.; Masoumi, R.; Marzban, A.; Mohajeri, S.A.; Ramezani-Jolfaie, N.; Salehi-Abargouei, A. Effect of saffron (*Crocus sativus* L.) on lipid profile, glycemic indices and antioxidant status among overweight/obese prediabetic individuals: A double-blinded, randomized controlled trial. *Clin. Nutr. ESPEN* **2019**, *34*, 130–136. [CrossRef]
44. Moravej Aleali, A.; Amani, R.; Shahbazian, H.; Namjooyan, F.; Latifi, S.M.; Cheraghian, B. The effect of hydroalcoholic Saffron (*Crocus sativus* L.) extract on fasting plasma glucose, HbA1c, lipid profile, liver, and renal function tests in patients with type 2 diabetes mellitus: A randomized double-blind clinical trial. *Phytother. Res.* **2019**, *33*, 1648–1657. [CrossRef]
45. Rajaei, Z.; Hadjzadeh, M.A.; Nemati, H.; Hosseini, M.; Ahmadi, M.; Shafiee, S. Antihyperglycemic and antioxidant activity of crocin in streptozotocin-induced diabetic rats. *J. Med. Food* **2013**, *16*, 206–210. [CrossRef] [PubMed]
46. Yaribeygi, H.; Mohammadi, M.T.; Sahebkar, A. Crocin potentiates antioxidant defense system and improves oxidative damage in liver tissue in diabetic rats. *Biomed. Pharmacother.* **2018**, *98*, 333–337. [CrossRef] [PubMed]
47. Shirali, S.; Zahra Bathaie, S.; Nakhjavani, M. Effect of crocin on the insulin resistance and lipid profile of streptozotocin-induced diabetic rats. *Phytother. Res.* **2013**, *27*, 1042–1047. [CrossRef]
48. Razavi, B.M.; Hosseinzadeh, H. Saffron: A promising natural medicine in the treatment of metabolic syndrome. *J. Sci. Food Agric.* **2017**, *97*, 1679–1685. [CrossRef] [PubMed]
49. Farkhondeh, T.; Samarghandian, S. The effect of saffron (*Crocus sativus* L.) and its ingredients on the management of diabetes mellitus and dislipidemia. *Afr. J. Pharm. Pharmacol.* **2014**, *8*, 541–549. [CrossRef]
50. Nemati, Z.; Harpke, D.; Gemicioglu, A.; Kerndorff, H.; Blattner, F.R. Saffron (*Crocus sativus*) is an autotriploid that evolved in Attica (Greece) from wild Crocus cartwrightianus. *Mol. Phylogenet. Evol.* **2019**, *136*, 14–20. [CrossRef]

51. Aleström, P.; D'Angelo, L.; Midtlyng, P.J.; Schorderet, D.F.; Schulte-Merker, S.; Sohm, F.; Warner, S. Zebrafish: Housing and husbandry recommendations. *Lab. Anim.* **2020**, *54*, 213–224. [CrossRef]
52. Livak, K.J.; Schmittgen, T.D. Analysis of relative gene expression data using real-time quantitative PCR and the 2(-Delta Delta C(T)) Method. *Methods* **2001**, *25*, 402–408. [CrossRef]

Sample Availability: Samples of the CRCs is available from the authors.

Publisher's Note: MDPI stays neutral with regard to jurisdictional claims in published maps and institutional affiliations.

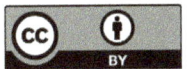 © 2020 by the authors. Licensee MDPI, Basel, Switzerland. This article is an open access article distributed under the terms and conditions of the Creative Commons Attribution (CC BY) license (http://creativecommons.org/licenses/by/4.0/).

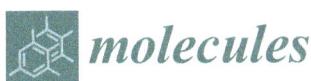

Review

Recent Advances on the Anticancer Properties of Saffron (*Crocus sativus* L.) and Its Major Constituents

Andromachi Lambrianidou, Fani Koutsougianni [†], Irida Papapostolou [†] and Konstantinos Dimas *

Department of Pharmacology, Faculty of Medicine, University of Thessaly, 41500 Larissa, Greece; mahilabrianidou@hotmail.com (A.L.); koutsfan@gmail.com (F.K.); papapostolou.iris@gmail.com (I.P.)
* Correspondence: kdimas@uth.gr
† These authors contributed equally to this work.

Abstract: Cancer is the second leading cause of death globally with an estimated 9.6 million deaths in 2018 and a sustained rise in its incidence in both developing and developed countries. According to the WHO, about 1 in 6 deaths is due to cancer. Despite the emergence of many pioneer therapeutic options for patients with cancer, their efficacy is still time-limited and noncurative. Thus, continuous intensive screening for superior and safer drugs is still ongoing and has resulted in the detection of the anticancer properties of several phytochemicals. Among the spices, *Crocus sativus* L. (saffron) and its main constituents, crocin, crocetin, and safranal, have attracted the interest of the scientific community. Pharmacological experiments have established numerous beneficial properties for this brilliant reddish-orange dye derived from the flowers of a humble crocus family species. Studies in cultured human malignant cell lines and animal models have demonstrated the cancer prevention and antitumor activities of saffron and its main ingredients. This review provides an insight into the advances in research on the anticancer properties of saffron and its components, discussing preclinical data, clinical trials, and patents aiming to improve the pharmacological properties of saffron and its major ingredients.

Keywords: *Crocus sativus*; saffron; cancer; anticancer activity; chemoprevention; clinical trials; patents

1. Introduction

Saffron, a plant product derived from the dried stigma of the *Crocus sativus* flower, is proposed to have useful biological properties [1]. Intensive research is ongoing on the importance of the health properties of saffron in its natural form [2], but a lot of interest has also been focused on the extraction, purification, and study of saffron's major bioactive constituents, including crocin, crocetin, picrocrocin, and safranal (Figure 1).

These phytochemicals have been reported to show beneficial effects against numerous diseases, such as diabetes [3], neurodegenerative diseases [4], cognitive problems [4], depression [5], inflammatory diseases [6], autoimmune diseases [7], digestive diseases [8], and cardiovascular inflammations [9]. The potential activity of saffron and its ingredients against cancer has been investigated as well and the results show saffron's potent anticancer activity in preclinical settings [10], importantly without adverse effects on normal cells [11,12]. Despite the intensive research, many details on the mechanism(s) of action of saffron and its components against the progression of cancer are still unknown. It seems that saffron and its major ingredients may have a pleiotropic mechanism of action against malignant cells. There are a plethora of studies that have analyzed the effect and the action mechanism of the different ingredients of saffron extract and how their action could be optimized [13,14]; of great interest is also the fact that saffron's major ingredients may act synergistically against malignant cells [15], suggesting that saffron extract may be more effective than its components alone. We need to note though that apart from the unique compounds that can be found only in saffron extracts, as already mentioned above, saffron possesses a plethora of other bioactive compounds, such as kaempferol and its glycosides, other flavonols such as quercetin, etc. [16].

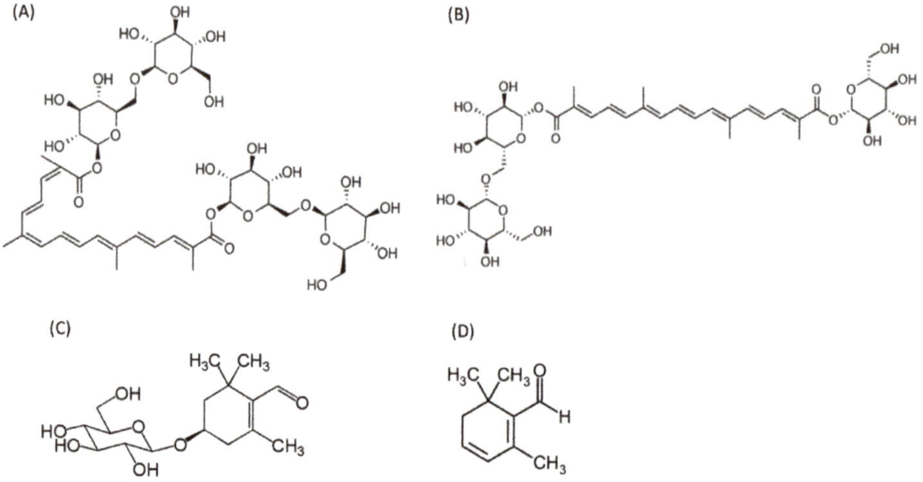

Figure 1. The chemical structure of the four major unique saffron ingredients. (**A**) Crocin and (**B**) crocetin are both are water-soluble carotenoid chemical compounds. (**C**) Picrocrocin is a monoterpene glycoside precursor of safranal (**D**).

In this review, we present and discuss from a critical point of view the most recent advances from the last five years on the anticancer properties of saffron extract and its major unique ingredients crocin, crocetin, picrocrocin, and safranal. We also discuss some critical issues that need to be urgently and properly addressed, such as harvesting and extraction conditions, storage parameters, and extract analyses, to safely and beyond any doubt come to a conclusion about the usefulness of this extract that has been a versatile medicine for the last 3500 years.

2. Anticancer Properties of Saffron and Its Major Ingredients

2.1. Effects of Saffron towards Preventing Carcinogenesis

Researchers put a great deal of effort into finding molecules that can delay carcinogenesis at the earliest possible stages of its development or even reverse cancer growth. In this context, it has been reported that saffron extract prevents tumor formation at an initial stage. In a recent study performed on hamsters that were treated with the carcinogen 7,12-dimethylbenz[a]anthracene (DMBA), oral administration of saffron at a dose of 100 mg/kg b.w./day, one week before the exposure to the carcinogen, completely prevented the formation of oral squamous cell carcinomas [17]. Similarly, the ingestion of 200 mg/kg b.w./day saffron by mice that received three topical applications of 100 nmol DMBA in 100 mL acetone delayed the onset of skin papilloma formation [18].

2.2. Saffron and Its Components as Anticancer Agents

In vitro and in vivo studies have demonstrated significant antitumor properties of saffron and its compounds. However, research is still ongoing to address questions about the particular mechanism of action of each saffron component against malignancies. The antitumor activity is mainly attributed to (i) inhibition of synthesis of DNA and RNA, (ii) inhibition or suppression of cancer cells proliferation, (iii) apoptosis, (iv) inhibition of metastasis and angiogenesis, and (v) changes in the expression pattern of oncogenes or tumor-suppressive genes (Table 1).

Table 1. Major studies on the anticancer effects of saffron extract and its major ingredients in cell lines and animal models of cancer.

Bioactive Compound	Cell Line/Animal Model	Suggested Mechanism of Action/Outcome	References
Saffron ethanol extract	Breast cancer cells MCF-7	Caspase activation, upregulation of Bax expression. Apoptosis.	Mousavi et al., 2009
		Downregulation of VEGFR expression. Cell proliferation and angiogenesis inhibition	Mousavi and Baharara, 2014
Safranal, crocin	Myelogenous leukemia cells K-562	Downregulation of Bcr-Abl expression	Geromichalos et al., 2014
Safranal, crocetin, crocin	Breast cancer cells MCF-7, MDA-MB 231	Cell proliferation inhibition	Chryssanthi et al., 2007
Crocetin	Breast cancer cells MCF-7, MDA-MB 231	Downregulation of metalloproteases expression. Cell invasion inhibition, apoptosis	Paper et al., 2000
Crocetin	Colon cancer cells SW480	Arrest of cells in the S phase, upregulation of P21 expression. Cell proliferation inhibition	Li et al., 2012
Crocetin	Leukemia cells HL60, K-562, L1210, NB4, P388	Activation of the intrinsic apoptotic pathway	Moradzadeh et al., 2019
Crocetin, crocin	Lung adenocarcinoma cells A549, SPC-A1	Upregulation of the p53 and Bax mRNA levels; downregulation of the f Bcl-2 mRNA levels. Apoptosis	Chen et al., 2015
Crocin	Breast cancer cells MCF-7	Caspase-8,9 and 3 activation, Bax/Bcl-2 ratio increase, mitochondrial membrane potential disruption, cytochrome c release. Cell proliferation inhibition, apoptosis	Lu et al., 2015; Bakshi et al., 2016; Mostafavinia et al., 2016
Crocin	Breast cancer cells HCC70, HCC1806	Microtubules depolymerization. Cell proliferation inhibition	Hire et al., 2017
Crocin	Ovarian cancer HO-8910 cells	Arrest of cells in the G0/G1, upregulation of p53, Fas/APO-1, and Caspase-3 expression. Apoptosis	Xia et al., 2015
Crocin	Gastric cancer cells AGS	p53 dependent and independent mechanisms. Apoptosis	Hoshyar et al., 2017
Crocin	Colorectal cancer cells HCT-116, SW-480, HT-29	p53 dependent action. Cell proliferation inhibition	Aung et al., 2007
Crocin	Colorectal cancer HCT116	p53 dependent action, arrest of cells in the G0/G1, down-regulation of Beclin 1, and Atg7 expression. Apoptosis	Amin et al., 2015
Crocin	Gastric cancer cells AGS, HGC-27	Downregulation of Krüppel-like factor 5 (KLF5) and hypoxia-inducible factor-1α (HIF-1α) expression. Cell proliferation inhibition	Zhou et al., 2019
Crocin	Gastric cancer cells AGS	Downregulation of OCT4, KLF, SOX2, NANOG, and Nucleostemin expression. Apoptosis	Akbarpoor et al., 2020
Crocin	Prostate cancer cells BPH-1, LnCaP, 22rv1, CWR22, PC3, and DU145, LAPC-4, C4–2B	Arrest of cells at the G0/G1, activation of the intrinsic apoptotic pathway	D'Alessandro et al., 2013
Saffron aqueous extract	4T1 cells were xenografted in mice	Changes in p53 expression. Inhibition of tumor progression	Nezamdoost et al., 2020
Crocin	Administration of N-Nitroso-N-Methyluria to female Wistar albino rats	Downregulation of cyclin D1 and p21 expression. Inhibition of tumor progression, apoptosis.	Ashrafi et al., 2015
Crocin	4T1 breast cancer cells were xenografted in mice	Controlling metastasis via Wnt/β-catenin pathway. Inhibition of tumor progression, antimetastatic effect	Arzi et al., 2018
Crocin	T24 cells xenografted in BALB/c nude mice	Downregulation of Survivin, Cyclin D1 and upregulation of the Bax/Bcl-2 ratio. Apoptosis	Zhao et al., 2008
Crocin	Azoxymethane and dextran sodium sulfate to induce chemical colitis associated with colorectal cancer in mice	Inhibition of tumor progression	Amerizadeh et al., 2018
Crocin	Adenomatous polyposis. ApcMin/+ mice: models for human familial adenomatous polyposis	Decrease in the number of intestinal polyps	Fujimoto et al., 2019
Crocin, crocetin	Prostate cancer cells PC3 and 22rv1 xenografted in male nude mice	Downregulation of N-cadherin and b-catenin expression, upregulation of E-cadherin expression. Inhibition of tumor progression, cell invasion and migration	Festuccia et al., 2014

2.3. Anticancer Activity of Saffron and Its Mmajor Ingredients

2.3.1. Breast Cancer

Mousavi et al. reported that saffron ethanol extract decreased MCF-7 cell viability with an IC50 of 400 ± 18.5 µg/mL after 48 h and induced apoptosis through caspase activation and Bax increment [19]. Mousavi and Baharara's analysis showed the inhibitory effect of saffron aqueous extract on the expression of two biomarkers of angiogenesis, VEGF-A and VEGFR-2, in the MCF-7 cell line [20].

It has also been demonstrated that crocin can significantly inhibit the proliferation of MCF-7 cells, and kill cells by inducing their apoptotic cell death through mitochondrial signaling pathways activating caspase-8,9 and 3, upregulating Bax expression and conversely downregulating Bcl-2 expression, disrupting the mitochondrial membrane potential (MMP), and releasing the cytochrome c [21–23]. It has also been reported that crocin shows antiproliferative activity on human breast cancer cells, such as HCC70 and HCC1806, through depolymerization of spindle microtubules and production of multipolar spindles resulting in chromosomes misalignment, also inhibiting the progression of mitosis. Further studies showed that vinblastine inhibits the binding of crocin on tubulin, which indicates that crocin has the same binding site as vinblastine [24]. It is important to note that crocin did not affect normal cells that were used as controls in the experiments [24].

Saffron constituents, i.e., *trans*-crocin-4, crocetin, and safranal, were also found to significantly inhibit the proliferation of MCF-7 and MDA-MB231 cells [25]. Crocetin inhibited the proliferation of MDA-MB231 cancer cells similarly to *trans*-crocin-4. They inhibited the proliferation of both cell lines at concentrations higher than 200 µM. Safranal inhibited the proliferation of MDA-MB231 at concentrations higher than 125 µM and the proliferation of MCF-7 at concentrations higher than 500 µM. The MCF-7 cells that were treated with crocetin showed apoptotic DNA fragmentation in electrophoresis. Crocetin was additionally reported to inhibit invasiveness by reducing the matrix metalloproteases expression [26].

Nezamdoost et al. [6] tested the effect of the aqueous extract of saffron in combination with high-intensity training in female BALB/C mice bearing 4T1 cells, a mouse breast tumor model. This study was based on the idea that training in combination with some herbal components could have an anticancer function. Oral administration of saffron extract in combination with the training indeed suppressed the tumor growth resulting in a lower growth rate of the tumors in this animal group as compared to the tumors of the animals that received only the saffron extract. However, the mechanisms that mediated this delay in tumor growth remain still elusive.

Ashrafi et al. administered N-Nitroso-N-Methyluria to female Wistar albino rats, a highly carcinogenic, mutagenic, and teratogenic agent, to induce breast cancer in rats and further studied the anticancer properties of crocin [27]. They showed that crocin led to tumor growth suppression and induced apoptosis and cell cycle arrest by downregulating cyclin D1 and p21 through the p53 pathway.

Arzin and his colleagues suggested crocin as a promoting complementary antimetastatic herbal medicine for the treatment of triple-negative breast cancer. In their study, 4T1 cells were xenografted to female BALB/c mice and 200 mg/kg of crocin injected in mice thrice a week. Crocin led to tumor growth suppression with no signs of metastasis in the liver and lung of the treated animal group as opposed to the animals in the control group. Crocin was additionally found to exhibit its antimetastatic effects by regulating the Wnt/β-catenin pathway [28].

2.3.2. Ovarian Cancer

Xia et al. tested the effect of crocin in the human ovarian cancer cell line HO-8910. Crocin significantly inhibited the growth rate of the cells [29]. Also, crocin raised the proportion of HO-8910 cells in the G0/G1 phase and increased the apoptosis rate. Crocin treatment was also found to increase p53 and Fas/APO-1 expression which subsequently led to the activation of the apoptotic pathway via caspase 3 activation [29].

2.3.3. Gastrointestinal Cancer

Gastrointestinal cancer is amongst the most studied cancers with regard to the potential anticancer activity of saffron and its ingredients [30–37]. Studies have shown that crocin can induce apoptotic cell death in colorectal cancer cells through p53 dependent and independent mechanisms [30].

The anticancer effect of crocin on three human colorectal cancer cells (HCT-116, SW-480, and HT-29) has been recently reported. Crocin reduced the rate of cell proliferation but HCT-116 showed higher sensitivity to crocin than the other two cell lines. The data indicate that the sensitivity of HCT-116 to crocin is due to the wild-type p53. SW-480 and HT-29 cells have a mutant p53 tumor suppressor gene, which suggests that the anticancer activity of crocin may be linked to p53 expression [31].

Amin et al. reported data supporting the notion that crocin initiates apoptosis in HCT 116 p53 mutant cells by damaging the DNA and thus that crocin can be used for sensitizing cancer cells for other chemotherapeutic agents [32]. Crocin could lead to a G0/G1 cell cycle arrest in HCT116 wild-type cells, functioning thus as a cytostatic agent. However, in HCT116 p53 mutant cells crocin led to a G2/M cell cycle arrest and apoptosis after 48-h incubation. Also, the treatment of wild-type HCT116 cells and HCT116 p53 mutant cells with crocin and Bafilomycin A1, a lysosome and autophagosome infusion inhibitor, showed that crocin leads to programmed cell death through apoptosis, independent of autophagy [32].

Crocin was further found to be associated with reduced expression of Krüppel-like factor 5 (KLF5) and hypoxia-inducible factor-1α (HIF-1α), two important transcription factors for the development of gastric cancer, following administration in human gastric cancer cell lines AGS and HGC-27 cells [33]. Crocin also inhibited the migration, invasion, and epithelial-to-mesenchymal transition (EMT) of gastric cancer cells. Other studies support the finding that crocin can lead to an increase of the Bax/Bcl-2 ratio, activation of caspases, and also the reduction of the expression of genes such as OTC4, SOX2, NANOG, KLF4, and NUCLEOSTEMIN in AGS cells. These genes are known to regulate the cell cycle and self-regeneration in stem cells [34].

Crocetin is also reported to inhibit the proliferation of SW480 cells in a concentration-dependent manner. Crocetin induced S-phase arrest through p53-independent mechanisms accompanied by P21 induction [35].

Amerizadeh et al. injected azoxymethane in C57BL/6 mice and administered dextran sodium sulfate to induce chemical colitis— as a model associated with cancer, and to evaluate the activity of orally administered crocin, 5-FU, and their combination. Crocin indeed decreased colorectal cancer growth in an animal model but was inferior to the 5-FU. Interestingly, the arrest of tumor growth was much higher in the combination group [36].

Fujimoto et al. administered saffron extract to adenomatous polyposis coli (APC)$^{Min/+}$ Mice (APC$^{Min/+}$) [37]. APC$^{Min/+}$ (C57BL/6J) mice are models for human familial adenomatous polyposis and human colon cancer. Mice were given food mixed with the saffron extract. The saffron extract (10 mg) was prepared in MeOH (10 mg/mL). In this study, it was found that saffron reduced the number of polyps in the area located next to the big intestine. This was also the area that seemed to have the highest sensitivity to the saffron extract. It is important to note that in this study the researchers administrated specific amounts of the saffron extract to the mice so that it could resemble daily intake dosage [15].

2.3.4. Prostate

In vitro experiments in prostate human carcinoma cells LnCaP, 22rv1, CWR22, PC3, and DU145 evaluated the antitumor activity of saffron aqueous extract and crocin. Both saffron extract and crocin reduced cell proliferation in all malignant cell lines tested in a time- and concentration-dependent manner, with IC50 values ranging between 0.4 and 4 mg/mL and 0.26 and 0.95 mg/mL, respectively [12].

Festuccia et al. xenografted PC3 and 22rv1 cells to investigate the antitumor effect of aqueous extract of saffron, crocin, and crocetin orally administered [38]. Crocetin was more effective in delaying tumor growth in comparison to saffron extract and crocin. The comparative effect of treatment with extract versus crocin in terms of tumor growth did not reach statistical significance. Immunohistochemistry analyses showed that crocetin and crocin led to a reduction of epithelial–mesenchymal transdifferentiation markers, such as vimentin, N-cadherin, and β-catenin, and to an increase of cell–cell adhesion markers, such as E-cadherin, in a time-dependent manner. Additionally, crocetin, crocin, and saffron extract inhibited malignant cell invasion and migration through the downmodulation of metalloproteinases MMP-9 and MMP-2.

2.3.5. Lung Cancer

Chen et al. compared the effect of crocin against the human lung cancer cell lines A549 and SPC-A1 [39]. Crocin inhibited cell proliferation and induced apoptosis in a concentration-dependent manner, accompanied by an increase of G0/G1 arrest. Crocin increased the mRNA levels of p53 and B-cell lymphoma 2-associated X protein (Bax), while it decreased B-cell lymphoma 2 (Bcl-2) mRNA expressions. Besides, crocin combined with cisplatin or pemetrexed had a stronger inhibitory effect than the single agent [39]. Thus, these results indicate that crocin could be used in combination with these chemotherapeutic agents for the treatment of lung cancer.

2.3.6. Leukemia

In vitro studies have been conducted to evaluate the effect of crocetin upon the growth of various leukemia cancer cell lines such as HL60, K-562, L1210, NB4, and P388, showing that crocetin has a cytotoxic effect [40]. Moradzadeh et al. investigated the apoptogenic potential of crocin and its underlying mechanism in acute human leukemia HL-60 cells versus normal human polymorph nuclear (PMN) cells [41]. The results showed that crocin decreased cell viability and increased sub-G1 cell population in HL-60 cells, in a concentration-dependent manner, without significant toxicity toward normal PMN cells. Also, the expression of the caspase 3,9 and Bax/Bcl-2 ratio was significantly increased in HL-60 cells, while caspase 8 remained unchanged. It was suggested that crocin promoted apoptosis through the induction of the intrinsic pathway. The researchers studied the effect of crocin on these cells in comparison with ATRA (all-*trans*-retinoic acid), an anticancer chemotherapy drug, and arsenic trioxide (As_2O_3), which have therapeutic effect on leukemia. The toxicity of ATRA and As_2O_3 remains an important limitation for its use at high therapeutical doses. So crocin may be utilized as an appropriate alternative drug against leukemia [40].

In a different study, Geromichalos et al. conducted in silico and in vitro experiments with imatinib, safranal, and crocin to study the anticancer effects of safranal and crocin in K-562 human chronic myelogenous leukemia (CML) cells [42]. Interestingly in silico studies indicated that crocin and safranal inhibit the Bcr-Abl gene expression and protein activity. Studies revealed that safranal can be attached to the Bcr-Abl protein, at the same place as the imatinib mesylate, the drug used in the treatment of CML. In vitro studies regarding the expression of the Bcr-Abl gene revealed that safranal inhibited the expression of the gene but to a lesser degree as compared to imatinib. Crocin, on the other hand, led to an increase of expression of the Bcr-Abl oncogene but also interacted with the Bcr-Abl protein and thus showed a toxic effect, through a different signal transduction pathway.

2.4. Use of Saffron Ingredients as Adjuvants to Chemotherapeutic Drugs

Apart from radiotherapy, chemotherapy, immunotherapy and surgery [43], scientists are also looking for alternative approaches to treat cancer and to improve the life quality of patients. Saffron's compounds are reported to be a safe and effective treatment to reduce the toxic side effects of some conventional chemotherapeutic drugs such as tamoxifen [44], cisplatin [45], and doxorubicin [46]. Also, besides the protective features mentioned above, several studies have highlighted that the combined treatment of saffron extracts with chemotherapeutic drugs had synergistic effects, enhancing the outcome of the applied treatment. A synergistic antiproliferative and apoptotic effect of crocin and cisplatin has been reported on human osteosarcoma and lung cancer cells, for example [45]. Pretreatment with saffron significantly inhibited the induction of DNA damage (strand breaks) by antitumor drugs, like cisplatin, cyclophosphamide, and mitomycin-C, and protected against the genotoxicity of these antitumor drugs in normal cells [47].

2.5. The Achilles' Heel: Bioavailability of Crocus sativus Active Compounds

The active compounds of *Crocus sativus* are considered to be quite beneficial for human health through their antidepressive, antioxidant, anticancer and antitumor effects, etc. [48]. However, all these compounds share major drawbacks, namely their lipophilic character and poor bioavailability. To start with, the effects of these bioactive constituents are related to the dose that is bioavailable and not to the dose that is ingested. Thus, bioavailability is crucial for the bioefficacy of the available drug [49].

In light of this, researchers put effort into improving the unfavorable features of the basic bioactive compounds of saffron, as they are characterized by their low bioavailability, stability, and absorption [50]. Better knowledge of the bioavailability of these ingredients could result in a more successful use against malignancies. There has indeed been an effort to increase the bioefficacy of the bioactive ingredients of saffron by advancing and implementing new drug delivery system methods [51,52].

Nanoparticles: this category can be divided into four subcategories due to the different kinds of carriers that have been used. There are polymeric, lipidic, inorganic, and selenium nanoparticles. At first, polymeric nanoparticles were used as encapsulating agents. The bioavailability, water solubility, stability, and targeted delivery of the encapsulated natural compounds were improved due to the small size of nanoparticles [53]. Rahaiee et al. showed enhanced crocin stability with biopolymers compared to the standard crocin [52]. Lamgroodi et al studied in MCF7 cells the effect of PLGA (poly . . . glycolide) upon delivering doxorubicn alone or co-delivering doxorubicin and crocetin. Co-delivey of doxorubicin and crocetin in PLGA nanoparticles resluted to higher cytotoxicity compared to other formulations or the free form of doxorubicin or crocetin [54]. Moreover, the bioavailability of crocin was demonstrated to be higher when it was encapsulated in chitosan-alginate nanoparticles [55].

Another form of lipid carriers, liposomes, have been used to improve the pharmacokinetic properties of saffron-derived phytochemicals. Liposomes have the benefit of being non-toxic, overcoming the poorly water-solubility limitations of the drugs and stabilizing them [56]. In 2011, Mousavi et al. showed that liposomal encapsulation of crocin enhanced the apoptogenic effects on MCF-7 and HeLa cells [57].

Another significant category of nanoparticles that have been used to improve saffron's bioactive efficacy are inorganic nanoparticles. Inorganic nanoparticles are non-toxic, hydrophilic, biocompatible, and highly stable particles compared to organic materials. Hoshyar et al. used crocin for the synthesis of gold nanoparticles (AuNPs). Spherical, stable, and uniform AuNPs were synthesized and used to prepare crocin-AuNPs. The data demonstrated that the proliferation rate of breast cancer cells was reduced by crocin-AuNPs compared to crocin alone [58]. Interestingly, silver nanoparticles (AgNPs) are a promising saffron carrier [59].

Finally, selenium nanoparticles have been studied with regard to their capacity to carry anticancer drugs [60]. Thottumugathu et al. tried using poly(ethylene glycol)-PEG selenium nanoparticles (SeNPs) to carry crocin as a drug delivery system. In vitro studies with A549 human lung cancer cells showed that PEG-SeNPs may be promising carriers for crocin, improving its antitumor activity.

Nanostructured lipid dispersions (NLDs): nanostructured lipid dispersions retain crocin's beneficial activity and control the release of the drug directly to the target. Specifically, NLDs can protect the crocin from degradation, control its skin diffusion, and prolong crocin's antioxidant activity, therefore suggesting the suitability of nanostructured lipid dispersions for crocin topical administration [61].

2.6. Patents Based on Saffron's (Crocus sativus) Pharmaceutical Effects in Cancer Treatment

Besides the drug delivery systems already mentioned, several patents have also been granted based on ways to improve the pharmacokinetic profiles of the saffron-derived agents. We focused on the patents that have been invented to improve saffron's unique compounds' action against cancer (Table 2). These patents are based on formulations that contain bioactive phytochemicals, like crocin, crocetin, and safranal, which increase their bioavailability and/or optimize their action against malignancies.

Table 2. Patents based on saffron and its major ingredients and their intended applications.

Patent	Title of Patent	Saffron Component	Subject of the Patent/Application	Inventors (Year Patent Issued)
AU2019264659	Combination therapy for cancer (i.e., a TOP inhibitor)	Safranal	Potent method of treating, suppressing, or reducing the severity of a liver cancer	Amin, A. (2019)
AU2019264660	Method of liver cancer treatment with safranal-based formulations	Safranal	Potent method of treating, suppressing, or reducing the severity of a liver cancer	Ala'a Al Hrout, Amin, A. (2019)
US10568873	Safranal–Sorafenib combination therapy for liver cancer	Safranal	Potent effective treatment for liver cancer	Amin, A., Al Mansoori, A., Baig, B. (2020)
US20200276133	Prevention of liver cancer with safranal-based formulations	Safranal	Potent method of preventing the formation of liver cancer in a subject	Amin, A. (2020)
US20130337068	Carotenoid particles and uses thereof	Crocetin or crocin	Increase of the bioavailability of the delivery molecules	Petyaev, I. (2013)
US9889105	In vivo method for treating, inhibiting, and/or prophylaxis of cancer, such as pancreatic cancer	Crocetin or crocin	Possible inhibition of tumorigenesis in vivo	Dhar, A., Gutheil, G.W. (2018)
US20040116729	Bipolar *trans*-carotenoid salts and their uses	Crocetin or crocin	Improvement of crocin's and crocetin's efficacies	Gainer, J., Grabiak, R. (2013)
US6060511	*Trans*-sodium crocetinate (TSC), methods of making and methods of use thereof	Crocetin	Enhancement of crocin's solubility and increase of bioavailability and radio-sensitizer in in vivo studies	Gainer, J.L. (2000)
US2015352068	Oral formulations of bipolar *trans*-carotenoids (BTCs)	Crocetin	Oral dosage forms of BTCs in chemotherapy	Gainer, J.L., Murray, R. (2015)

One of the main goals of these patents is the increase of the bioavailability and bioefficacy of their cargo. The inventors of patent US20130337068 report the use of carotenoids, such as lycopene, to increase the bioavailability of crocin or crocetin, and thus reduce the dose required to achieve efficacy [62]. In another patent, a purified fraction of crude crocetin, including crocetinic acid, was administered orally or intravenously for prevention, treatment, and therapy of pancreatic cancer [63]. In recent years new patents have been issued, suggesting that administration of safranal may prevent tumor formation or restrict cancer development. In these patents, safranal was reported to be administered alone or in combination with established drugs (i.e., Sorafenib, topoisomerase-1 inhibitors, etc.) [64–67].

Crocin and crocetin have been reported to be most effective when incorporated into bipolar *trans*-carotenoids (BTCs) with a *trans*-carotenoid skeleton [68,69]. These bipolar *trans*-carotenoid salts (BTCS) are useful in improving the diffusivity of oxygen between red blood cells and body tissues. Trans isomer of sodium crocetinate indeed belongs to bipolar *trans*-carotenoid salts. It bears beneficial effects for crocetin, enhancing its solubility, and has been reported to be used to reduce hypoxia, a characteristic of malignancies [70].

2.7. Clinical Trials

As is clear from what has been presented above, a plethora of studies have been conducted upon the anticancer properties of saffron and its unique constituents, like crocin, crocetin, and safranal. Moreover, preclinical in vitro and in vivo data support the findings that the activity of these substances is targeted on malignant cells, sparing normal cells, making these natural agents ideal for developing a human therapeutic approach. However, despite this, little research has been undertaken on humans. So far only two clinical trials report the use of saffron for the treatment of cancer. There is one reported clinical study, published in the Avicenna Journal of Phytomedicine (AJP), which demonstrated the anticancer effect of saffron in combination with chemotherapy in cancer patients suffering from liver metastasis [71]. This clinical study took place in Mashhad, Iran, and it is reported to have been approved by the Ethics Committee of Mashhad University of Medical Sciences with grant number 87432. The 13 patients who participated had primary cancer, including esophagus, stomach, colon, ovarian, and breast cancers, and consumed capsules containing 50 mg of dried saffron stigma. The efficacy of this treatment was evaluated based on CT scan results. The number and size of metastatic lesions were calculated according to the guidelines of the National Cancer Institute (probably that of the USA as it is not mentioned in the publication of the trial). It is reported that 14.3% of the group showed a complete response to saffron treatment, an important outcome towards establishing the proof-of-concept for the anticancer properties of saffron. However, a larger sample size is required, as the placebo and saffron groups included only three and four patients, respectively.

Another clinical trial, referred to as the "Safety and Efficacy Study of trans sodium crocetinate (TSC) with concomitant radiation therapy and temozolomide in newly diagnosed glioblastoma (GBM)", coordinated by INC Research, Raleigh, North Carolina, and conducted in 2013, examined the properties of trans sodium crocinate as a radio-sensitizer [72]. The trial is registered with the ClinicalTrials.gov database (http://www.clinicaltrials.gov) and its registration number is NCT01465347. A total of 59 patients with newly diagnosed GBM participated in this trial. The trial began with a Phase I run-in period to establish the safety of dosing TSC concurrently with radiation therapy and temozolomide. After a safety monitoring committee (SMC) had determined that the TSC caused no dose-limiting toxicity, Phase II was begun. In Phase II, 50 additional patients were enrolled, all receiving the established safe regimen of 0.25 mg/kg TSC, intravenously, three times a week, about 45 min before radiation therapy. Four weeks after the completion of radiation therapy, patients began chemotherapy with TMZ (150–200 mg/m^2) for five days of the first week of a four-week cycle, continuing for six such cycles. No TSC was administered during this period of chemotherapy. During the patient visits (every eight weeks), data consisting of contrast MRI, Karnofsky Performance Status (KPS) scores, and answers to two quality of life questionnaires, were collected. Comparative tumor areas were determined based on the maximum diameters and lengths shown on the MR images. Patients were followed up for two years after their treatment began. The overall survival was analyzed using Kaplan–Meier statistics at two years, and the results were compared with the results that arose from another clinical trial in which the patients received radiotherapy plus TMZ without TSC [73]. These results strongly suggest that adding TSC during radiation therapy is beneficial for the treatment of newly diagnosed glioblastoma.

3. Discussion

Scientists have striven to take advantage of nature's armamentarium and discover the beneficial properties of medicinal plants that may play an important role in human health for centuries [74]. Among such plants is *Crocus sativus* L., commonly known as saffron crocus. Studies report the beneficial action of the components of saffron against a variety of diseases and especially cancer. These findings suggest that saffron's compounds could have potent cancer-preventing effects and antitumor activity with selective toxicity against cancer cells, without affecting the normal cells and without causing any adverse effects, such as conventional cancer treatment drugs do, or drug resistance [75].

As researchers are focused on clarifying the mechanisms through which each compound acts [76], there are plenty of data from in vitro and in vivo studies shedding light on the mechanism of their action, as has been presented above. Signaling pathways and molecules that are involved in the inhibition of cancer cell proliferation, in the triggering of programmed cell death, in the prevention of metastasis, and in the blocking of angiogenesis are the major subjects of all the research [77]. Despite the promising results that have emerged from these extremely important and sound studies, we have to underline that there is a lack of human clinical trials. We cannot draw any definite conclusions so far, as the information about the beneficial effects of saffron's unique ingredients against malignancies is still at the preclinical level. A study conducted in Iran by Hosseini and his colleagues [71] reported encouraging results in patients with liver metastases, but without examining the course of primary cancer after saffron administration, and the authors emphasized the small sample size of their study. The second and maybe most important clinical trial, as we mentioned above, was carried out based on the crocinate patents, with a sufficient number of participants, and reported encouraging results for administration of trans sodium crocetinate during radiation therapy in patients with glioblastoma [72]. What is certain is that more human clinical studies with a sufficient number of participants are required to confirm both the actions of saffron and its main ingredients and the safest dose of saffron administration with the best outcome against cancer.

Besides the need for clinical trials, another urgent need is the determination of specific protocols and approved guidelines regarding some practical but extremely important issues that are required to ensure consistency and repeatability of the results of all conducted studies.

Since 2011, guidelines for the analysis of saffron's major bioactive compounds have been established by the International Standards Organization (ISO 3632). According to ISO 3632, crocin, picrocrocin and safranal are responsible for the color, the flavor, and the aroma of saffron, respectively. This ISO defines specific procedures to determine the concentration of these compounds by spectrophotometric analyses and the variations in concentrations of substances by which saffron quality can be classified have been established. These values are defined as a direct reading of the absorbance of a 1% aqueous solution of dried saffron at 257, 330, and 440 nm using a 1 cm pathway quartz cell [78]. From the analysis of the literature we undertook, it seems that so far the majority of researchers have not followed the ISO guidelines. Thus, a strong recommendation to classify all the saffron samples to be studied, according to ISO trade specifications and quality parameters [79], so that the results obtained are comparable, should be made. By adapting and applying these techniques as established by ISO, wrong labeling and fraud with low-quality saffron material could be militated and limited. Besides, if the isolation and characterization of the main components of saffron are carried out according to the ISO specifications, it will be much easier to analyze bioavailability and the bioefficacy because it will be more consistent with their pharmacokinetic properties.

Analyses of the accurate determination of saffron's composition are however only a piece of a bigger puzzle. *Crocus sativus* L. is a 20–30 cm tall flower blooming in autumn. Generally, saffron is adaptable to temperature and can grow on soils varying from sandy to well-drained clay loams. It blooms in autumn and spends a long period of dormancy in the summer. The flowering period is usually between 15 October and 20 November and may vary depending on the temperature. This period is also the harvest period of saffron. Saffron produces stigmas annually and these parts of the plant are the ones used for medical purposes. The Mediterranean environment is considered worldwide as the best region to produce saffron with regard to its quality, which is attributed to many factors [78,80]. The little available information on flowering phenology in saffron has related it to environmental conditions like temperature radiation, water availability, or nutrients [81]. Temperature and soil water content trigger flowering whereas unitary stigma weights negatively correlate with the flower number per area unit. Higher air temperature and no excessive rain during the flowering period generate the best high-quality stigma yield [82]. Saffron yield is a parameter that also depends on agronomic aspects [83]. For example, soil preparation before planting is necessary. The field should be plowed four to five times to a depth of 30–35 cm to bring the soil into fine tilth. Planting time with the appropriate crop density is important for better yield performance. In Greece, for example, corms are planted in furrows at a distance of 25 × 12 cm, whereas, in Italy, where saffron is planted annually, the best yields of flower and corm productions were obtained by planting corms in furrows at a spacing of 2–3 cm. Recommended planting depths for corms vary from 7.5–10 to 15–22 cm. Finally, harvesting the flowers and separating the stigmas from the flower is a difficult operation. The flowers should be picked exactly when they are fully bloomed. The harvesting must begin shortly after dawn because upon exposure to the sun stigmas lose color and flavor. A two-year study recently published evaluated the effect of soil texture and chemical properties (pH, electrical conductivity, organic carbon, organic matter, total, and active lime) on saffron growth, yield, and quality [82]. The soil conditions were found to be essential for the high quality characteristics of the spice. The best performance, in terms of stigma, observed in soils characterized by sandy loam or loam texture, respectively with neutral-sub alkaline pH and a good amount of organic matter. Similar results were also observed by Khorramdel et al., who reported that stigma yield in sandy loam soil was 49% higher than in greenhouse experiments [84]. It is thus obvious that pedoclimatic factors may impact the quality of the final product i.e., saffron extract, which will further affect the outcome of any bioefficacy studies that follow.

Postharvest treatment is necessary to convert stigmas into saffron spice. Three molecules are the major determinants of the properties of saffron i.e., crocin, picrocrocin and safranal, responsible for the color, the flavor, and the aroma of saffron, respectively [85]. However, the concentrations of these saffron ingredients (and therefore the aroma, the color, and the flavor of saffron) depend on the drying and storage conditions, which are decisive for the quality of the spice [86,87]. For example, saffron stigmas that have been dried in an oven will not have the same properties as others that have been dried in the sun or an airy place in the shade [88]. The highest coloring strength is obtained when saffron is treated at higher temperatures and lower times. Also, a higher amount of safranal (aroma) and crocin (color) is obtained at high temperatures. Picrocrocin concentration was not found to be affected at different temperatures in drying methods [86]. Tong et al. concluded that drying treatment at lower microwave power and over a longer time benefitted the quality of saffron. In this work, the authors suggested that the highest quality of saffron is obtained when fresh saffron is dried at a high temperature, no more than 70 °C, using an electric or vacuum oven [89].

Saffron is well known to be very hygroscopic, oxidizing, darkening, and losing its aroma when exposed to moisture, so storage conditions are essential to preserve the quality of the product if it needs to be stored and not used immediately. The studies by Tsimidou and Biliaderis [90] and Bolandi and Ghoddusi [91] reported high humidity results in the degradation of crocin and picrocrocin. Sereshti et al. concluded that the storage time/duration affects the saffron quality [92]. In this study, the relative concentration of the saffron metabolites in freshly dried and two-year-stored saffron samples prepared with ISO 3632 were evaluated. Freshly dried samples had higher levels of crocin and picrocrocin, while the stored samples were more abundant in safranal as the main saffron aroma agent, reflecting a negative correlation between them.

The biocomponent quality of saffron, also depends on the extraction methods: duration, solvents, and extraction temperature may significantly affect the composition and the quality of the extract [93]. In this study, it was reported that a long-lasting extraction, e.g., 24 h, caused the loss of coloring strength. With alcoholic extracts, a better coloring strength was obtained as compared to aqueous extraction. The highest coloring strength values were obtained with extracts prepared with 50% water: ethanol solvent. A water/ethanol solvent was found to be better than water/methanol, and this last to be better than water alone because the polar carotenoids of saffron are not easily soluble in cold water, while they are soluble in alcoholic solutions. Notably, the concentrations of the molecules in the solutions were determined according to the ISO 3632 standards. In agreement with these findings, Gazerani and his colleagues [94] showed that the optimal parameters to extract the compounds from saffron were an extraction solvent of 50% aqueous ethanol and extraction condition of 5 h at 25 °C. The authors subsequently determined the crocin, picrocrocin, and safranal contents of the extract, following the ISO 3632 guidelines. Under these conditions, the absorbances for crocin, picrocrocin, and safranal were 423.9, 49.51, and 133.1, respectively, as compared to 125.4, 24.99, and 67.18, respectively, for distilled water, which was the control, suggesting a much higher concentration in the 50% aqueous ethanol extract [94]. Generally, conventional extraction methods, which include Soxhlet extraction, vapor or hydrodistillation and maceration or solvent extraction, use huge amounts of organic hazardous solvents, are not selective, have long extraction times, and in some cases extirpate thermolabile/heat sensitive compounds. To overcome these drawbacks, novel extraction methods have been developed, known as "green methods". Enzyme-assisted extraction, ultrasound-assisted extraction or sonication, microwave-assisted extraction, and emulsion liquid membrane extraction are examples of green extraction techniques, which exhibit appropriate potentials to extract saffron bioactive compounds [95]. For example, it is reported that under optimized emulsion liquid membrane extraction, more than 90% of saffron bioactives (i.e., safranal, picrocrocin and crocins) were collected into the aqueous phase, thus underlining the importance of a proper extraction method.

Low absorption of saffron's active compounds is another significant obstacle and thus the method of their administration may greatly affect its bioavailability and biodistribution [96]. To address the low bioavailability, new delivery methods with the aid of advanced drug delivery systems are being developed, so that saffron's bioactives can be delivered with increased efficacy. In this context, many patents focused on methods to improve the efficacy of saffron's ingredients against cancer have been issued.

In conclusion, we herein reviewed advances over the last five years with regard to the anticancer properties of saffron and its major ingredients, crocin, crocetin, picrocrocin, and safranal, recent improvements addressing their poor pharmacokinetic properties, patents, and clinical trials geared towards evaluating their use as potential agents to fight cancer. Major improvements have been achieved with the aid of pharmaceutical technology and the use of novel drug delivery systems. In general, all the results that emerge continue to be very encouraging, especially these from the two clinical trials. In our opinion, this is precisely the next major step that must be emphasized and toward which more effort from the scientific community should be directed: more clinical trials should be set up to get the final proof-of-concept for the potential of saffron and its ingredients as anticancer agents. However, these clinical trials should be conducted only after adopting strict and very specialized protocols for the preparation, storage, and use of saffron and its ingredients to ensure the use of only high-quality saffron material and its consistency.

Funding: This research received no external funding.

Data Availability Statement: Not applicable.

Conflicts of Interest: The authors declare no conflict of interest.

References

1. Bagur, M.J.; Salinas, G.L.A.; Jiménez-Monreal, A.M.; Chaouqi, S.; Llorens, S.; Martínez-Tomé, M.; Alonso, G.L. Saffron: An old medicinal plant and a potential novel functional food. *Molecules* **2018**, *23*, 30. [CrossRef] [PubMed]
2. Rahmani, A.H.; Khan, A.A.; Aldebasi, Y.H. Saffron (Crocus sativus) and its active ingredients: Role in the prevention and treatment of disease. *Pharmacogn. J.* **2014**, *9*, 873–879. [CrossRef]
3. Giannoulaki, P.; Kotzakioulafi, E.; Chourdakis, M.; Hatzitolios, A.; Didangelos, T. Impact of Crocus sativus L. on metabolic profile in patients with diabetes mellitus or metabolic syndrome: A systematic review. *Nutrients* **2020**, *12*, 1424. [CrossRef] [PubMed]
4. Shaterzadeh-Yazdi, H.; Samarghandian, S.; Farkhondeh, T. Effects of crocins in the management of neurodegenerative pathologies: A review. *Neurophysiology* **2018**, *50*, 302–308. [CrossRef]
5. Hassani, F.V.; Naseri, V.; Razavi, B.M.; Mehri, S.; Abnous, K.; Hosseinzadeh, H. Antidepressant effects of crocin and its effects on transcript and protein levels of CREB, BDNF, and VGF in rat hippocampus. *DARU J. Pharm. Sci.* **2014**, *22*, 16. [CrossRef] [PubMed]

6. Pashirzad, M.; Shafiee, M.; Avan, A.; Ryzhikov, M.; Fiuji, H.; Bahreyni, A.; Khazaei, M.; Soleimanpour, S.; Hassanian, S.M. Therapeutic potency of crocin in the treatment of inflammatory diseases: Current status and perspective. *J. Cell. Physiol.* **2019**, *234*, 14601–14611. [CrossRef]
7. Korani, S.; Korani, M.; Sathyapalan, T.; Sahebkar, A. Therapeutic effects of crocin in autoimmune diseases: A review. *BioFactors* **2019**, *45*, 835–843. [CrossRef]
8. Faramarzpour, A.; Tehrani, A.A.; Tamaddonfard, E.; Imani, M. The effects of crocin, mesalazine and their combination in the acetic acid-induced colitis in rats. *Vet. Res. Forum* **2019**, *10*, 227–234. [CrossRef]
9. Rahim, V.B.; Khammar, M.T.; Rakhshandeh, H.; Samzadeh-Kermani, A.; Hosseini, A.; Askari, V.R. Crocin protects cardiomyocytes against LPS-Induced inflammation. *Pharmacol. Rep.* **2019**, *71*, 1228–1234. [CrossRef]
10. Gezici, S. Comparative anticancer activity analysis of saffron extracts and a principle component, crocetin for prevention and treatment of human malignancies. *J. Food Sci. Technol.* **2019**, *56*, 5435–5443. [CrossRef]
11. Bathaie, S.Z.; Hoshyar, R.; Miri, H.; Sadeghizadeh, M. Anticancer effects of crocetin in both human adenocarcinoma gastric cancer cells and rat model of gastric cancer. *Biochem. Cell Biol.* **2013**, *91*, 397–403. [CrossRef] [PubMed]
12. D'Alessandro, A.M.; Mancini, A.; Lizzi, A.R.; De Simone, A.; Marroccella, C.E.; Gravina, G.L.; Tatone, C.; Festuccia, C. Crocus sativus stigma extract and its major constituent crocin possess significant antiproliferative properties against human prostate cancer. *Nutr. Cancer* **2013**, *65*, 930–942. [CrossRef] [PubMed]
13. Rameshrad, M.; Razavi, B.M.; Hosseinzadeh, H. Saffron and its derivatives, crocin, crocetin and safranal: A patent review. *Expert Opin. Ther. Pat.* **2018**, *28*, 147–165. [CrossRef] [PubMed]
14. Tong, Y.; Jiang, Y.; Guo, D.; Yan, Y.; Jiang, S.; Lu, Y.; Bathaie, S.Z.; Wang, P. Homogenate extraction of crocins from saffron optimized by response surface methodology. *J. Chem.* **2018**, *2018*. [CrossRef]
15. Makhlouf, H.; Diab-Assaf, M.; Alghabsha, M.; Tannoury, M.; Chahine, R.; Saab, A.M. In vitro antiproliferative activity of saffron extracts against human acute lymphoblastic T-cell human leukemia. *Indian J. Tradit. Knowl.* **2016**, *15*, 16–21.
16. Zeka, K.; Ruparelia, K.C.; Continenza, M.A.; Stagos, D.; Vegliò, F.; Arroo, R.R.J. Petals of Crocus sativus L. as a potential source of the antioxidants crocin and kaempferol. *Fitoterapia* **2015**, *107*, 128–134. [CrossRef]
17. Manoharan, S.; Wani, S.A.; Vasudevan, K.; Manimaran, A.; Prabhakar, M.M.; Karthikeyan, S.; Rajasekaran, D. Saffron reduction of 7,12-dimethylbenz[a]anthracene-induced hamster buccal pouch carcinogenesis. *Asian Pac. J. Cancer Prev.* **2013**, *14*, 951–957. [CrossRef]
18. Das, I.; Das, S.; Saha, T. Saffron suppresses oxidative stress in DMBA-induced skin carcinoma: A histopathological study. *Acta Histochem.* **2010**, *112*, 317–327. [CrossRef]
19. Mousavi, S.H.; Tavakkol-Afshari, J.; Brook, A.; Jafari-Anarkooli, I. Role of caspases and Bax protein in saffron-induced apoptosis in MCF-7 cells. *Food Chem. Toxicol.* **2009**, *47*, 1909–1913. [CrossRef]
20. Mousavi, M.; Baharara, J. Effect of Crocus sativus L. on expression of VEGF-A and VEGFR-2 genes (angiogenic biomarkers) in MCF-7 cell line. *Zahedan J. Res. Med. Sci.* **2014**, *16*, 8–14.
21. Lu, P.; Lin, H.; Gu, Y.; Li, L.; Guo, H.; Wang, F.; Qiu, X. Antitumor effects of crocin on human breast cancer cells. *Int. J. Clin. Exp. Med.* **2015**, *8*, 20316–20322. [PubMed]
22. Bakshi, H.A.; Hakkim, F.L.; Sam, S. Molecular mechanism of crocin induced caspase mediated MCF-7 cell death: In vivo toxicity profiling and ex vivo macrophage activation. *Asian Pac. J. Cancer Prev.* **2016**, *17*, 1499–1506. [CrossRef] [PubMed]
23. Mostafavinia, S.E.; Khorashadizadeh, M.; Hoshyar, R. Antiproliferative and proapoptotic effects of crocin combined with hyperthermia on human breast cancer cells. *DNA Cell Biol.* **2016**, *35*, 340–347. [CrossRef] [PubMed]
24. Hire, R.R.; Srivastava, S.; Davis, M.B.; Konreddy, A.K.; Panda, D. Antiproliferative activity of crocin involves targeting of microtubules in breast cancer cells. *Sci. Rep.* **2017**, *7*, 44984. [CrossRef]
25. Chryssanthi, D.G.; Lamari, F.N.; Iatrou, G.; Pylara, A.; Karamanos, N.K.; Cordopatis, P. Inhibition of breast cancer cell proliferation by style constituents of different crocus species. *Anticancer Res.* **2007**, *27*, 357–362.
26. Chryssanthi, D.G.; Dedes, P.G.; Karamanos, N.K.; Cordopatis, P.; Lamari, F.N. Crocetin inhibits invasiveness of MDA—MB—231 breast cancer cells via downregulation of matrix metalloproteinases. *Planta Med.* **2011**, *77*, 146–151. [CrossRef]
27. Ashrafi, M.; Bathaie, S.Z.; Abroun, S.; Azizian, M. Effect of crocin on cell cycle regulators in N-Nitroso-N-Methylurea-Induced breast cancer in rats. *DNA Cell Biol.* **2015**, *34*, 684–691. [CrossRef]
28. Arzi, L.; Farahi, A.; Jafarzadeh, N.; Riazi, G.; Sadeghizadeh, M.; Hoshyar, R. Inhibitory effect of crocin on metastasis of triple-negative breast cancer by interfering with Wnt/β-catenin pathway in murine model. *DNA Cell Biol.* **2018**, *37*, 1068–1075. [CrossRef]
29. Xia, D. Ovarian cancer HO-8910 cell apoptosis induced by crocin in vitro. *Nat. Prod. Commun.* **2015**, *10*, 249–252. [CrossRef]
30. Hoshyar, R.; Mollaei, H. A comprehensive review on anticancer mechanisms of the main carotenoid of saffron, crocin. *J. Pharm. Pharmacol.* **2017**, *69*, 1419–1427. [CrossRef]
31. Aung, H.H.; Wang, C.Z.; Ni, M.; Fishbein, A.; Mehendale, S.R.; Xie, J.T.; Shoyama, A.Y.; Yuan, C.S. Crocin from crocus sativus possesses significant anti-proliferation effects on human colorectal cancer cells. *Exp. Oncol.* **2007**, *29*, 175–180. [PubMed]
32. Amin, A.; Bajbouj, K.; Koch, A.; Gandesiri, M.; Schneider-Stock, R. Defective autophagosome formation in p53-null colorectal cancer reinforces crocin-induced apoptosis. *Int. J. Mol. Sci.* **2015**, *16*, 1544–1561. [CrossRef] [PubMed]
33. Zhou, Y.; Xu, Q.; Shang, J.; Lu, L.; Chen, G. Crocin inhibits the migration, invasion, and epithelial-mesenchymal transition of gastric cancer cells via miR-320/KLF5/HIF-1α signaling. *J. Cell. Physiol.* **2019**, *234*, 17876–17885. [CrossRef] [PubMed]

34. Akbarpoor, V.; Karimabad, M.N.; Mahmoodi, M.; Mirzaei, M.R. The saffron effects on expression pattern of critical self-renewal genes in adenocarcinoma tumor cell line (AGS). *Gene Reports* **2020**, *19*, 100629. [CrossRef]
35. Li, C.Y.; Huang, W.F.; Wang, Q.L.; Wang, F.; Cai, E.; Hu, B.; Du, J.C.; Wang, J.; Chen, R.; Cai, X.J.; et al. Crocetin induces cytotoxicity in colon cancer cells via p53-independent mechanisms. *Asian Pac. J. Cancer Prev.* **2012**, *13*, 3757–3761. [CrossRef] [PubMed]
36. Amerizadeh, F.; Rezaei, N.; Rahmani, F.; Hassanian, S.M.; Moradi-Marjaneh, R.; Fiuji, H.; Boroumand, N.; Nosrati-Tirkani, A.; Ghayour-Mobarhan, M.; Ferns, G.A.; et al. Crocin synergistically enhances the antiproliferative activity of 5-flurouracil through Wnt/PI3K pathway in a mouse model of colitis-associated colorectal cancer. *J. Cell. Biochem.* **2018**, *119*, 10250–10261. [CrossRef] [PubMed]
37. Fujimoto, K.; Ohta, T.; Yamaguchi, H.; Tung, N.H.; Fujii, G.; Mutoh, M.; Uto, T.; Shoyama, Y. Suppression of Polyps formation by saffron extract in adenomatous polyposis coli Min / + Mice. *Pharmacogn. Res.* **2019**, *11*, 98–101. [CrossRef]
38. Festuccia, C.; Mancini, A.; Gravina, G.L.; Scarsella, L.; Llorens, S.; Alonso, G.L.; Tatone, C.; Cesare, E.D.; Jannini, E.A.; Lenzi, A.; et al. Antitumor effects of saffron-derived carotenoids in prostate cancer cell models. *Biomed. Res. Int.* **2014**, *2014*. [CrossRef]
39. Chen, S.; Zhao, S.; Wang, X.; Zhang, L.; Jiang, E.; Gu, Y.; Shangguan, A.J.; Zhao, H.; Lv, T.; Yu, Z. Crocin inhibits cell proliferation and enhances cisplatin and pemetrexed chemosensitivity in lung cancer cells. *Transl. Lung Cancer Res.* **2015**, *4*, 775–783. [CrossRef]
40. Moradzadeh, M.; Kalani, M.R.; Avan, A. The antileukemic effects of saffron (Crocus sativus L.) and its related molecular targets: A mini review. *J. Cell. Biochem.* **2019**, *120*, 4732–4738. [CrossRef]
41. Moradzadeh, M.; Tabarraei, A.; Ghorbani, A.; Hosseini, A.; Sadeghnia, H.R. Short-Term in vitro exposure to crocetin promotes apoptosis in human leukemic HL-60 cells via intrinsic pathway. *Acta Pol. Pharm. Drug Res.* **2018**, *75*, 445–451.
42. Geromichalos, G.D.; Papadopoulos, T.; Sahpazidou, D.; Sinakos, Z. Safranal, a Crocus sativus L constituent suppresses the growth of K-562 cells of chronic myelogenous leukemia. In silico and in vitro study. *Food Chem. Toxicol.* **2014**, *74*, 45–50. [CrossRef] [PubMed]
43. Miller, K.D.; Nogueira, L.; Mariotto, A.B.; Rowland, J.H.; Yabroff, K.R.; Alfano, C.M.; Jemal, A.; Kramer, J.L.; Siegel, R.L. Cancer treatment and survivorship statistics, 2019. *CA Cancer J. Clin.* **2019**, *69*, 363–385. [CrossRef] [PubMed]
44. Mir, M.A.; Ganai, S.A.; Mansoor, S.; Jan, S.; Mani, P.; Masoodi, K.Z.; Amin, H.; Rehman, M.U.; Ahmad, P. Isolation, purification and characterization of naturally derived Crocetin beta-D-glucosyl ester from Crocus sativus L. against breast cancer and its binding chemistry with ER-alpha/HDAC2. *Saudi J. Biol. Sci.* **2020**, *27*, 975–984. [CrossRef] [PubMed]
45. Li, S.; Shen, X.Y.; Ouyang, T.; Qu, Y.; Luo, T.; Wang, H.Q. Synergistic anticancer effect of combined crocetin and cisplatin on KYSE-150 cells via p53/p21 pathway. *Cancer Cell Int.* **2017**, *17*, 1–11. [CrossRef] [PubMed]
46. Chahine, N.; Chahine, R. *Protecting Mechanisms of Saffron Extract Against Doxorubicin Toxicity in Ischemic Heart*; Elsevier Inc.: Amsterdam, The Netherlands, 2020; ISBN 9780128184622.
47. Premkumar, K.; Thirunavukkarasu, C.; Abraham, S.K.; Santhiya, S.T.; Ramesh, A. Protective effect of saffron (Crocus sativus L.) aqueous extract against genetic damage induced by anti-tumor agents in mice. *Hum. Exp. Toxicol.* **2006**, *25*, 79–84. [CrossRef] [PubMed]
48. Shahi, T.; Assadpour, E.; Jafari, S.M. Main chemical compounds and pharmacological activities of stigmas and tepals of 'red gold'; Saffron. *Trends Food Sci. Technol.* **2016**, *58*, 69–78. [CrossRef]
49. Holst, B.; Williamson, G. Nutrients and phytochemicals: From bioavailability to bioefficacy beyond antioxidants. *Curr. Opin. Biotechnol.* **2008**, *19*, 73–82. [CrossRef]
50. Puglia, C.; Santonocito, D.; Musumeci, T.; Cardile, V.; Graziano, A.C.E.; Salerno, L.; Raciti, G.; Crascì, L.; Panico, A.M.; Puglisi, G. Nanotechnological approach to increase the antioxidant and cytotoxic efficacy of crocin and crocetin. *Planta Med.* **2019**, *85*, 258–265. [CrossRef]
51. Dehcheshmeh, M.A.; Fathi, M. Production of core-shell nanofibers from zein and tragacanth for encapsulation of saffron extract. *Int. J. Biol. Macromol.* **2019**, *122*, 272–279. [CrossRef]
52. Rahaiee, S.; Shojaosadati, S.A.; Hashemi, M.; Moini, S.; Razavi, S.H. Improvement of crocin stability by biodegradeble nanoparticles of chitosan-alginate. *Int. J. Biol. Macromol.* **2015**, *79*, 423–432. [CrossRef] [PubMed]
53. Sheth, U.; Nagane, R.; Bahadur, P.; Bahadur, A. Salt effect on solubilization of hydrophobic drugs in block copolymeric micelles and investigation of their in vitro and in vivo oral efficiency. *J. Drug Deliv. Sci. Technol.* **2017**, *39*, 531–541. [CrossRef]
54. Alibolandi, M.; Ebrahimian, M.; Hashemi, M. Evaluation of the effect of crocetin on antitumor activity of doxorubicin encapsulated in PLGA nanoparticles. *Nanomed. J.* **2016**. [CrossRef]
55. Rahaiee, S.; Hashemi, M.; Shojaosadati, S.A.; Moini, S.; Razavi, S.H. Nanoparticles based on crocin loaded chitosan-alginate biopolymers: Antioxidant activities, bioavailability and anticancer properties. *Int. J. Biol. Macromol.* **2017**. [CrossRef]
56. Akbarzadeh, A.; Rezaei-sadabady, R.; Davaran, S.; Joo, S.W.; Zarghami, N. Liposome: Classification, preparation, and applications. *Nanoscale Res. Lett.* **2013**, *8*, 1. [CrossRef]
57. Mousavi, S.H.; Moallem, S.A.; Mehri, S.; Shahsavand, S.; Nassirli, H.; Malaekeh-nikouei, B. Improvement of cytotoxic and apoptogenic properties of crocin in cancer cell lines by its nanoliposomal form. *Pharm. Biol.* **2011**, *49*. [CrossRef]
58. Hoshyar, R.; Khayati, G.R.; Poorgholami, M.; Kaykhaii, M. A novel green one-step synthesis of gold nanoparticles using crocin and their anti-cancer activities. *JPB* **2016**. [CrossRef]
59. Prashob, P. Multi-Functional Silver Nanoparticles for Drug Delivery: A Review. *Int. J. Cur. Res. Rev.* **2017**, *9*, 1–5.
60. Thottumugathu, A.M.; Krishnamurthy, S.; Vimala, K.; Kannan, S. PEG functionalized selenium nanoparticles as a carrier of crocin to achieve anticancer synergism. *RSC Adv.* **2016**. [CrossRef]

61. Esposito, E.; Drechsler, M.; Mariani, P.; Panico, M.A.; Cardile, V.; Crascì, L.; Carducci, F.; Graziano, A.C.E.; Cortesi, R.; Puglia, C. Nanostructured lipid dispersions for topical administration of crocin, a potent antioxidant from saffron (Crocus sativus L.). *Mater. Sci. Eng.* **2017**, *71*, 669–677. [CrossRef]
62. Petyaev, I. Carotenoid Particles and Uses Thereof. U.S. Patent US2013337068 (A1), 19 December 2013.
63. Dhar, A.; Gutheil, W.G. In Vivo Method for Treating, Inhibiting, and/ or Prophylaxis of Cancer, Such as Pancreatic Cancer. U.S. Patent US9889105 (B2), 13 February 2018.
64. Amin, A. Combination Therapy for Cancer. Australian Patent AU2019264659 (A1), 15 November 2019.
65. Hrout, A.A.; Amin, A. Method of Liver Cancer Treatment with Safranal-Based Formulations. Australian Patent AU2019264660 (A1), 27 August 2020.
66. Amin, A.; AlMansoori, A.; Baig, B. Safranal- Sorafenib Combination Therapy for Liver Cancer. U.S. Patent US10568873 (B1), 25 February 2020.
67. Amin, A. Prevention of Liver Cancer with Safranal-Based Formulations. U.S. Patent US20200276133 (A1), 20 September 2020.
68. Gainer, J.L.; Grabiak, R.C. Bipolar Trans Carotenoid Salts and Their Uses. U.S. Patent US20040116729 (A1), 20 July 2013.
69. Gainer, J.L. Trans-Sodium Crocetinate, Methods of Making and Methods of Use Thereof. U.S. Patent US6060511 (A), 9 May 2000.
70. Lapchak, P.A. Efficacy and safety profile of the carotenoid trans sodium crocetinate administered to rabbits following multiple infarct ischemic strokes: A combination therapy study with tissue plasminogen activator. *Brain Res.* **2010**, *1309*, 136–145. [CrossRef] [PubMed]
71. Hosseini, A.; Mousavi, S.H.; Ghanbari, A.; Shandiz, F.H.; Raziee, H.R.; Rad, M.P.; Mousavi, S.H. Effect of saffron on liver metastases in patients suffering from cancers with liver metastases: A randomized, double blind, placebo-controlled clinical trial. *Avicenna J. Phytomedicine* **2015**, *5*, 434–440. [CrossRef]
72. Gainer, J.L.; Sheehan, J.P.; Larner, J.M.; Jones, D.R. Trans sodium crocetinate with temozolomide and radiation therapy for glioblastoma multiforme. *J. Neurosurg.* **2017**, *126*, 460–466. [CrossRef] [PubMed]
73. Stupp, R.; Mason, W.P.; van den Bent, M.J.; Weller, M.; Fisher, B.; Taphoorn, M.J.B.; Belanger, K.; Brandes, A.A.; Marosi, C.; Bogdahn, U.; et al. Radiotherapy plus concomitant and adjuvant temozolomide for glioblastoma. *N. Engl. J. Med.* **2005**, *352*, 987–996. [CrossRef]
74. Benetou, V.; Lagiou, A.; Lagiou, P. Chemoprevention of cancer: Current evidence and future prospects. *F1000Research* **2015**, *4*, 916. [CrossRef]
75. Bostan, H.B.; Mehri, S.; Hosseinzadeh, H. Toxicology effects of saffron and its constituents: A review. *Iran. J. Basic Med. Sci.* **2017**, *20*, 110–121. [CrossRef]
76. Shakeri, M.; Tayer, A.H.; Shakeri, H.; Jahromi, A.S.; Moradzadeh, M.; Hojjat-Farsangi, M. Toxicity of saffron extracts on cancer and normal cells: A review article. *Asian Pac. J. Cancer Prev.* **2020**, *21*, 1867–1875. [CrossRef]
77. Milajerdi, A.; Djafarian, K.; Hosseini, B. The toxicity of saffron (Crocus satious L.) and its constituents against normal and cancer cells. *J. Nutr. Intermed. Metab.* **2016**. [CrossRef]
78. Lage, M.; Cantrell, C.L. Scientia horticulturae quantification of saffron (Crocus sativus L.) metabolites crocins, picrocrocin and safranal for quality determination of the spice grown under different environmental Moroccan conditions. *Sci. Hortic.* **2009**, *121*, 366–373. [CrossRef]
79. Consonni, R.; Ordoudi, S.A.; Cagliani, L.R.; Tsiangali, M.; Tsimidou, M.Z. On the traceability of commercial saffron samples using 1H-NMR and FT-IR metabolomics. *Molecules* **2016**, *21*, 286. [CrossRef]
80. Renau-Morata, B.; Nebauer, S.G.; Sánchez, M.; Molina, R.V. Effect of corm size, water stress and cultivation conditions on photosynthesis and biomass partitioning during the vegetative growth of saffron (Crocus sativus L.). *Ind. Crops Prod.* **2012**, *39*, 40–46. [CrossRef]
81. Gresta, F.; Avola, G.; Lombardo, G.M.; Siracusa, L.; Ruberto, G. Analysis of flowering, stigmas yield and qualitative traits of saffron (Crocus sativus L.) as affected by environmental conditions. *Sci. Hortic. (Amsterdam).* **2009**, *119*, 320–324. [CrossRef]
82. Cardone, L.; Castronuovo, D.; Perniola, M.; Scrano, L.; Cicco, N.; Candido, V. The influence of soil physical and chemical properties on saffron (Crocus sativus L.) growth, yield and quality. *Agronomy* **2020**, *10*, 1154. [CrossRef]
83. Kumar, R.; Singh, V.; Devi, K.; Sharma, M.; Singh, M.K.; Ahuja, P.S. State of art of saffron (Crocus sativus L.) agronomy: A comprehensive review. *Food Rev. Int.* **2008**, *25*. [CrossRef]
84. Khorramdel, S.; Gheshm, R.; Ghafori, A.A.; Esmaielpour, B. Evaluation of soil texture and superabsorbent polymer impacts on agronomical characteristics and yield of saffron. *J. Saffron Res.* **2014**, *1*, 120–135.
85. Moratalla-López, N.; Bagur, M.J.; Lorenzo, C.; Martínez-Navarro, M.E.; Salinas, M.R.; Alonso, G.L. Bioactivity and bioavailability of the major metabolites of Crocus sativus L. Flower. *Molecules* **2019**, *24*, 2827. [CrossRef]
86. Maghsoodi, V.; Kazemi, A.; Akhondi, E. Effect of different drying methods on saffron (Crocus sativus L.) quality. *Iran. J. Chem. Chem. Eng.* **2012**, *31*, 85–89.
87. Gregory, M.J.; Menary, R.C.; Davies, N.W. Effect of drying temperature and air flow on the production and retention of secondary metabolites in saffron. *J. Agric. Food Chem.* **2005**, *53*, 5969–5975. [CrossRef]
88. Raina, B.L.; Agarwal, S.G.; Bhatia, A.K.; Gaur, G.S. Changes in pigments and volatiles of saffron (Crocus sativus L.) during processing and storage. *J. Sci. Food Agric.* **1996**, *71*, 27–32. [CrossRef]
89. Tong, Y.; Zhu, X.; Yan, Y.; Liu, R.; Gong, F.; Zhang, L.; Hu, J.; Fang, L.; Wang, R.; Wang, P. The influence of different drying methods on constituents and antioxidant activity of saffron from China. *Int. J. Anal. Chem.* **2015**, *2015*. [CrossRef]

90. Tsimidou, M.; Biliaderis, C.G. Kinetic studies of saffron (Crocus sativus L.) quality deterioration. *J. Agric. Food Chem.* **1997**, *45*, 2890–2898. [CrossRef]
91. Bolandi, M.; Ghoddusi, H.B. Flavour and colour changes during processing and storage of saffron (Crocus sativus L.). *Dev. Food Sci.* **2006**, *43*, 323–326. [CrossRef]
92. Sereshti, H.; Ataolahi, S.; Aliakbarzadeh, G.; Zarre, S.; Poursorkh, Z. Evaluation of storage time effect on saffron chemical profile using gas chromatography and spectrophotometry techniques coupled with chemometrics. *J. Food Sci. Technol.* **2018**, *55*, 1350–1359. [CrossRef] [PubMed]
93. Atyane, L.H.; Caid, M.B.E.; Serghini, M.A.; Elmaimouni, L. Influence of different extraction methods and the storage time on secondary metabolites of saffron. *Int. J. Eng. Res. Technol.* **2017**, *6*, 65–69.
94. Gazerani, S.; Sani, A.; Tajalli, F. Effect of solvent extraction on qualitative parameters of saffron edible extract Regular Paper. *Res. Rev. Biosci.* **2013**, *7*, 2–6.
95. Garavand, F.; Rahaee, S.; Vahedikia, N.; Jafari, S.M. Different techniques for extraction and micro/nanoencapsulation of saffron bioactive ingredients. *Trends Food Sci. Technol.* **2019**, *89*, 26–44. [CrossRef]
96. Christodoulou, E.; Grafakou, M.E.; Skaltsa, E.; Kadoglou, N.; Kostomitsopoulos, N.; Valsami, G. Preparation, chemical characterization and determination of crocetin's pharmacokinetics after oral and intravenous administration of saffron (Crocus sativus L.) aqueous extract to C57/BL6J mice. *J. Pharm. Pharmacol.* **2019**, *71*, 753–764. [CrossRef]

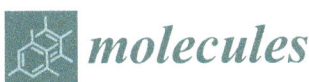

Article

Saffron and Its Major Ingredients' Effect on Colon Cancer Cells with Mismatch Repair Deficiency and Microsatellite Instability

Amr Amin [1,2], Aaminah Farrukh [1], Chandraprabha Murali [1], Akbar Soleimani [3], Françoise Praz [4], Grazia Graziani [5], Hassan Brim [3] and Hassan Ashktorab [3,*]

1. Biology Department, College of Science, United Arab Emirates University, Al-Ain 15551, United Arab Emirates; a.amin@uaeu.ac.ae (A.A.); 201870123@uaeu.ac.ae (A.F.); chandra_prabha@uaeu.ac.ae (C.M.)
2. The College, The University of Chicago, Chicago, IL 60637, USA
3. Department of Pathology and Cancer Center, College of Medicine, Howard University College of Medicine, Washington, DC 20059, USA; hooman1350@yahoo.com (A.S.); hbrim@howard.edu (H.B.)
4. INSERM UMR_S 938, Centre de Recherche Saint-Antoine (CRSA), Sorbonne Université and Centre National de la Recherche Scientifique (CNRS), CEDEX 12, 75012 Paris, France; Francoise.Praz@inserm.fr
5. Department of Systems Medicine, University of Rome Tor Vergata, Via Montpellier 1, 00133 Rome, Italy; graziani@uniroma2.it
* Correspondence: hashktorab@howard.edu

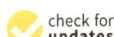

Citation: Amin, A.; Farrukh, A.; Murali, C.; Soleimani, A.; Praz, F.; Graziani, G.; Brim, H.; Ashktorab, H. Saffron and Its Major Ingredients' Effect on Colon Cancer Cells with Mismatch Repair Deficiency and Microsatellite Instability. *Molecules* 2021, 26, 3855. https://doi.org/10.3390/molecules26133855

Academic Editors: Nikolaos Pitsikas and Konstantinos Dimas

Received: 30 April 2021
Accepted: 14 June 2021
Published: 24 June 2021

Publisher's Note: MDPI stays neutral with regard to jurisdictional claims in published maps and institutional affiliations.

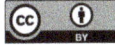

Copyright: © 2021 by the authors. Licensee MDPI, Basel, Switzerland. This article is an open access article distributed under the terms and conditions of the Creative Commons Attribution (CC BY) license (https://creativecommons.org/licenses/by/4.0/).

Abstract: Background: Colorectal cancer (CRC) is one of the most common cancers worldwide. One of its subtypes is associated with defective mismatch repair (dMMR) genes. Saffron has many potentially protective roles against colon malignancy. However, these roles in the context of dMMR tumors have not been explored. In this study, we aimed to investigate the effects of saffron and its constituents in CRC cell lines with dMMR. Methods: Saffron crude extracts and specific compounds (safranal and crocin) were used in the human colorectal cancer cell lines HCT116, HCT116+3 (inserted MLH1), HCT116+5 (inserted MSH3), and HCT116+3+5 (inserted MLH1 and MSH3). CDC25b, p-H2AX, TPDP1, and GAPDH were analyzed by Western blot. Proliferation and cytotoxicity were analyzed by MTT. The scratch wound assay was also performed. Results: Saffron crude extracts restricted (up to 70%) the proliferation in colon cells with deficient MMR (HCT116) compared to proficient MMR. The wound healing assay indicates that deficient MMR cells are doing better (up to 90%) than proficient MMR cells when treated with saffron. CDC25b and TDP1 downregulated (up to 20-fold) in proficient MMR cells compared to deficient MMR cells, while p.H2AX was significantly upregulated in both cell types, particularly at >10 mg/mL saffron in a concentration-dependent manner. The reduction in cellular proliferation was accompanied with upregulation of caspase 3 and 7. The major active saffron compounds, safranal and crocin reproduced most of the saffron crude extracts' effects. Conclusions: Saffron's anti-proliferative effect is significant in cells with deficient MMR. This novel effect may have therapeutic implications and benefits for MSI CRC patients who are generally not recommended for the 5-fluorouracil-based treatment.

Keywords: colorectal cancer; saffron; safranal; crocin; HCT116; MLH1; MSH3; DNA damage and repair; apoptosis

1. Introduction

Colorectal cancer (CRC) is one of the leading causes of cancer-related mortality and the third most prevalent cancer among both genders [1,2]. Most CRCs (60–85%) occur sporadically through acquired genetic mutations. About 5% of the cases consist of genetic cancer syndromes such as hereditary non-polyposis CRC (also called Lynch syndrome) caused by defective mismatch repair (MMR) enzymes such as MLH1 [3].

Microsatellite instability (MSI) in sporadic CRC is frequently caused by promoter hyper-methylation of the mismatch repair gene MLH1 and is highly associated with the CpG methylator phenotype (CIMP) [4,5].

The DNA mismatch repair system is an evolutionary conserved process responsible for fixing errors occurring during replication of proliferating cells. MMR is necessary to ensure the stability of the genetic information and to avoid future genetic diseases. This DNA repair machinery is regulated by different proteins such as: H2AX, PARP, TDP1, TOP1, etc. [6].

The use of natural compounds as therapeutics especially in combination with chemotherapeutic agents is attractive. There are many benefits of using natural compounds compared to the present-day medicine. Natural compounds have much lesser side effects and are nutritionally beneficial and cost-effective. One of the most studied natural compounds is *Crocus sativus*, commonly known as saffron. Saffron has been used as an analgesic, anti-spasmodic, and anti-depressant agent for quite some time [7]. Saffron and its constituents, especially safranal and crocin, have been studied owing to their therapeutic properties [8–12]. Saffron has reportedly served as an anti-cancer agent by inhibiting the DNA/RNA synthesis of malignant lung tumor cells and inhibiting proliferation of cancerous cells by apoptosis in Hela (human cervical carcinoma) and HepG2 (human hepatocellular carcinoma, HCC) cells [12].

Amin et al. have successfully reported the anticancer effect of saffron in mouse models of HCC. On treatment with saffron, the nodule formation of DEN-treated mice had been suppressed. This suppression was correlated with apoptosis and reduced the cell proliferation and oxidative stress [11].

Similarly, safranal which is given for the odor of saffron, has been extensively studied for its anti-cancerous and anti-tumor activities. Safranal's mechanisms of action include DNA double strand breakage (DSBs), induction of apoptosis, and inhibition of epithelial-mesenchymal transition (EMT). Safranal has shown similar pro-apoptotic and anti-proliferative properties in Hela cells, A549 (human lung cancer) and PC-3 (human prostate cancer) cells [8,12]. Crocin, that confers saffron's bright color, has reported pro-apoptotic properties in Hela and two different human skin cancer cell lines (A431 and SCL-1) [13]. Crocin has also reportedly exhibited selective cytotoxicity against HepG2, HL60 (promyelocytic leukemia), and different CRC cell lines [12]. The chemical structure of Saffron and its constituents, safranal and crocin is shown in Figure 1.

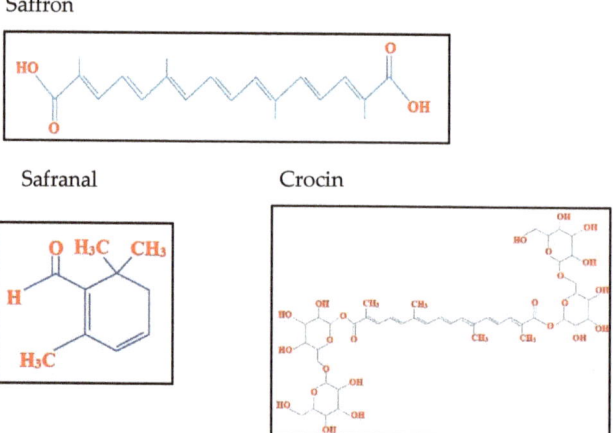

Figure 1. Chemical structure of saffron, safranal and crocin.

In this study, we assessed saffron and its major components on HCT116 cells. Previously, two similar studies were conducted wherein HCT116 cells with different p53 (a tumor suppressor protein) variants, were subjected to the treatment with crocin and saffron. These studies revealed that saffron and crocin have an anti-proliferative and pro-apoptotic effect and induced cell cycle arrest. Saffron had also resulted in autophagic cell death, but such pro-autophagic effect was not observed on the treatment with crocin [10,14]. The regulation of cell cycle is an important mechanism for cell survival. Abnormalities in this mechanism are frequently reported in most cancers. An important protein in this mechanism is CDC25b, which allows the cell to proceed from G2 to M phase of the cell cycle [8]. CDC25b can serve as an important therapeutic biomarker in research, to evaluate the effectiveness achieved against malignant cells by novel compounds.

Our proposed study is performed using the same cells HCT116 which will be supplemented with the two missing MMR genes (MLH1 and MSH3) to assess saffron and the associated compounds' effects in the context of an MMR-deficient (dMMR) or -proficient genotype (pMMR).

2. Results

2.1. Saffron and Crocin Decrease the Viability of pMMR HCT116 Compared to MSH3, MLH1, and Parental HCT116

The effect of saffron and its derivatives on the viability of HCT116 cells was determined using a cell viability assay, wherein the cells were treated with 0–8 mg/mL of saffron for 24 h. The whole saffron treatment showed a dose dependent decrease in cell viability in parental HCT116 cells (25 to 70%) compared to +3, +5 or +3+5 cells (Figure 2).

Viability was lowest at 8 mg/mL in all cell types while the gradual viability decrease was observed in HCT116+3+5 then HCT116+3, HCT116+5, and HCT116 parental. This result indicates the impact of MMR genes, MSH3, and MLH1, in the sensitivity of cell viability to the whole saffron treatment.

Safranal showed a dose dependent inhibition (0–900 µM) in all cell lines with the most significant effect observed in HCT116 (50–70%) and HCT116 +3 (25–90%) cells at 100 µM (Figure 3).

To determine the effect of crocin, cells were treated with different doses, 0–1000 µM for 24 h. Out of all the treated cells, +3 and +3+5 cells showed a significant inhibitory effect in a dose-dependent manner (Figure 4). Viability was lowest at 1000 µM crocin in all cell types while the gradual viability decrease was observed in HCT116+3+5 (10 to 40%) then HCT116+3 (25 to 40%), HCT116+5 (5 to 25%), and HCT116 parental (20% at 1000 µM). This result indicates the impact of MMR genes, MSH3 and MLH1, in sensitivity of cell viability to the crocin treatment.

2.2. Effect of Saffron and Its Derivatives on the Migration of HCT116 Cells and MMR Genes, MSH3, MLH12 Proficient Subtypes

The migration assay provides an important insight in the progression of cancer, hence after validating the effect of saffron and its derivatives on the viability of HCT116 cells, the effect on migration was determined. All cells were treated with the following doses: Saffron 5 mg/mL, safranal 300 µM, and crocin 600 µM for 24 h and compared with the control (Figure 5). The doses were selected conservatively to minimize their effects on the cells' morphology.

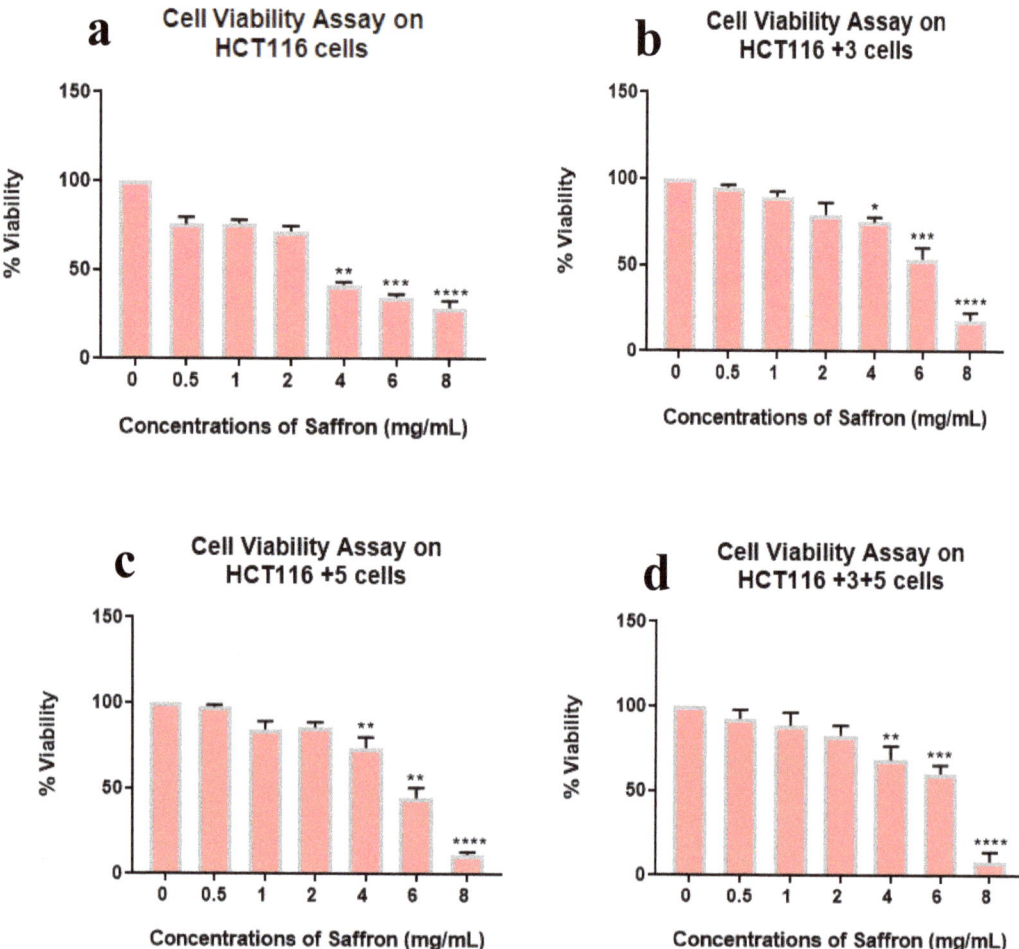

Figure 2. Cell viability assay of saffron-treated cells. Percentage of viability shown vs. concentration of saffron. (**a–d**) show the effect of saffron treatment on the viability of HCT116, HCT116+3, HCT116+5 and HCT116+3+5 cells respectively. (* $p < 0.05$, ** $p < 0.01$, *** $p < 0.001$ and **** $p < 0.0001$).

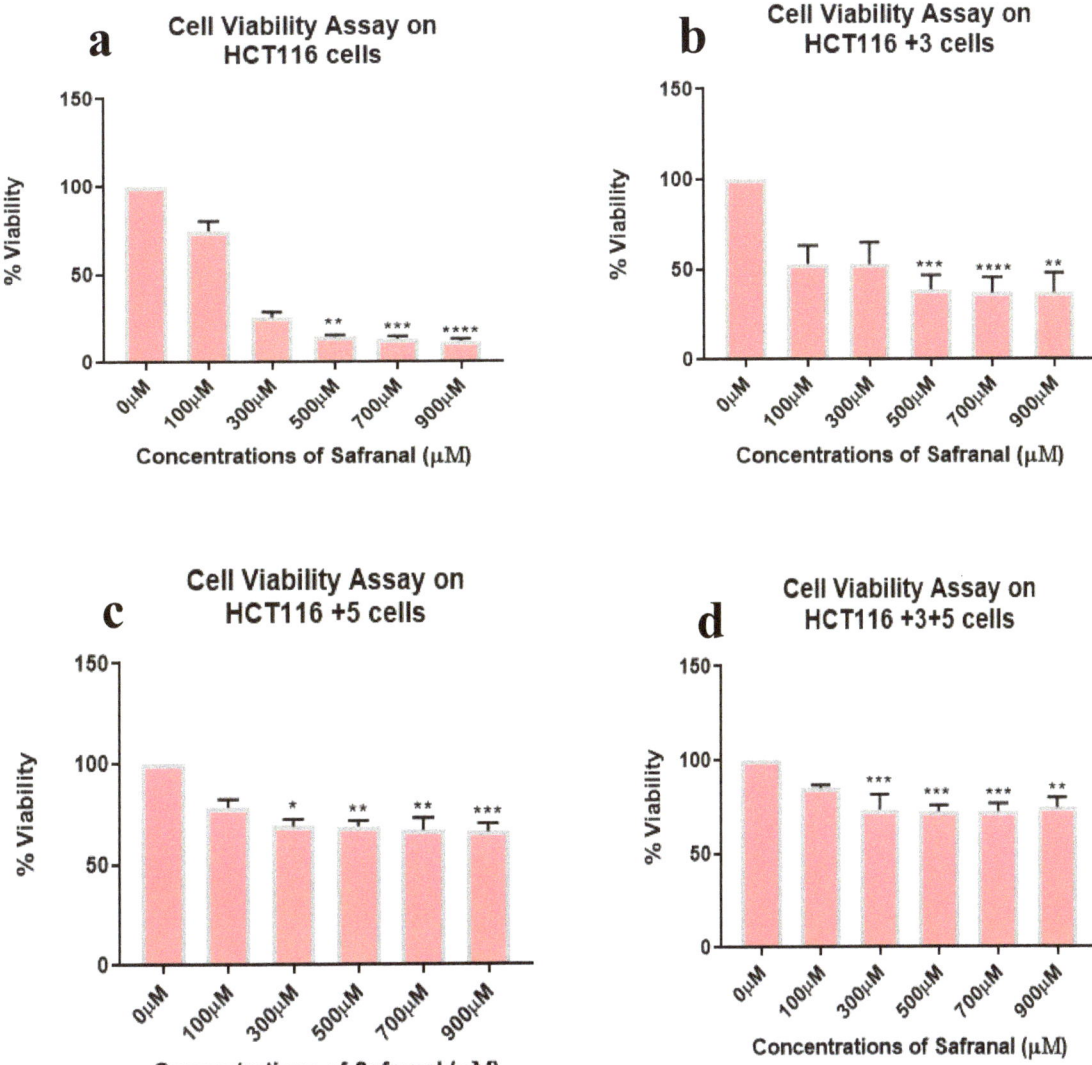

Figure 3. Cell viability assay of safranal-treated cells. Percentage of viability shown vs. concentration of safranal. (**a–d**) show the effect of safranal treatment on the viability of HCT116, HCT116+3, HCT116+5 and HCT116+3+5 cells respectively. (* $p < 0.05$, ** $p < 0.01$, *** $p < 0.001$ and **** $p < 0.0001$).

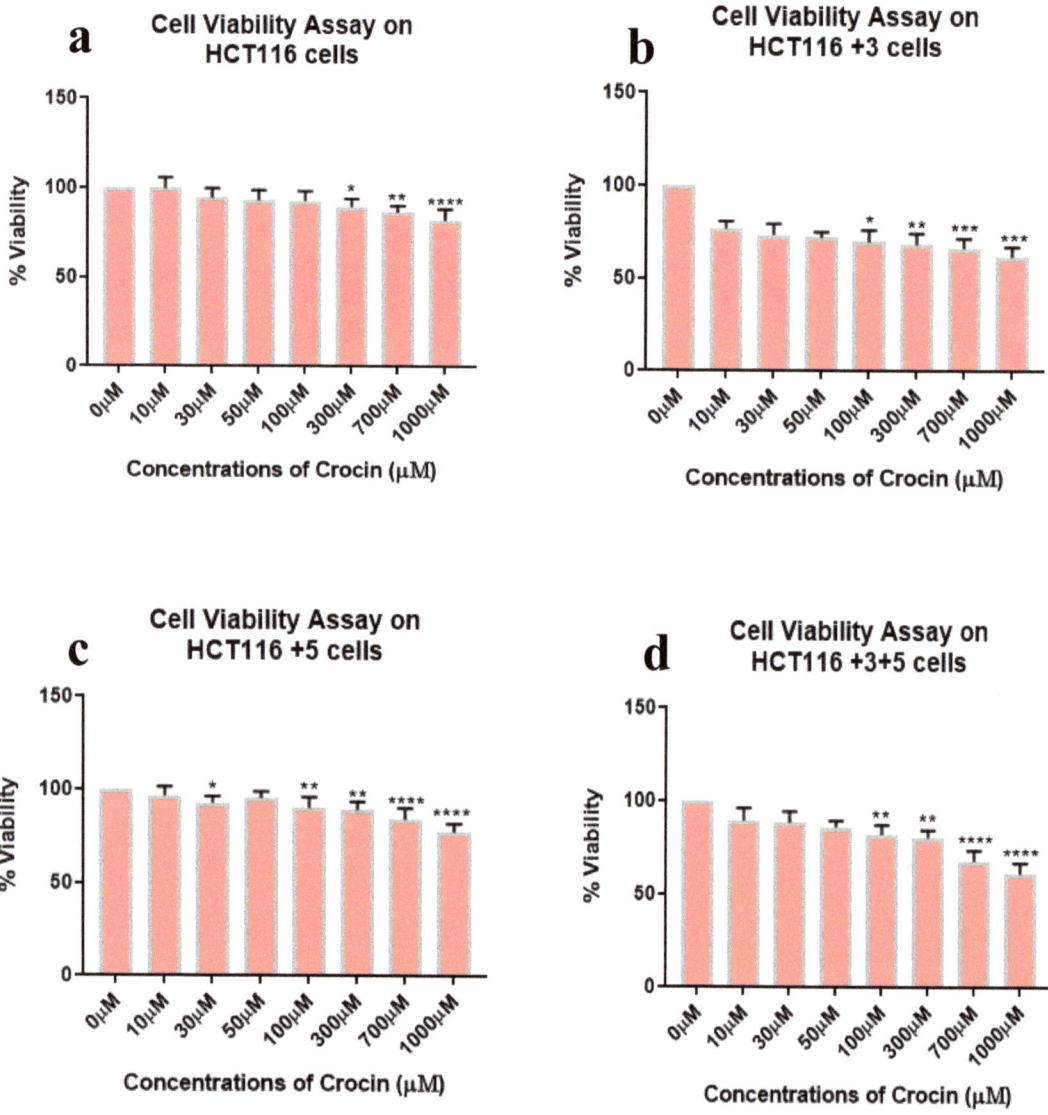

Figure 4. Cell viability assay of crocin-treated cells. Percentage of viability shown vs. concentration of crocin. (**a**–**d**) show the effect of crocin treatment on the viability of HCT116, HCT116+3, HCT116+5 and HCT116+3+5 cells respectively. (* $p < 0.05$, ** $p < 0.01$, *** $p < 0.001$ and **** $p < 0.0001$).

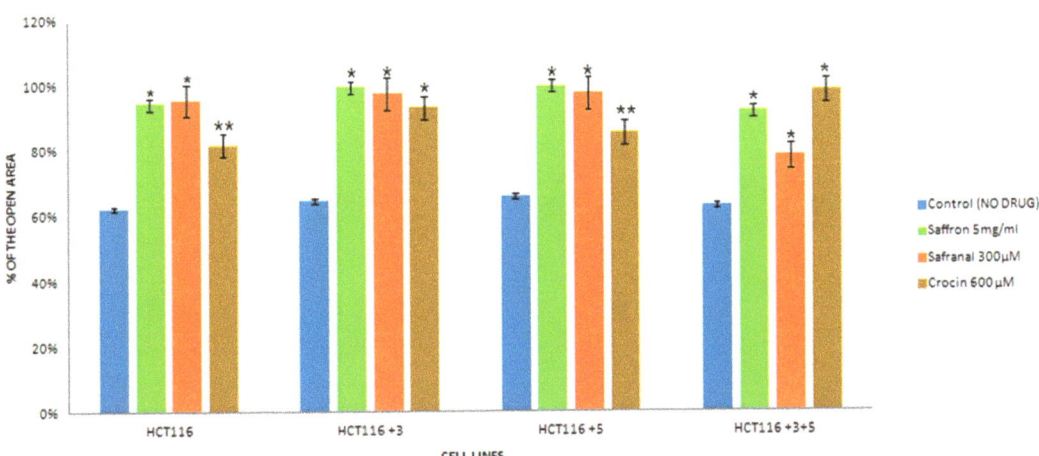

Figure 5. Quantification histogram of the wound healing assay. The assay was performed in triplicates. (* $p < 0.05$, ** $p < 0.01$).

The images were captured at 0 and 24 h for the control and treated cells. For saffron-treated cells, the 0 h image is not available due to the interference of saffron's bright color. The treatment with saffron showed a significant decrease (90% open wound area) in the migratory and invasive capacity of proficient MMR in HCT116+3+5 cells (Figure 5) compared to the parental HCT-116. Safranal had its most significant effect in +3+5 cells (80% open wound area) where it inhibited the migration of cells considerably 24 h post-treatment compared to the control (Figure 5).

2.3. Cell Cycle and DNA Repair Machinery Are Affected by Saffron and Its Derivatives

In order to determine the pathway involved in the cytotoxic nature of saffron and its derivatives, markers of DNA damage and repair and cell cycle were analyzed. Immunoblots of p.H2AX and TDP1 (involved in the repair of stalled Topoisomerase I-DNA complexes) were analyzed for DNA damage and repair. A key cell cycle checkpoint regulator CDC25b was also analyzed.

To determine the effect of saffron, cells were treated with 5, 10, and 15 mg/mL of saffron for 24 h. Expression of CDC25b decreased at 15 mg/mL of saffron in mutant cells but not consistent in a dose dependent manner (Figure 6). The DDR markers, p.H2AX and TDP1 showed an increase and decrease in protein expression, respectively at a dose of 15 mg/mL saffron in all cell lines (Figure 6). The fold change of relative expression compared to the control is mentioned below each band.

For safranal's treatment, the cells were treated with 300, 500, and 700 µM for 24 h (Figure 7). The expression of CDC25b decreased with the increase in safranal concentration for parental HCT116 cells. There was a relative decrease in protein expression in +3 and +3+5 cells, compared to the control at 500 µM. The expression of p.H2AX increased in HCT116 cells at 300 and 500 µM, and in HCT116+3 cells at 300 and 700 µM TDP1 expression decreased at the 500 µM treatment of HCT116 cells, at 300 µM in +3 and +5 cells, and constantly decreased with all doses in HCT116+3+5 cells (Figure 7). The fold change of the relative expression compared to the control is mentioned below each band.

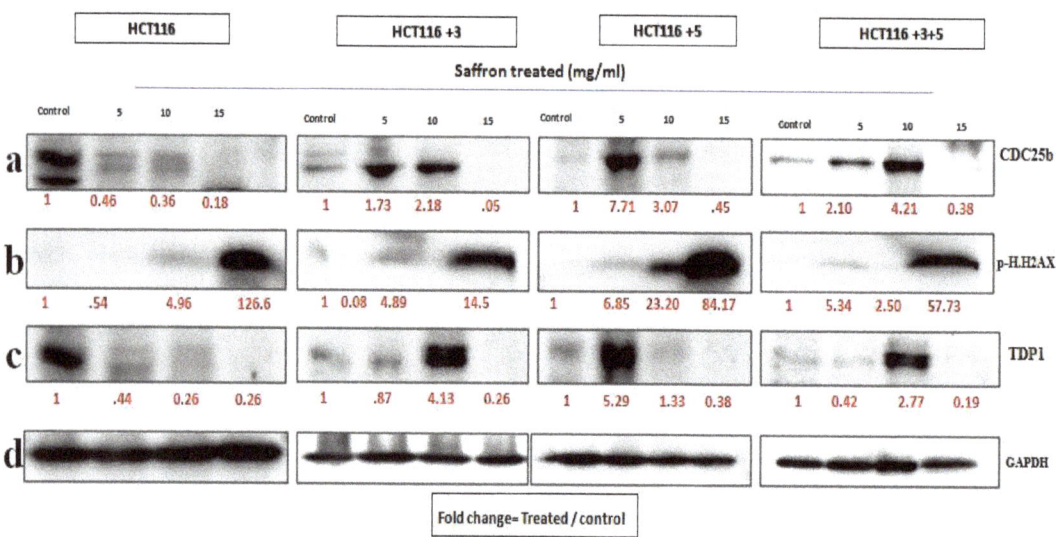

Figure 6. Saffron's effect on cell cycle and DNA repair machinery [15]. Cells were treated with saffron 5, 10, and 15 mg/mL for 24 h. (**a–c**) show the effect of Saffron treatment on CDC25b, p.H2AX and TDP1 respectively. (**d**). GAPDH was used as loading control. Red font represents the fold change value.

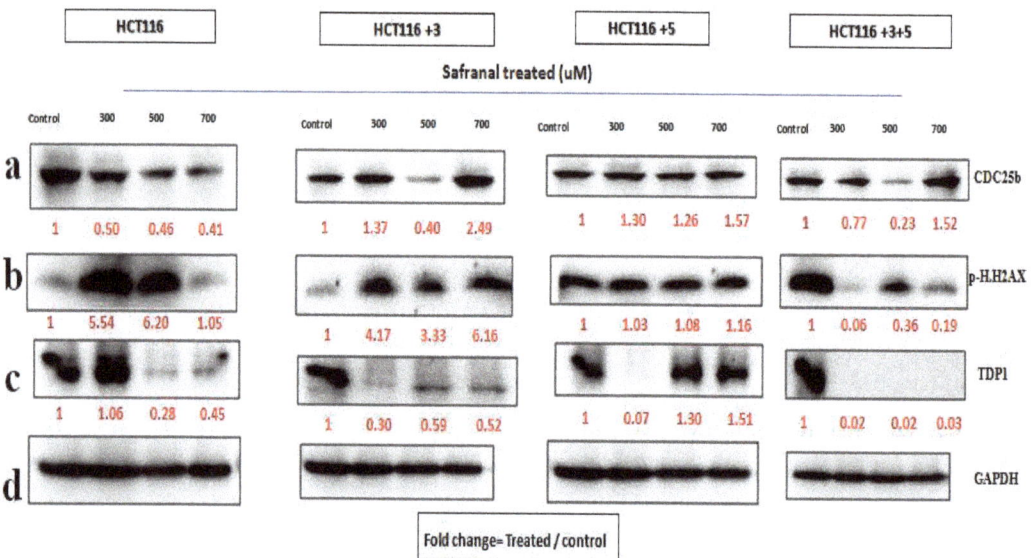

Figure 7. Safranal's effect on cell cycle and DNA repair machinery. (**a–d**) Cells were treated with safranal 300, 500, and 700 μM for 24 h. (**a–c**) show the effect of Safranal treatment on CDC25b, p.H2AX and TDP1 respectively. (**d**). GAPDH was used as loading control. Red font represents the fold change value.

To evaluate the effects of crocin, the cells were treated with 300, 600, and 900 μM crocin for 24 h. The CDC25b expression in HCT116 cells on the treatment with 300 μM and in +3 cells on the treatment with 900 μM was decreased. The p.H2AX expression increased on the treatment with 600 μM in +3 cells and on the treatment with 600 and 900 μM in

+5 cells (Figure 8). The fold change of the relative expression compared to the control is mentioned below each band.

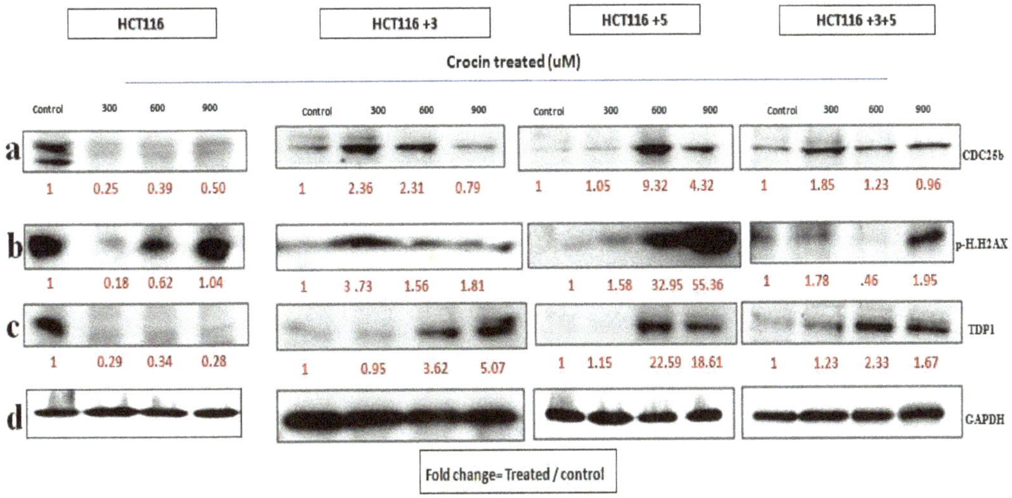

Figure 8. Crocin's effect on cell cycle and DNA repair machinery. (**a**–**d**) Cells were treated with crocin 300, 600, and 900 µM for 24 h. (**a**–**c**) show the effect of Crocin treatment on CDC25b, p.H2AX and TDP1 respectively. (**d**). GAPDH was used as loading control. Red font represents the fold change value.

To sum up, the expression of CDC25b was completely downregulated in both HCT116 parental and mutant cells at a dose of 15 mg/mL saffron. Safranal and crocin were not as consistent on the CDC25b protein, with crocin showing a steady effect only on the HCT116 parental. In the HCT116 parental, the protein levels of p.H.H2AX were upregulated in a dose dependent manner by saffron (15 mg/mL), safranal (300 and 500 µM), and crocin (600 and 900 µM) at the stated doses. Crocin (900 µM) had a persistent upregulation of p.H2AX in mutant cells where as safranal and saffron showed irregular results. Meanwhile, crocin, saffron, and safranal inhibited the TDP1 protein in parental HCT116 cells in a dose dependent manner. Safranal reduced the expression of TDP1 in HCT116+3 and HCT116+3+5 cells, whereas, crocin and saffron did not have a constant effect on TDP1 in mutant cells.

2.4. Saffron, Crocin, and Safranal Induce Apoptosis

The effect of saffron and its compounds on apoptosis was analyzed. The activity and expression of caspase 3 and 7 were analyzed, since they are the executioner caspases of apoptosis. A Western blot analysis was performed to determine the expression of pro-caspase 3 in saffron-treated cells (Figure 9). For safranal and crocin-treated cells, the caspase 3/7 activity was also measured. The caspase activity for saffron-treated cells was not measured since saffron's color interfered with the assay.

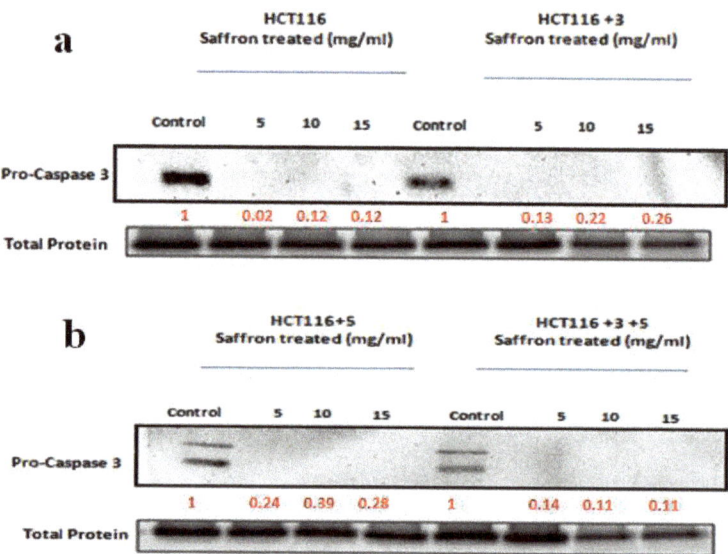

Figure 9. Saffron activates the caspase pathway. A Western blot analysis was performed to determine the expression of pro-caspase 3 in saffron-treated cells. The indicated cells were treated with 5, 10, and 15 mg/mL of saffron for 24 h. Pro-caspase 3, which cleaves to caspase 3, was analyzed. The saffron treatment led to a decrease in the expression of pro-caspase 3, which was visible in the control cells. The fold change of relative expression compared to the control is mentioned below each band. Red font represents the fold change value. (**a**,**b**) show the effect of saffron treatment on caspase pathway in HCT116, HCT116+3 and HCT116+5, HCT116+3+5 cells respectively.

To study the effect of saffron on apoptosis, cells were treated with 5, 10, and 15 mg/mL of saffron for 24 h (Figure 9). Pro-caspase 3, which cleaves to caspase 3, was analyzed. The saffron treatment led to a decrease in the expression of pro-caspase 3, which was visible in the control cells. The fold change of the relative expression compared to the control is mentioned below each band.

The activity of executioner caspases, caspase 3 and 7, was measured after treating the cells with safranal 300, 500, and 700 µM (Figure 10). All cell lines showed an increase in caspase activity with the increase in dose, with the most significant effect observed at 700 µM compared to the control. Safranal showed an increased caspase 3/7 activity in HCT116+3+5 (approx. 300-fold), HCT116+3 (approx. 400-fold) then HCT116+5 (approx. 200-fold). These results suggest that MSH3 and MLH1 play an important role in processes involving saffron and apoptosis.

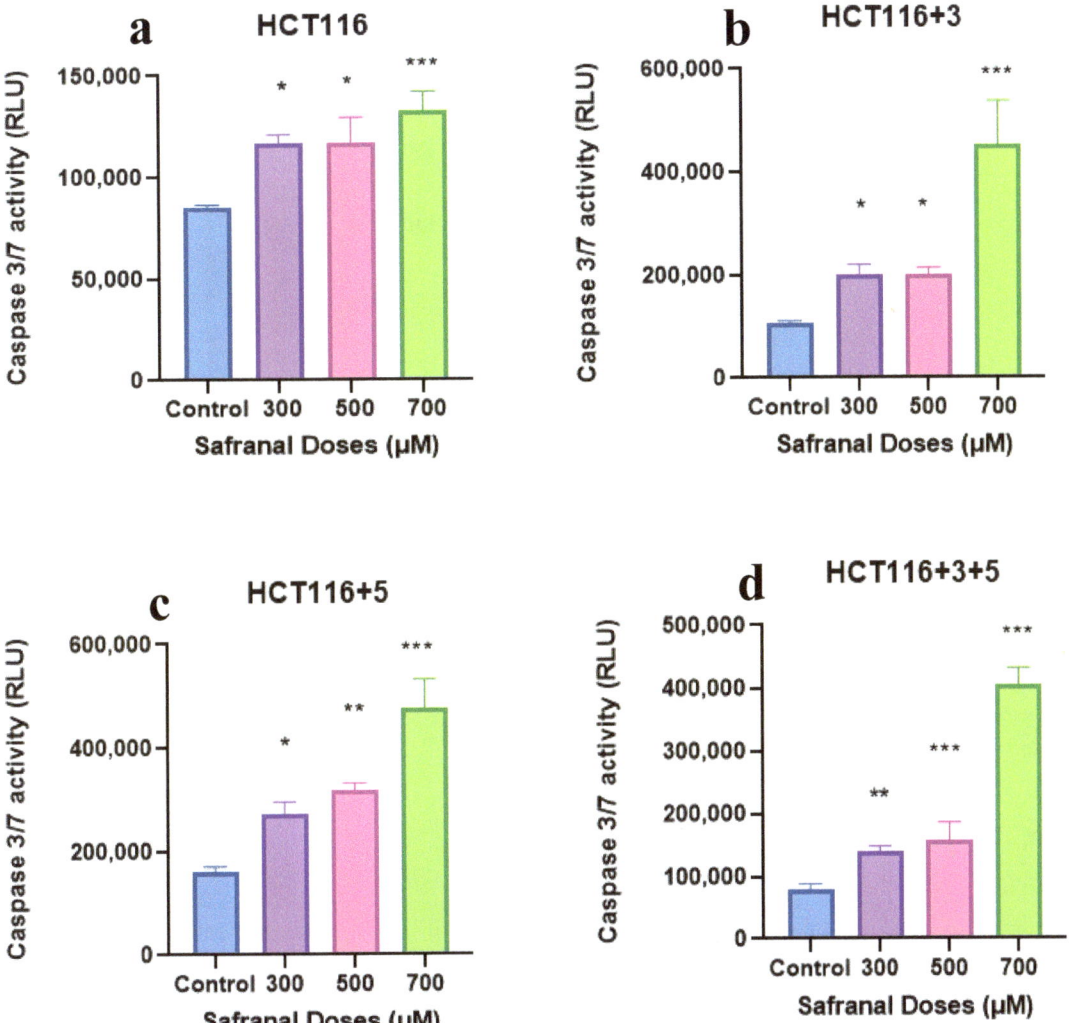

Figure 10. Effect of safranal on the caspase pathway (caspase activity measured in the relative light unit (RLU). (**a–d**) show the effect of Safranal on the caspase activity in HCT116, HCT116+3, HCT116+5 and HCT116+3+5 cells respectively. An ANOVA (Analysis of Variance) test was carried out (≥ 0.05 NS, ≤ 0.01 *, < 0.01 **, ≤ 0.001 ***).

To evaluate the effect of crocin, cells were treated with 300, 600, and 900 µM following the protocol. The cells showed an increase in caspase activity on the treatment with 300 µM in HCT116 +3, HCT116 +5, and HCT116+3+5 cells (approx. 50-fold) (Figure 11). The effect was not consistent and significant when compared to the same as imparted by safranal on these cells.

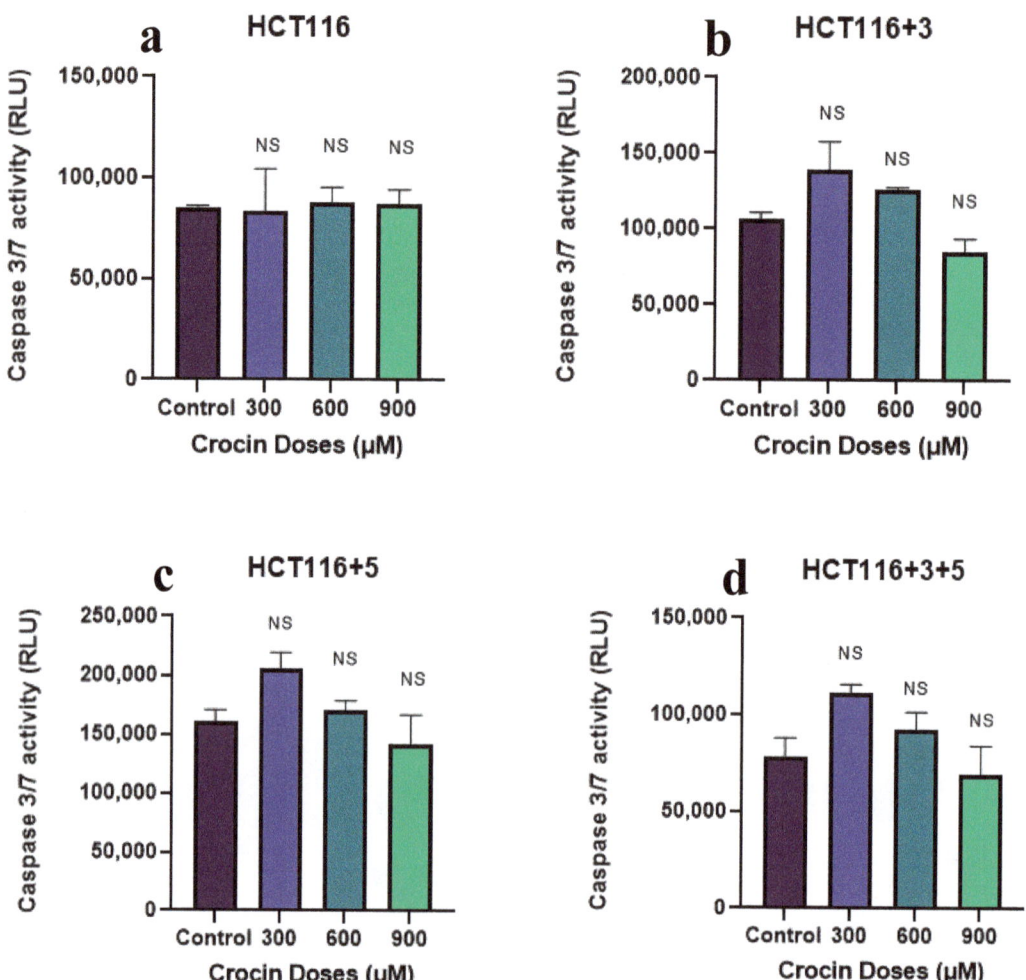

Figure 11. Effect of crocin on caspase pathway (caspase activity measured in the relative light unit (RLU). (**a–d**) show the effect of crocin on the caspase activity in HCT116, HCT116+3, HCT116+5 and HCT116+3+5 cells respectively. An ANOVA (Analysis of Variance) test was carried out (≥ 0.05 NS).

3. Discussion

Colorectal cancer is one of the leading causes of cancer-related deaths worldwide. Different environmental and genetic factors are responsible for its development. Different CRC subtypes such as MSI and microsatellite stable (MSS) tumors may have different outcomes due to their different molecular and pathological characteristics. Patients with MSI tumors have better prognosis than MSS ones. While those with EMAST tumors have different immunological and pathological features and poor prognosis, as well. The CRC treatment based on MMR deficiency is a key approach for better outcome and the need for healthier and long-lasting treatments remain pivotal [16]. In this study, we showed that saffron's anti-proliferative effect is significant in cells with deficient MMR.

Saffron has long been used as a traditional medicine. It has shown anti-tumor properties in vitro in different cancer cell lines such as those from liver and prostate. The therapeutic efficacy of saffron has also been observed with its derivatives: Safranal and crocin. Saffron and its derivatives have shown no detrimental effects on normal cells, hence making it a model curative agent that can be used as an adjuvant therapy [8]. Indeed, we recently showed that it can affect the action of MACC1, a metastasis-associated gene in CRC [17]. In the present study, we analyzed its effects within the context of MMR genes deficiency in HCT116 cell lines.

HCT116 cells with different MLH1 and/or MSH3 gene supplements were treated with different doses of saffron, ranging from 0–10 mg/mL for 24 h, to assess cell viability. All cells had shown significant dose-dependent inhibition on the treatment with saffron (Figure 2). This dose-dependent inhibition is consistent with the results previously published by Bajbouj et al. where HCT116 cells (with or without p53) were studied for saffron's effect [14]. Saffron caused DNA damage and promoted apoptosis in both tested cell lines. An interesting observation was the delayed apoptosis in cells that lacked p53 [14]. Saffron has previously been reported to inhibit cell viability at lower doses (100–150 μg/mL) in other cancer cell lines, suggesting that HCT116 cells have higher resistance to this compound [12]. On treatment with safranal and crocin, the cells exhibited a dose-dependent cell viability inhibition pattern, similar to saffron (Figures 3 and 4). Safranal and crocin dose ranges in our study are close to the effective doses published for other cancers [9,18,19]. Malaekeh-Nikouei et al. have reported safranal's effective dose range to be much higher for other cells suggesting that HCT116 cells have a higher susceptibility [20]. Cancer cells migration and invasion are critical features for metastasis [21]. Saffron, safranal, and crocin treatments showed a significant decrease in migration as compared to the control. Safranal has been previously shown to have anti-migration properties on other cell lines including HepG2 (liver cancer cells) and HSC-3 (prostate cancer cells). Although the effective concentration for HSC-3 cells was lower, the concentration is closer to what is reported for HepG2 cells [8]. The results of crocin treatment are also consistent with the previous findings where the crocin treatment has inhibited invasion of different cell lines including HUVEC (human umbilical vein endothelial cells), AGS and HGS-27 (gastric cancer cells), and MG63 (osteosarcoma) [22,23]. Interestingly, Wang et al. reported crocin's inability to inhibit the invasion of HCT116 cells, at 271.18 μM, but comparing it with the present findings suggests that a higher dose is required to inhibit invasiveness (Figure 5) [19]. In patients with CRC, recurrence and metastasis are the most common causes of cancer-related death. The ability of saffron and its derivatives to minimize migration of HCT116 cells provides a novel course of action that can be used as an adjuvant therapy, especially in patients with MSI tumors.

In order to determine the effect of treatment on the cells, with altered MLH1 and/or MSH3 genes, immunoblots of two DNA damage markers, p.H2AX and TDP1, together with CDC25b, a cell cycle checkpoint regulator, were analyzed (Figures 6–8). To our knowledge, the effect of crocin on these particular markers is reported here for the first time, making it a novel finding in the saffron mechanistic action.

As mentioned earlier, DNA MMR is required to ensure genetic stability. A commonly occurring error in DNA replication is DNA DSBs. H2AX, a histone, is phosphorylated to p.H2AX in response to DSB and hence is a marker for studying DNA damage [8]. In this study, saffron and its derivatives upregulated the expression of p.H2AX. Saffron up regulated the expression at 15 mg/mL across all the different cells (Figure 6), indicating a DNA damage as a result of the treatment. Similar findings were also reported by Bajbouj et al. where the treatment with saffron had shown increased expression of p.H2AX in HCT116 cells [14]. p.H2AX was also reported to have been induced by saffron at a lower dose, 6 mg/mL, in HepG2 cells [8]. Safranal upregulated the expression in HCT116 and HCT116 +3 cells, compared to the untreated control (Figure 7). The effective concentrations observed in this study are closer to a previously mentioned effective concentration, where safranal at 500 μM had similar effects on HepG2 cells [8].

TDP1, such as p.H2AX, is involved in the DNA repair. It protects against DNA strands breakage by repairing stalled Topoisomerase I-DNA complexes, occurring as a result of DSBs [8]. All cells treated with saffron and its derivatives displayed downregulated the TDP-1 expression. The most notable response for saffron treated cells was observed at

15 mg/mL (Figure 6). This downregulation of TDP-1 is likely the result of a cellular decision to allow such DNA-damaged cells to undergo apoptosis rather than repairing them.

In the case of damage to DNA, the cell cycle comes to an arrest and induces apoptosis or cell death. After establishing the effect of treatment on DNA damage, its effect on cell cycle was evaluated. CDC25b, is a key cell cycle regulator and also an oncogene with an over-expression observed in breast cancer, lung cancer, and CRC [6]. Saffron showed a dose-dependent inhibition of CDC25b in HCT116 cells while for the other cells an inhibition was observed at 15 mg/m. Doxorubicin, a widely used chemotherapeutic agent, had no effect on CDC25b in HCT116 cells [24], while saffron inhibited the expression of CDC25b. The treatment with safranal showed a similar pattern of dose dependent inhibition, for HCT116 cells (Figure 7). The treatment with crocin showed varying results, but overall, the expression was downregulated as compared to the untreated controls.

Cells undergo apoptosis in the case of irreparable damage. Our results indicated DNA damage and cell cycle arrest in response to the saffron treatment. To further confirm the apoptotic property of saffron, executioner caspases of apoptosis, caspase 3 and 7, were studied. Immunoblots for saffron-treated cells showed the absence of pro-caspase 3, suggesting its cleavage to its active form (Figure 9). Saffron has also exhibited such pro-apoptotic properties in liver and breast cancer cells [25,26]. The activity of caspase 3 and 7 for safranal and crocin-treated cells was measured using the Caspase-Glo® 3/7 Assay kit (Figure 10. Effect of safranal on the caspase pathway (caspase activity measured in the relative light unit (RLU). An ANOVA (Analysis of Variance) test was carried out (≥ 0.05 NS, ≤ 0.01 *, ≤ 0.001 ***).

Both saffron compounds showed a significant increase of caspase activity post-treatment compared to the control suggesting an increase in apoptotic activity. Safranal has also shown such caspase activity, previously, on HepG2 cells. These findings are in concordance with the previously available data where safranal has shown similar pro-apoptotic properties in A549 (alveolar human lung cancer) and PC-3 (human prostate cancer) cell lines, as reported by Al-Hrout et al. [8]. Crocin has previously displayed pro-apoptotic properties across different cell lines, including liver, breast, skin, and gastric cancer cells [13,22,27,28] but the effective dose was lower compared to the one used in this study.

4. Materials and Methods

4.1. Cell Lines

The isogenic HCT116 cell line that is deficient in both MLH1 and MSH3 genes was used in this study [29,30]. This cell line was complemented for these MMR gene deficiencies by transfecting chromosomes 3 and 5 separately to create HCT116+3 and HCT116+5 and together to create HCT116+3+5 cell lines. Briefly, MSH3-deficient/MLH1-proficient colorectal cancer HCT116 (MLH1) cells were transfected with the MLH1 cDNA cloned into the pcDNA3.1 (−) vector [30]. MSH3/MLH1-deficient HCT116, carrying MLH1 and MSH3 mutations on chromosome 3 and 5, respectively, and HCT116 in which parental MLH1 (HCT116 +3), MSH3 (HCT116 +5) or both genes (HCT116 +3+5) were introduced by the chromosome transfer by the microcell transfer of normal human chromosome 3 and/or 5 (Table 1) [29–31].

Table 1. HCT-116 with and without MMR genes and the corresponding phenotypes.

CRC Cell Line	MLH1	MSH3	Tumor Type
HCT116	−	−	MSI and EMAST
HCT116 +3	+	−	EMAST
HCT116 +5	−	+	MSI with no EMAST
HCT116 +3+5	+	+	MSS

MSI: Microsatellite instable; EMAST: Elevated microsatellite alterations at selected tetranucleotide repeat; MSS: microsatellite stable.

4.2. Cell Cultures

The HCT116 cells were cultured in the RPMI 1640 Medium (Hyclone, Marlborough, MA, USA) while HCT116 +3, HCT116 +5, and HCT116 +3+5 cells were cultured in McCoy's Medium (Hyclone, Marlborough, MA, USA). Both media were supplemented with 10% fetal bovine serum (Sigma Aldrich, St. Louis, MO, USA) and containing 1% of 100 U/mL penicillin and 100 µg/mL streptomycin (Sigma Aldrich, St. Louis, MO, USA) at 37 °C in a humidified 5% CO2 atmosphere. Cells were sub-cultured every 3–5 days using Trypsin 0.25% (Hyclone, Marlborough, MA, USA).

Saffron, safranal, and crocin preparations: Saffron crude extracts (Gulf Pearls SPRL Brussels, Belgium, www.gp-food.com, accessed on 3 May 2021) and specific compounds (safranal and crocin (Sigma Aldrich, St. Louis, MO, USA)) were used as previously described [7,17]. Saffron was grinded by a pestle and mortar and dissolved in water at a final concentration of 20 mg/mL and mixed on an orbital shaker in the dark for 1 h then used at different concentrations.

4.3. Cell Viability Assay

All cells were seeded at a density of 5000 cells/well in 96-well plates in 100 µL of complete growth medium. Cells were allowed to attach for 24 h before being treated with different concentrations of saffron, safranal, and crocin for 24 h. Cells were then treated with 3-[4,5-dimethylthiazol-2-yl]-2,5-diphenyltratrazolium bromide (MTT) (Sigma Aldrich, St. Louis, MO, USA) and incubated for 3 h. The formed formazan crystals were dissolved using DMSO (Sigma Aldrich, St. Louis, MO, USA) and the absorbance of the resulting product was measured at 570 nm using GloMax Microplate Reader (Promega, Madison, WI, USA). Cell viability is presented as the percent of viable cells = (Abs. of treated cells/Abs. of control cells) × 100. The experiment was carried out in triplicates.

4.4. Wound Healing Assay

For the wound healing assay, cells were seeded in 6-well plates. When cells were confluent, a scratch was made with a 200 µL sterile pipette tip, generating a cell-free area of approximately 1 mm in width. Cellular debris was removed by gentle washing with the culture medium and the photos of the wounds (0 h) were taken. Afterwards, the medium was replaced by the culture medium with different concentrations of the drugs and the cells were allowed to migrate for 24 h. At the end of migration experiment, another set of photos was taken, from the same regions using Phase Contrast Fluorescence microscopy (Olympus, Tokyo, Japan). The gap size was analyzed using the Image-J software (LOCI, Madison, WI, USA). To assess the migration ability of cultured cells, cell-free areas of the scratches at 24 h after scratching were subtracted from the area of the scratches at 0 h and calculated as a percentage of untreated (0 h) cultures. The experiment was carried out in triplicates.

4.5. Caspase 3 and 7 Activity

Caspase 3 and 7 activities were detected using the Caspase-Glo® 3/7 Assay kit (Promega, Madison, WI, USA) following the manufacturer's protocol. Briefly, the cells were seeded at a density of 5000 cells/well in 100 µL media for 24 h. Next, the cells were treated with saffron (0.5–8 mg/mL), crocin (100–900 µM) or safranal (10–1000 µM) for 24 h. The next day, the Caspase-Glo reagent (Promega, Madison, WI, USA) was added to the cells and incubated for 4 h. The control which was composed of untreated cells and a blank control, containing media with the reagent, was also included to subtract the background. The luminescence was measured using the GloMax Microplate Reader (Promega, Madison, WI, USA).

4.6. Western Blot

Cells were seeded at a density of 1×10^6 cells/100 mm plate and allowed to attach before being treated with saffron, safranal, and crocin for 24 h. Whole cell extracts were isolated using the RIPA buffer (Sigma Aldrich, St. Louis, MO, USA) and protease inhibitors (Sigma Aldrich, St. Louis, MO, USA). The concentration of the isolated proteins was determined using the BCA Protein Assay Reagent (Bio-Rad, Hercules, CA, USA). Thirty micrograms of protein were separated using 10–15% SDS Polyacrylamide gel electrophoresis in our lab. Proteins were transferred onto PVDF membranes (Bio-Rad, Hercules, CA, USA). Membranes were then blocked using 5% BSA (Bovine Serum Albumin) (Sigma Aldrich, St. Louis, MO, USA) followed by incubation with various primary antibodies against CDC25b, p.H2AX, TDP1, and Pro-caspase 3 (1:2000) (Cell Signaling Technology, Danvers, MA, USA) and appropriate secondary antibodies, HRP conjugated (Cell Signaling Technology, Danvers, MA, USA). GAPDH (1:10,000) (Abcam, Cambridge, UK) was used as the loading control. Protein bands were detected using the Westernsure Chemiluminescent Substrate (LI-COR, Lincoln, NE, USA). The experiment was carried out in triplicates.

4.7. Statistical Analysis

An ANOVA (Analysis of Variance) test was carried out (<0.05). All statistical analyses were conducted using the GraphPad Prism 8 software (San Diego, CA, USA).

5. Conclusions

In this study, the colorectal cell line HCT116 and derivatives with MLH1 and/or MSH3 added genes were treated with saffron and its main compounds, safranal and crocin. The treatment inhibited cell proliferation and blocked cell invasion. On further investigation, it was deduced that the mechanism of action for inhibiting the proliferation was by modulating the cell cycle and DNA damage and repair system. The treatment had also manifested pro-apoptotic properties. It is noteworthy, that the different cells did not respond in a particular manner to the different treatments conducted, nor had the compounds expressed any pattern for a particular cell type. The differential effects of saffron and its main components safranal and crocin in the different tested cell lines, might be capitalized on to develop specific compound protocols in patients with different types of genetic instability in their tumors. In vivo testing in mice models of MSI and MSS CRC is needed to potentially translate these findings in human subjects with such tumors. If confirmed, saffron as an adjuvant therapy might even be recommended for patients' MSI tumors regardless of the nature of the primary cancer.

Author Contributions: Conceptualization, H.A. and A.A.; methodology, A.S., A.A., C.M., G.G. and F.P.; data curation, A.S., A.F., A.A., C.M.; writing—review and editing, H.A., A.A., H.B., G.G., F.P.; supervision, H.A., A.A.; project administration, H.A.; funding acquisition, H.A., A.A. All authors have read and agreed to the published version of the manuscript.

Funding: This research and the APC was funded for A.A. by Zayed Center for Health Sciences grant number 31R174, Terry Fox grant number 21S103 and (in part) by the National Institute on Minority Health and Health Disparities of the National Institutes of Health under Award Number G12MD007597. The funders had no role in study design, data collection and analysis, decision to publish, or preparation of the manuscript.

Institutional Review Board Statement: Not applicable.

Informed Consent Statement: Not applicable.

Data Availability Statement: All data are presented in this study.

Acknowledgments: We would like to thank Michael Surette and his laboratory for the support in the microbiota work. We also thank all saffron growers and gp-food.com (http://www.gp-food.com/index.php/about-us.html) (accessed on 3 May 2021) for providing saffron.

Conflicts of Interest: The authors declare no conflict of interest. The funders had no role in the design of the study; in the collection, analyses, or interpretation of data; in the writing of the manuscript, or in the decision to publish the results.

Sample Availability: Not Applicable.

References

1. Ashktorab, H.; Kupfer, S.S.; Brim, H.; Carethers, J.M. Racial Disparity in Gastrointestinal Cancer Risk. *Gastroenterology* **2017**, *153*, 910–923. [CrossRef]
2. Jung, G.; Hernández-Illán, E.; Moreira, L.; Balaguer, F.; Goel, A. Epigenetics of colorectal cancer: Biomarker and therapeutic potential. *Nat. Rev. Gastroenterol. Hepatol.* **2020**, *17*, 111–130. [CrossRef]
3. Keum, N.; Giovannucci, E. Global burden of colorectal cancer: Emerging trends, risk factors and prevention strategies. *Nat. Rev. Gastroenterol. Hepatol.* **2019**, *16*, 713–732. [CrossRef] [PubMed]
4. Ashktorab, H.; Azimi, H.; Varma, S.; Tavakoli, P.; Nickerson, M.L.; Brim, H. Distinctive DNA mismatch repair and APC rare variants in African Americans with colorectal neoplasia. *Oncotarget* **2017**, *8*, 99966–99977. [CrossRef]
5. Zhang, J.; Roberts, T.M.; Shivdasani, R.A. Targeting PI3K Signaling as a Therapeutic Approach for Colorectal Cancer. *Gastroenterology* **2011**, *141*, 50–61. [CrossRef]
6. Takemasa, I.; Yamamoto, H.; Sekimoto, M.; Ohue, M.; Noura, S.; Miyake, Y.; Matsumoto, T.; Aihara, T.; Tomita, N.; Tamaki, Y.; et al. Overexpression of CDC25B phosphatase as a novel marker of poor prognosis of human colorectal carcinoma. *Cancer Res.* **2000**, *60*, 3043–3050. [PubMed]
7. Ashktorab, H.; Soleimani, A.; Singh, G.; Amin, A.; Tabtabaei, S.; Latella, G.; Stein, U.; Akhondzadeh, S.; Solanki, N.; Gondré-Lewis, M.C.; et al. Saffron: The Golden Spice with Therapeutic Properties on Digestive Diseases. *Nutrients* **2019**, *11*, 943. [CrossRef] [PubMed]
8. Al-Hrout, A.; Chaiboonchoe, A.; Khraiwesh, B.; Murali, C.; Baig, B.; El-Awady, R.; Tarazi, H.; Alzahmi, A.; Nelson, D.R.; Greish, Y.E.; et al. Safranal induces DNA double-strand breakage and ER-stress-mediated cell death in hepatocellular carcinoma cells. *Sci. Rep.* **2018**, *8*, 16951. [CrossRef] [PubMed]
9. Amin, A.; AHamza, A.; Daoud, S.; Khazanehdari, K.; Al Hrout, A.; Baig, B. Saffron-Based Crocin Prevents Early Lesions of Liver Cancer: In vivo, In vitro and Network Analyses. *Recent Pat. Anti Cancer Drug Discov.* **2016**, *11*, 121–133. [CrossRef] [PubMed]
10. Amin, A.; Bajbouj, K.; Koch, A.; Gandesiri, M.; Schneider-Stock, R. Defective autophagosome formation in p53-null colorectal cancer reinforces crocin-induced apoptosis. *Int. J. Mol. Sci.* **2015**, *16*, 1544–1561. [CrossRef] [PubMed]
11. Amin, A.; Hamza, A.A.; Bajbouj, K.; Ashraf, S.S.; Daoud, S. Saffron: A potential candidate for a novel anticancer drug against hepatocellular carcinoma. *Hepatology* **2011**, *54*, 857–867. [CrossRef] [PubMed]
12. Milajerdi, A.; Djafarian, K.; Hosseini, B. The toxicity of saffron (*Crocus sativus* L.) and its constituents against normal and cancer cells. *J. Nutr. Intermed. Metab.* **2016**, *3*, 23–32.
13. Wang, G.; Zhang, B.; Wang, Y.; Han, S.; Wang, C. Crocin promotes apoptosis of human skin cancer cells by inhibiting the JAK/STAT pathway. *Exp. Ther. Med.* **2018**, *16*, 5079–5084. [CrossRef] [PubMed]
14. Bajbouj, K.; Schulze-Luehrmann, J.; Diermeier, S.; Amin, A.; Schneider-Stock, R. The anticancer effect of saffron in two p53 isogenic colorectal cancer cell lines. *BMC Complement. Altern. Med.* **2012**, *12*, 69. [CrossRef]
15. Feehan, A.K.; Velasco, C.; Fort, D.; Burton, J.H.; Price-Haywood, E.G.; Katzmarzyk, P.T. Racial and Workplace Disparities in Seroprevalence of SARS-CoV-2, Baton Rouge, Louisiana, USA. *Emerg. Infect. Dis.* **2021**, *27*, 314. [CrossRef]
16. Thanikachalam, K.; Khan, G. Colorectal Cancer and Nutrition. *Nutrients* **2019**, *11*, 164. [CrossRef]
17. Güllü, N.; Kobelt, D.; Brim, H.; Rahman, S.; Timm, L.; Smith, J.; Soleimani, A.; Di Marco, S.; Bisti, S.; Ashktorab, H.; et al. Saffron Crudes and Compounds Restrict MACC1-Dependent Cell Proliferation and Migration of Colorectal Cancer Cells. *Cells* **2020**, *9*, 1829. [CrossRef]
18. Jabini, R.; Ehtesham-Gharaee, M.; Dalirsani, Z.; Mosaffa, F.; Delavarian, Z.; Behravan, J. Evaluation of the Cytotoxic Activity of Crocin and Safranal, Constituents of Saffron, in Oral Squamous Cell Carcinoma (KB Cell Line). *Nutr. Cancer* **2017**, *69*, 911–919. [CrossRef]
19. Wang, J.; Ke, Y.; Shu, T. Crocin has pharmacological effects against the pathological behavior of colon cancer cells by interacting with the STAT3 signaling pathway. *Exp. Ther. Med.* **2020**, *19*, 1297–1303. [CrossRef]
20. Malaekeh-Nikouei, B.; Mousavi, S.H.; Shahsavand, S.; Mehri, S.; Nassirli, H.; Moallem, S.A. Assessment of Cytotoxic Properties of Safranal and Nanoliposomal Safranal in Various Cancer Cell Lines. *Phytother. Res.* **2013**, *27*, 1868–1873. [CrossRef]
21. Feng, B.; Dong, T.T.; Wang, L.L.; Zhou, H.M.; Zhao, H.C.; Dong, F.; Zheng, M.H. Colorectal cancer migration and invasion initiated by microRNA-106a. *PLoS ONE* **2012**, *7*, e43452. [CrossRef]
22. Li, X.; Huang, T.; Jiang, G.; Gong, W.; Qian, H.; Zou, C. Synergistic apoptotic effect of crocin and cisplatin on osteosarcoma cells via caspase induced apoptosis. *Toxicol. Lett.* **2013**, *221*, 197–204. [CrossRef] [PubMed]
23. Zhou, Y.; Xu, Q.; Shang, J.; Lu, L.; Chen, G. Crocin inhibits the migration, invasion, and epithelial-mesenchymal transition of gastric cancer cells via miR-320/KLF5/HIF-1α signaling. *J. Cell. Physiol.* **2019**, *234*, 17876–17885. [CrossRef] [PubMed]
24. Dalvai, M.; Mondesert, O.; Bugler, B.; Manenti, S.; Ducommun, B.; Dozier, C. Doxorubicin promotes transcriptional upregulation of Cdc25B in cancer cells by releasing Sp1 from the promoter. *Oncogene* **2012**, *32*, 5123–5128. [CrossRef]
25. Mousavi, S.H.; Tavakkol-Afshari, J.; Brook, A.; Jafari-Anarkooli, I. Role of caspases and Bax protein in saffron-induced apoptosis in MCF-7 cells. *Food Chem. Toxicol.* **2009**, *47*, 1909–1913. [CrossRef]
26. Tavakkol-Afshari, J.; Brook, A.; Mousavi, S.H. Study of cytotoxic and apoptogenic properties of saffron extract in human cancer cell lines. *Food Chem. Toxicol.* **2008**, *46*, 3443–3447. [CrossRef] [PubMed]
27. Hoshyar, R.; Bathaie, S.Z.; Sadeghizadeh, M. Crocin Triggers the Apoptosis Through Increasing the Bax/Bcl-2 Ratio and Caspase Activation in Human Gastric Adenocarcinoma, AGS, Cells. *DNA Cell Biol.* **2013**, *32*, 50–57. [CrossRef] [PubMed]

28. Vali, F.; Changizi, V.; Safa, M. Synergistic Apoptotic Effect of Crocin and Paclitaxel or Crocin and Radiation on MCF-7 Cells, a Type of Breast Cancer Cell Line. *Int. J. Breast Cancer* **2015**, *2015*, 1–7. [CrossRef]
29. Koi, M.; Umar, A.; Chauhan, D.P.; Cherian, S.P.; Carethers, J.M.; Kunkei, T.A.; Boland, C.R. Human chromosome 3 corrects mismatch repair deficiency and microsatellite instability and reduces N-methyl-N'-nitro-N-nitrosoguanidine tolerance in colon tumor cells with homozygous hMLH1 mutation. *Cancer Res.* **1994**, *54*, 4308–4312.
30. Jacob, S.; Aguado, M.; Fallik, D.; Praz, F. The role of the DNA mismatch repair system in the cytotoxicity of the topoisomerase inhibitors camptothecin and etoposide to human colorectal cancer cells. *Cancer Res.* **2001**, *61*, 6555–6562.
31. Tentori, L.; Muzi, A.; Dorio, A.S.; Dolci, S.; Campolo, F.; Vernole, P.; Lacal, P.M.; Praz, F.; Graziani, G. MSH3 expression does not influence the sensitivity of colon cancer HCT116 cell line to oxaliplatin and poly(ADP-ribose) polymerase (PARP) inhibitor as monotherapy or in combination. *Cancer Chemother. Pharmacol.* **2013**, *72*, 117–125. [CrossRef] [PubMed]

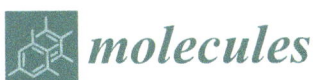

Article

Phytochemical Differentiation of Saffron (*Crocus sativus* L.) by High Resolution Mass Spectrometry Metabolomic Studies

Evangelos Gikas [1], Nikolaos Stavros Koulakiotis [2] and Anthony Tsarbopoulos [2,3,*]

1. Department of Chemistry, National and Kapodistrian University of Athens, 15771 Athens, Greece; vgikas@chem.uoa.gr
2. GAIA Research Center, Bioanalytical Department, The Goulandris Natural History Museum, 14562 Kifissia, Greece; koulak13@gmail.com
3. Department of Pharmacology, Medical School, National and Kapodistrian University of Athens, 11527 Athens, Greece
* Correspondence: atsarbop@med.uoa.gr; Tel.: +30-210-7462-702

Abstract: The metabolite profiling of saffron (*Crocus sativus* L.) from several countries was measured by using ultra-performance liquid chromatography combined with high resolution mass spectrometry (UPLC-HR MS). Multivariate statistical analysis was employed to distinguish among the several samples of *C. sativus* L. from Greece, Italy, Morocco, Iran, India, Afghanistan and Kashmir. The results of this study showed that the phytochemical content in the samples of *C. sativus* L. were obviously diverse in the different countries of origin. The metabolomics approach was deemed to be the most suitable in order to evaluate the enormous array of putative metabolites among the saffron samples studied, and was able to provide a comparative phytochemical screening of these samples. Several markers have been identified that aided the differentiation of a group from its counterparts. This can be important for the selection of the appropriate saffron sample, in view of its health-promoting effect which occurs through the modulation of various biological and physiological processes.

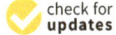

Keywords: *Crocus sativus* L. (Iridaceae); saffron; reversed-phase UPLC; metabolomics; HR MS

Citation: Gikas, E.; Koulakiotis, N.S.; Tsarbopoulos, A. Phytochemical Differentiation of Saffron (*Crocus sativus* L.) by High Resolution Mass Spectrometry Metabolomic Studies. *Molecules* **2021**, *26*, 2180. https://doi.org/10.3390/molecules26082180

Academic Editor: Nikolaos Pitsikas

Received: 6 March 2021
Accepted: 5 April 2021
Published: 10 April 2021

Publisher's Note: MDPI stays neutral with regard to jurisdictional claims in published maps and institutional affiliations.

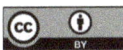

Copyright: © 2021 by the authors. Licensee MDPI, Basel, Switzerland. This article is an open access article distributed under the terms and conditions of the Creative Commons Attribution (CC BY) license (https://creativecommons.org/licenses/by/4.0/).

1. Introduction

Crocus sativus L. is a species of flowering plant of the Crocus genus which grows in the Mediterranean, east Asia and the Irano-Turanian region. *Crocus sativus* L. is a member of the Iridaceae family, and is cultivated worldwide due to the use of its dried styles (the uppermost colored part of which is referred to as stigma), not only as a spice (saffron), but also in health management since ancient times [1,2]. Saffron is a perennial spicy herb which is difficult to be cultivated since it demands a special climate and soil conditions. The earliest apparent reference to *Crocus sativus* L. cultivation goes back to around 2300 BC, and a saffron harvest is shown in a Minoan fresco painting in the Knossos palace of Minoan Crete dated from 1600–1500 BC [3]. It is also seen in a fresco in Akrotiri on the Greek island of Thera dated back in 1627 BC [4], which depicts the flowers being picked by young girls and monkeys. The most plausible ancestor of *Crocus sativus* L. was *Crocus cartwrightianus* [5–7], as derived from morphological [5], cytological [8] and molecular analyses [9].

Saffron is the spice derived from the flower of *Crocus sativus* which is comprised of the three red stigmas included in the flower that are consequently collected and dried under special conditions to produce the final saffron as a spice. Crocus contains more than 150 volatile aromatic substances that afford its distinctive aroma, and a large number of non-volatiles such as carotenoids including zeaxanthin, lycopene, as well as various α- and β-carotenes, glycosides, monoterpenes, aldehydes, flavonoids, anthocyanins, vitamins (especially riboflavin and thiamine) and amino acids [10]. The four main bioactive constitutes of saffron stigma are crocetin, crocins, picrocrocin and safranal [11]. In previous studies, the volatile compounds of saffron samples have been characterized by gas chromatography–mass spectrometry (GC–MS) methods [12,13], and have been evaluated as markers of geographic differentiation [14]. In a recent study, the metabolite profiling of three different parts of *Crocus sativus* L., i.e., tepals, stigmas and stamens, was measured by ultra-performance liquid chromatography (UPLC) coupled to hybrid quadrupole time-of-flight mass spectrometry (QqTOF MS), which provided the diverse chemical characteristics of the parts of the flower [15]. In the last 20 years, there has been an increasing amount of scientific data on saffron extract or its constituent's biological activity and health-promoting properties, including use as an anticonvulsant [16], anti-inflammatory [17], anti-tumor [18], anti-oxidant [19], antiatherogenic [20] and has shown antidepressant [21] activity, as well as enhancement of learning and memory capacity [22,23]. Therefore, saffron and its ingredients can be useful in the treatment of a variety of diseases such as neurodegenerative disorders, blood pressure abnormalities, acute and/or chronic inflammatory disease and coronary artery disease. The main bioactive constituents in saffron are the crocins existing mainly in the stigmas, and they are mono- and bis-esters of crocetin with glucose, gentiobiose and/or gentiotriose [24]. The esterification of crocetin with varying number of hydrophilic gentiobiose(s), or any other sugar precursors, renders the carotenoid derivative water soluble, a property that gives crocus its pigmentation properties. The complexity of crocins may result from the incorporation of various sugars connected to crocetin such as glucose, gentiobiose, gentiotriose and neapolitanose, the number carbohydrate units (1–5), the number of glycosylation sites (1,), their linkage to the acid moiety of the carotenoid, or even by the varying number of repeating units in crocin [25]. Therefore, there is a huge range of crocins, with most of them being found only in trace amounts. To date, the majority of studies performed support the therapeutic potential of crocins in treating aging and age-related neurodegenerative disorders. The major crocin component, *trans*-crocin-4 (TC4; bis-gentiobiosyl-E-crocetin) possesses numerous pharmacological activities including antihypertensive [26], anxiolytic [27] and neuroprotective [28] activity. In particular, TC4 has shown the highest inhibitory potential towards reducing or even preventing amyloid oligomerization [29], which is considered as one of the main causes of Alzheimer disease (AD) progression [30]. Conversely, the characteristic flavor of saffron is due to picrocrocin, the glucoside of the terpene aldehyde safranal, which comprises more than 4% of the dry weight of saffron. Safranal is produced by the oxidative cleavage of the carotenoid zeaxanthine, and accounts for more than 70% of the volatile fraction of the spice. Saffron is likely the most expensive spice, owing to its very limited geographical spread and the difficulty of its collection. The higher content of the analyzed saffron samples in crocin, picrocrocin and safranal indicates the higher value of saffron.

We know that plant secondary metabolites are a group of naturally occurring compounds biosynthesized by differing biochemical pathways, and their plant content and regulation is strongly amenable to environmental influences as well as to potential herbal predators [31–33]. Moreover, the level and type of secondary metabolites is strongly influenced by the geoclimatic characteristics of the cultivation area as well as the preparation procedures and traditions followed in that area. Therefore, there is a necessity to identify the content of bioactive compounds in collected saffron samples and explore whether there is any correlation between different geographical regions and the contents of the bioactive compounds.

The aim of the current study is to explore the chemical space of *Crocus sativus* L. from different geographical regions in order to spot chemotaxonomic differences in the indigenous species. This could potentially aid towards our understanding of the plant's biochemistry but also the precise evaluation of its cultivation in diverse environments. We employ a metabolomics methodology based on UPLC high resolution mass spectrometry (HR–MS) in order to provide detailed information on the metabolite profiling of several samples of *C. sativus* L. from Greece and six other countries/areas: Italy, Morocco, Iran, India, Afghanistan and Kashmir. The metabolomics approach was deemed to be the most suitable choice in order to evaluate the enormous array of putative metabolites among the saffron samples studied, and thus provide a comparative phytochemical screening of the saffron samples studied.

2. Results and Discussion

2.1. UPLC-MS Analysis

A representative base peak LC–MS chromatogram of the stigma extract is shown in Figure 1. Several peaks have been annotated in the early eluting part of the chromatogram with the names of the putative metabolites shown in Table 1.

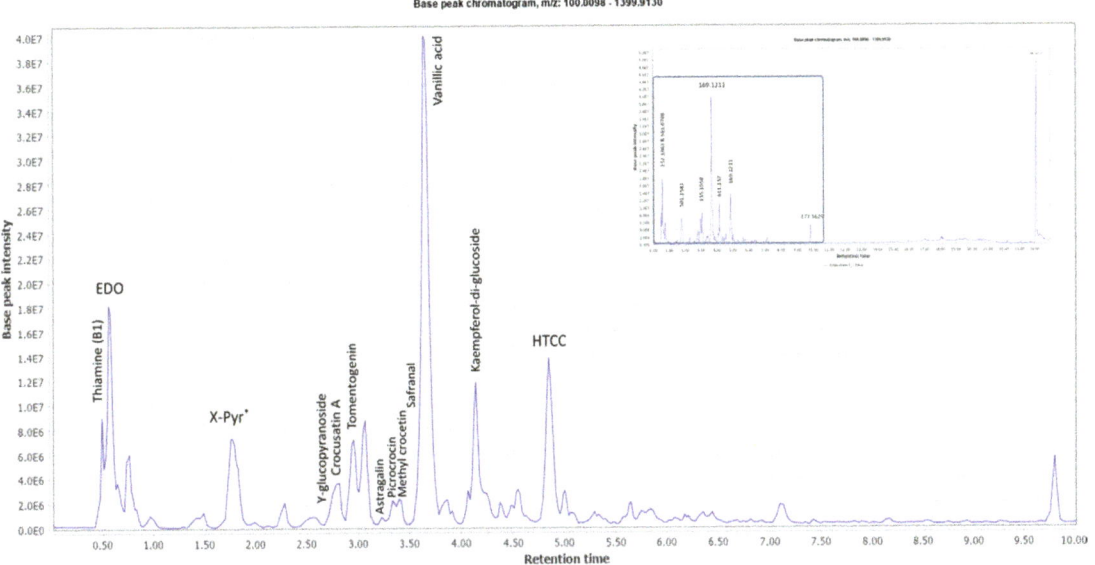

Figure 1. Characteristic ultra-performance liquid chromatography coupled to high resolution mass spectrometry (UPLC-HR MS) base peak chromatogram of the stigma extract from the *C. sativus* L. sample from India. This represents the early eluting part of the chromatogram shown in the inset. Several peaks have been annotated in the early eluting part of the chromatogram with the names of the putative metabolites shown in Table 1. * X-Pyr: 3,4,5-Trimethoxyphenol-1-O-[β-D-apiofuranosyl-(1→6)]]-β-D-glucopyranoside.

The mapping of the chemical potential of saffron according to its geographical spread is of significant importance in the effort to understand evolutional pressure exerted on the species, as well as to provide a chemotaxonomic tool towards the distribution of variants around the world (Figure 2). The content of the active secondary metabolites has an apparent effect on the quality as well as the medical properties of saffron. Furthermore, the extreme cost of the *Crocus sativus* L. stigmas, considered as the most valuable spice, mandates their accurate fingerprinting in order to control its quality. In order to capture the chemical space involved, as well as to compare the species in a holistic manner, an HRMS metabolomics approach was taken.

Specimens from seven representative regions capturing saffron's biodiversity around the world, namely Iran, Greece, Italy, Afghanistan, Kashmir, Morocco, and India were analyzed. The pairwise comparison of all possible combinations of the saffron specimen was employed, as this approach effectively highlights the differences between species regardless of their magnitude. In the case of a "total" comparison, the model would be dominated by the largest variance, and therefore would be biased towards the species with the largest pairwise differences. Figure 2 depicts the regions of collected specimens of saffron samples. The associated clusters are illustrated and interconnected in different colors, such as those between Greece and Morocco with saffron samples in orange, whereas those between India and Afghan specimens are indicated by green. These interconnections have been revealed in the multivariate statistical analysis (Figure 3).

Table 1. Cumulative table of the **A.** Multivariate statistics **B.** Identifying discriminating features and **C.** Putative metabolite annotation with the calculated protonated molecular ion (MH+) or the adduct ion mass signals shown in parenthesis, whereas the fragment ions are denoted in curly brackets.

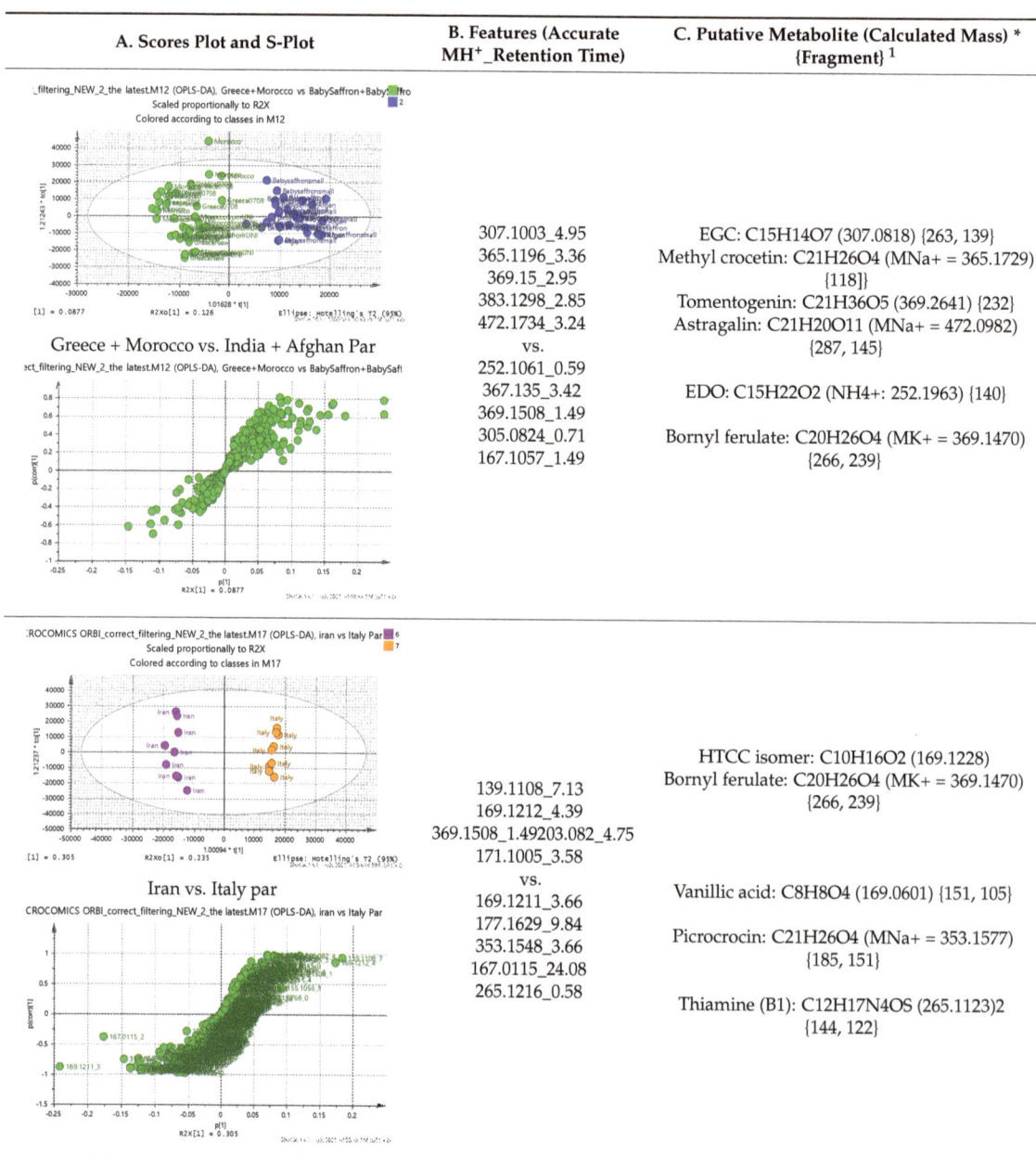

A. Scores Plot and S-Plot	B. Features (Accurate MH+_Retention Time)	C. Putative Metabolite (Calculated Mass) * {Fragment} [1]
Greece + Morocco vs. India + Afghan Par	307.1003_4.95 365.1196_3.36 369.15_2.95 383.1298_2.85 472.1734_3.24 vs. 252.1061_0.59 367.135_3.42 369.1508_1.49 305.0824_0.71 167.1057_1.49	EGC: C15H14O7 (307.0818) {263, 139} Methyl crocetin: C21H26O4 (MNa+ = 365.1729) {118]} Tomentogenin: C21H36O5 (369.2641) {232} Astragalin: C21H20O11 (MNa+ = 472.0982) {287, 145} EDO: C15H22O2 (NH4+: 252.1963) {140} Bornyl ferulate: C20H26O4 (MK+ = 369.1470) {266, 239}
Iran vs. Italy par	139.1108_7.13 169.1212_4.39 369.1508_1.49203.082_4.75 171.1005_3.58 vs. 169.1211_3.66 177.1629_9.84 353.1548_3.66 167.0115_24.08 265.1216_0.58	HTCC isomer: C10H16O2 (169.1228) Bornyl ferulate: C20H26O4 (MK+ = 369.1470) {266, 239} Vanillic acid: C8H8O4 (169.0601) {151, 105} Picrocrocin: C21H26O4 (MNa+ = 353.1577) {185, 151} Thiamine (B1): C12H17N4OS (265.1123)2 {144, 122}

Table 1. Cont.

A. Scores Plot and S-Plot	B. Features (Accurate MH+_Retention Time)	C. Putative Metabolite (Calculated Mass) * {Fragment} [1]
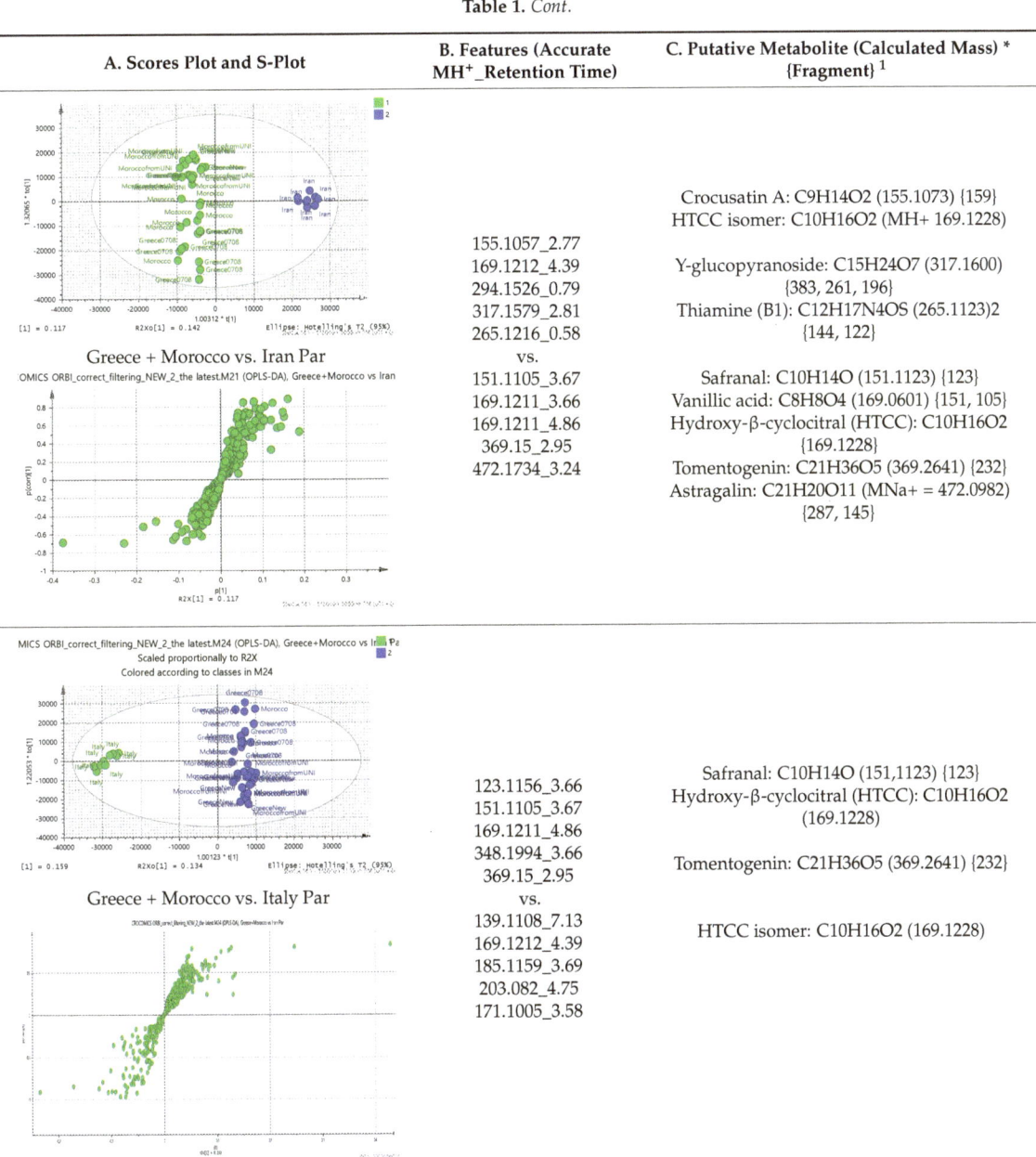 Greece + Morocco vs. Iran Par	155.1057_2.77 169.1212_4.39 294.1526_0.79 317.1579_2.81 265.1216_0.58 vs. 151.1105_3.67 169.1211_3.66 169.1211_4.86 369.15_2.95 472.1734_3.24	Crocusatin A: C9H14O2 (155.1073) {159} HTCC isomer: C10H16O2 (MH+ 169.1228) Y-glucopyranoside: C15H24O7 (317.1600) {383, 261, 196} Thiamine (B1): C12H17N4OS (265.1123)2 {144, 122} Safranal: C10H14O (151.1123) {123} Vanillic acid: C8H8O4 (169.0601) {151, 105} Hydroxy-β-cyclocitral (HTCC): C10H16O2 {169.1228} Tomentogenin: C21H36O5 (369.2641) {232} Astragalin: C21H20O11 (MNa+ = 472.0982) {287, 145}
Greece + Morocco vs. Italy Par	123.1156_3.66 151.1105_3.67 169.1211_4.86 348.1994_3.66 369.15_2.95 vs. 139.1108_7.13 169.1212_4.39 185.1159_3.69 203.082_4.75 171.1005_3.58	Safranal: C10H14O (151,1123) {123} Hydroxy-β-cyclocitral (HTCC): C10H16O2 (169.1228) Tomentogenin: C21H36O5 (369.2641) {232} HTCC isomer: C10H16O2 (169.1228)

Table 1. *Cont.*

A. Scores Plot and S-Plot	B. Features (Accurate MH+_Retention Time)	C. Putative Metabolite (Calculated Mass) * {Fragment} [1]
India + Afghan vs. Iran Par	252.1061_0.59 294.1526_0.79 280.1373_0.73 265.1216_0.58 606.229_4.15 vs. 151.1105_3.67 169.1211_3.66 169.1211_4.86369.15_2.95 472.1734_3.24	EDO: C15H22O2 (NH4+: 252.1963) {140} Thiamine (B1): C12H17N4OS (265.1123)2 {144, 122} Safranal: C10H14O (151.1123) Vanillic acid: C8H8O4 (169.0601) {151, 105} Hydroxy-β-cyclocitral (HTCC): C10H16O2 (169.1228) Tomentogenin: C21H36O5 (369.2641) {232} Astragalin: C21H20O11 (MNa+ = 472.0982) {287, 145}
India + Afghan vs. Italy Par	139.1108_7.13 169.1212_4.39 252.1061_0.59 369.1508_1.49 203.082_4.75 vs. 151.1105_3.67 169.1211_3.66 353.1548_3.66 365.1196_3.36 369.15_2.95	HTCC isomer: C10H16O2 (169.1228) EDO: C15H22O2 (MNH4+ = 252.1963) {140} Bornyl ferulate: C20H26O4 (MK+ = 369.1470) {266, 239} Safranal: C10H14O (151.1123) Vanillic acid: C8H8O4 (169.0601) {151, 105} Picrocrocin: C21H26O4 (MNa+ = 353.1577) {185, 151} Methyl crocetin: C21H26O4 (MNa+ = 365.1729) {118} Tomentogenin: C21H36O5 (369.2641) {232}

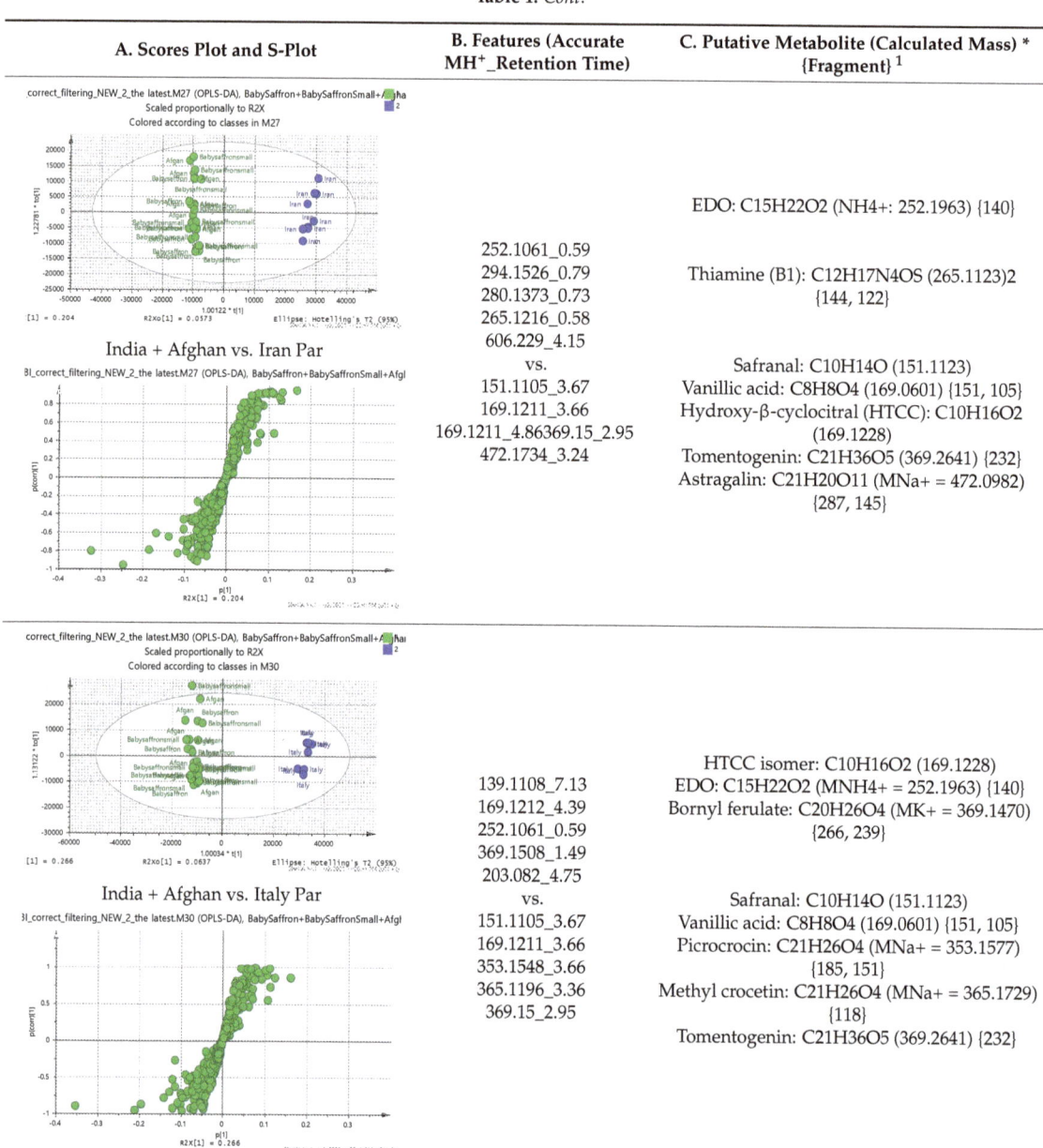

Table 1. Cont.

A. Scores Plot and S-Plot	B. Features (Accurate MH⁺_Retention Time)	C. Putative Metabolite (Calculated Mass) * {Fragment} [1]
Afghan + India vs. Kashmir Par	155.1057_2.77 307.1003_4.95 317.1579_2.81 331.173_3.66 364.1944_2.96 vs. 151.1105_3.67 151.1105_4.86 169.1211_3.66 169.1211_4.86 611.157_4.14	Crocusatin A: C9H14O2 (155.1073) EGC: C15H14O7 (307.0818) {263, 139} Y-glucopyranoside: C15H24O7 (317.1600) Picrocrocin: C16H26O7 (331.1757) {185, 151} Methyl crocetin-C21H26O4 (MNa+ = 365.1729) {118} Safranal: C10H14O (151.1123) {123} Vanillic acid: C8H8O4 (169.0601) {151, 105} Hydroxy-β-cyclocitral (HTCC): C10H16O2 (169.1228) Kaempferol-di-glucoside: C27H30O16 (611.1611) {287}
Greece + Morocco vs. Kashmir Par	155.1057_2.77 183.1005_3.33 307.1003_4.95 317.1579_2.81 331.173_3.66 vs. 151.1105_3.67 151.1105_4.86 169.1211_3.66 169.1211_4.86 611.157_4.14	Crocusatin A: C9H14O2 (155.1073) EGC: C15H14O7 (307.0818) {263, 139} Y-glucopyranoside: C15H24O7 (317.1600) Picrocrocin: C16H26O7 (331.1757) {185, 151} Safranal: C10H14O (151.1123) {123} Vanillic acid: C8H8O4 (169.0601) {151, 105} Hydroxy-β-cyclocitral (HTCC): C10H16O2 (169.1228) Kaempferol-di-glucoside: C27H30O16 (611.1611) {287}

Table 1. Cont.

A. Scores Plot and S-Plot	B. Features (Accurate MH+_Retention Time)	C. Putative Metabolite (Calculated Mass) * {Fragment} [1]
Italy vs. Kashmir Par	169.1211_3.66 307.1003_4.95 331.173_3.66 353.1548_3.66 369.15_2.95 vs. 169.1212_4.39 252.1061_0.59 369.1508_1.49 203.082_4.75 611.157_4.14	Vanillic acid: C8H8O4 (169.0601) {151, 105} EGC: C15H14O7 (307.0818) {263, 139} Picrocrocin: C16H26O7 (331.1757) {185, 151} Picrocrocin: C16H26O7 (MNa+ = 353.1577) {185, 151} Tomentogenin: C21H36O5 (369.2641) {232} HTCC isomer: C10H16O2 (169.1228) EDO: C15H22O2 (MNH4+ = 252.1963) {140} Bornyl ferulate: C20H26O4 (MK+ = 369.1470) {266, 239} Kaempferol-di-glucoside: C27H30O16 (611.1611) {287}
Iran vs. Kashmir Par	169.1211_3.66 307.1003_4.95 331.173_3.66 369.15_2.95 511.1749_4.94 vs. 252.1061_0.59 294.1526_0.79 280.1373_0.73 265.1216_0.58 611.157_4.14	Vanillic acid: C8H8O4 (169.0601) {151, 105} EGC: C15H14O7 (307. 0818) {263, 139} Picrocrocin: C16H26O7 (331.1757) {185, 151} Tomentogenin: C21H36O5 (369.2641) {232} EDO: C15H22O2 (MNH4+ = 252.1963) {140} Thiamine (B1): C12H17N4OS (265.1123)[2] {144, 122} Kaempferol-di-glucoside: C27H30O16 (611.1611) {287}

* The calculated mass values correspond to the protonated molecular ion (MH+) ion or the adduct ion (e.g., with Na or K) shown in parenthesis. [1] The fragment ions for the selected precursor ions are shown in curly brackets. [2] In case of thiamine, the M+ ion is observed instead of MH+, as the compound has a fixed positive charge. Abbreviations: HTCC: Hydroxy-β-cyclocitral; EGC: Epigallocatechin; EDO: Epoxybisabola-7(14),10-dien-2-one.

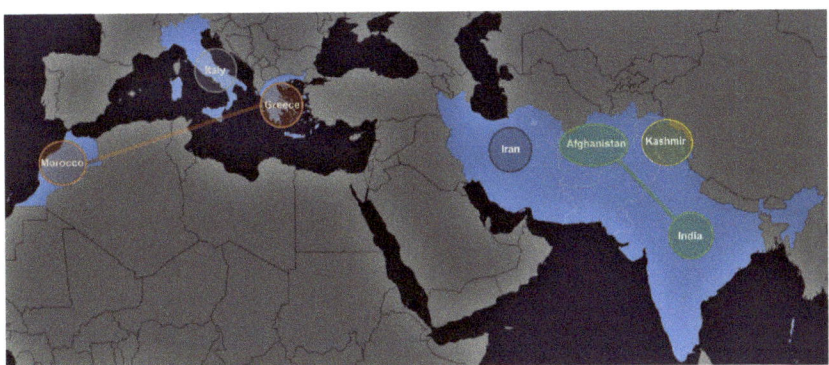

Figure 2. Regions of collected specimens of saffron samples along with their associated cluster.

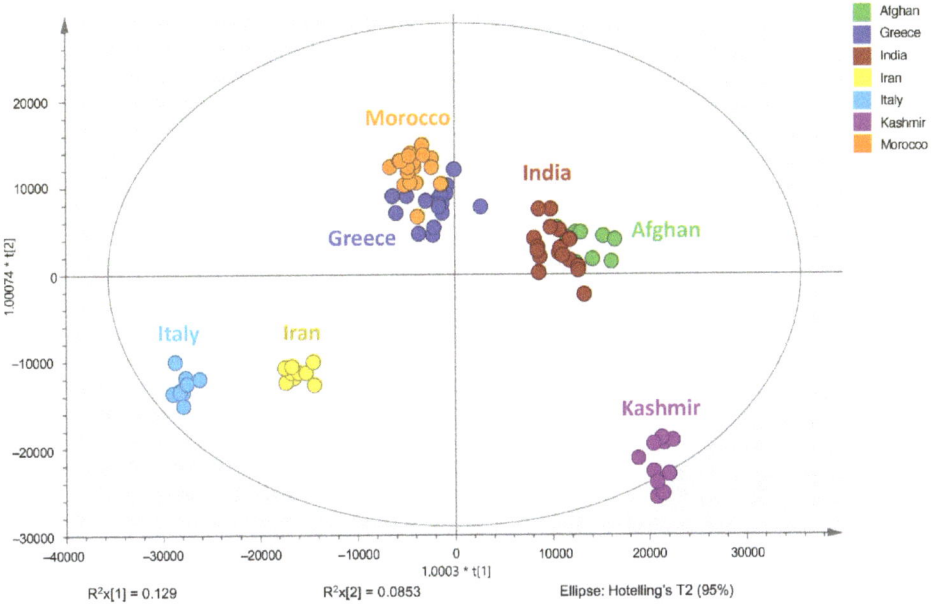

Figure 3. Orthogonal Projections to Latent Structures Discriminant Analysis (oPLS-DA) (**Par scaling**) of the seven saffron species examined.

2.2. Multivariate Statistical Analysis

In order to gain insight into the chemical space covered by the genus, as well as to discover trends and spot any possible outliers, a Principal Component Analysis (PCA) analysis was performed employing Pareto scaling. No significant clustering was apparent, but also no outlier values were detected. The R^2 was 0.707 with the Q^2 being 0.49 (7-fold cross validation). In order to further explore potentially significant markers among the samples, orthogonal Projections to Latent Structures Discriminant Analysis (oPLS-DA) was applied to enhance separation among the groups in PCA. The oPLS-DA algorithm was used in order to explore for underlying associations existing in the data, as it is considered a more efficient discriminating algorithm. Using Par scaling, clear clustering has been observed showing five clusters of samples, as depicted in Figure 3.

Thus, each one of the species found in Italy Iran and Kashmir were allocated to unique clusters as their only members, while Greece formed a cluster with Morocco, and Indian and Afghan saffron species formed another cluster. The model exhibited excellent fitting ($R^2 = 0.896$) and predictive power ($Q^2 = 0.688$).

In order to focus on differentiating metabolites between species, all pairwise oPLS-DA models between the five groups were constructed. Ten models were constructed as shown in Table 1. All models were validated by permutation testing, whereas ANalysis Of VAriance testing of Cross-Validated predictive residuals (CV-ANOVA) was used to verify the statistical significance of the model ($p < 0.05$). To verify the validity of the multivariate analysis concerning the generated models, the Hottelings T2 and the DModX were evaluated, and were considered as valid when no value exceeds the d-critical level set to 0.05. The residuals normality was also considered and examined for values deviating from normality. In order to discover the most influential features for the construction of each model, the corresponding S-plot was evaluated in every case, where the most differentiated metabolites for each compared group can be distinguished. Therefore, the Paretto based models were considered, whereas the VIP values were also considered in the process. As a rule of thumb, the five major features from each group of each pairwise comparison were investigated. All features identified in the manuscript are at identification level four [34]. The big three MS methodologies employed (MS, MS/MS and HR MS) gave access to corresponding fragmentation used for the assignment of probable structure through MS/MS. Features were attributed to metabolites based on multiple criteria, i.e., that the accurate mass should not deviate more than 10 ppm from its theoretical value, the isotopic pattern should show a score of >90, while the MS/MS fragments should be present with unit resolution (as they were acquired in the linear ion trap using a parallel scan). The second column in Table 1 lists the accurate protonated molecular ions MH^+ with their respective retention times, whereas the third column lists the putative metabolites and the corresponding fragment ions (in brackets) obtained in the linear ion trap using a parallel scan. The metabolites tabulated in Table 1 are the ones that are upregulated in the first pair (e.g., Greece and Morocco) and downregulated in the counterpart pair of the comparison (e.g., India and Afghan). It should be noted that there was no need to employ crocin standards available in our laboratory for the identification of putative metabolites, because none of them was identified to be significantly differentiated between the saffron samples analyzed, thus not assisting the discrimination of their geographical origin.

2.3. Geographical Region Differentiation

The results show that saffron samples were differentiated according to the geographical region of their collection. Interestingly, crocus from distant areas e.g., Greece and Morocco, exhibit more pronounced similarities compared to neighboring regions such as Greece and Italy. This could be attributed to the pivotal impact of microclimatic conditions rather than considering the wider geographical area of cultivation. The Moroccan climate is typically Mediterranean, resembling the Greek weather, even in the Atlantic coast of the country. Nevertheless, the proximity of Greece to Italy and the fact that they are both Mediterranean countries should indicate a large degree of similarity for the species. The Italian saffron shows the same degree of differentiation to the Greek, Moroccan and Iranian species. This reflects that the geoclimatic characteristics, along with the different preparation practices followed in the cultivation area determine the chemical composition of the final product [14,31]. The Greek saffron is collected in a very narrow area (a village in Macedonia province called Krokos from the name of the plant) where the conditions are likely to be the same when compared to the conditions in the collection area of Morocco. Indeed, this is also reflected to the Asian derived species. Thus, the Indian and Afghan saffron are more similar to the Greek and Moroccan species in terms of chemical profile when compared to either Kashmir region or their Iranian counterparts. It should be noted that the Iranian and Kashmir species are more differentiated in terms of chemical components content, despite their proximity.

Another issue that should be noted is the genetic profile of the species. Considering that they are cultivated plants rather than native, it seems that the phylogenetic association is more closely related to the human intervention than to their historically driven distribution. Thus, an assumption that needs further verification is that the Iranian or the Kashmir branch were transferred by merchants to the countries that were in financial contact. The Iranian/Middle East axis has a strong impact on the human financial relations, and it seems that the same holds true for the Kashmir/India branch. The *Crocus sativus* L. species were cultivated and integrated in the areas from the Mediterranean basin to Iran/Middle East and India/Kashmir, and both their similarities and differences clearly reflect the international trade and financial relations between countries that were geographically distant.

2.4. Saffron Components in the Saffron Samples from Various Regions

Saffron contains more than 150 volatile and aroma-yielding compounds. It also has a number of nonvolatile active components [10], many of which are carotenoids, including zeaxanthin, lycopene, and various α- and β-carotenes. The wealth (plethora) of chemical components in saffron poses complexity for its analysis. Several chromatographic and mass spectrometric methods have been developed for the quantitation of the main bioactive ingredients of saffron, such as crocins and picrocrocin [14,35–38]. The content of the active secondary metabolites has an effect on the quality and efficacy of saffron [14,26]. In view of the limitations of other techniques, ultra-performance liquid chromatography (UPLC-HR MS) has been considered to be the most suitable method to analyze the constituents of saffron extracts. In our study, UPLC-HR MS provided the metabolomic profile of the saffron samples affording high sensitivity and retention time reproducibility. The UPLC-HR MS and multivariate statistical analysis were combined to analyze saffron stigmas. Our results showed that chemical characteristics of saffron were apparently diverse, which mainly arose from the different geoclimatic characteristics inherent to the territory of cultivation. Moreover, changes in the preparation procedures, i.e., flower collection, separation/drying and conservation of stigmas, may strongly modify the final composition of chemical components present in the stigma.

2.5. Marker Discriminating Power

In order to discover generalized markers of discriminating the saffron species, the cross-tab (Table 2) has been created. The intention was to identify a single feature or even a couple that could differentiate a group from its counterparts. There were two clusters, those of Indian-Afghan and those in the Greek-Morocco saffron that were considered as belonging to the same group. Thus, no generalized marker was found for discriminating the Indian-Afghan saffron from the other groups, however the 252.1061_0.59 and 472.1734_3.24 ions could differentiate the four of the five groups. The former mass signal corresponds to the $(M+NH_4)^+$ adduct ion of 3,4-Epoxybisabola-7(14),10-dien-2-one (EDO; $C_{15}H_{22}O_2$) marker, whereas the latter corresponds to the $(M+Na)^+$ adduct ion of astragalin ($C_{21}H_{20}O_{11}$). Conversely, the putative metabolite of tomentogenin [12] with MH^+ signal 369.15_2.95 could be used to discriminate three of the five groups in the case of the Iranian stigmas. In the case of the Greek-Morocco saffron, the results were even less general, and no molecular species was found to show such a capacity. The Italian varieties could be clearly separated from the others using the 169.1211_3.66 and 353.1548_3.66 ions corresponding to the MH^+ of vanillic acid and the $(M+Na)^+$ adduct ion of picrocrocin, respectively. Finally, the 611.157_4.14 ion corresponding to the MH^+ ion of kaempferol-di-glucoside was found it can be employed to distinguish the Kashmir saffron. These results indicate that a combination of markers should be employed which necessitates the use of hyphenated separation methodologies (e.g., LC–MS) for achieving the screening of *saffron* extracts, as well as probing the *saffron* for the presence of adulterants [26].

Table 2. Markers discovered towards the differentiation of the *Crocus sativus* L. stigmas from various destination sources. In bold are marked the common metabolites across at least two destination sources whereas underlined are the ones that could differentiate between all species.

	IND_AFG	GR_MOR	IR	IT	KSH
IND_AFG		307.1003_4.95	151.1105_3.67	151.1105_3.67	151.1105_3.67
		365.1196_3.36	169.1211_3.66	169.1211_3.66	151.1105_4.86
		369.15_2.95	169.1211_4.86	353.1548_3.66	169.1211_3.66
		383.1298_2.85	369.15_2.95	365.1196_3.36	169.1211_4.86
		472.1734_3.24	472.1734_3.24	369.15_2.95	611.157_4.14
GR_MOR	252.1061_0.59		123.1156_3.66	169.1211_3.66	151.1105_3.67
	367.135_3.42		151.1105_3.67	177.1629_9.84	151.1105_4.86
	369.1508_1.49		169.1211_3.66	353.1548_3.66	169.1211_3.66
	305.0824_0.71		169.1211_4.86	167.0115_24.08	169.1211_4.86
	167.1057_1.49		369.15_2.95	265.1216_0.58	611.157_4.14
IR	252.1061_0.59	155.1057_2.77		169.1211_3.66	252.1061_0.59
	294.1526_0.79	169.1212_4.39		177.1629_9.84	294.1526_0.79
	280.1373_0.73	294.1526_0.79		353.1548_3.66	611.157_4.14
	265.1216_0.58	317.1579_2.81		167.0115_24.08	280.1373_0.73
	606.229_4.15	265.1216_0.58		265.1216_0.58	265.1216_0.58
IT	139.1108_7.13	123.1156_3.66	139.1108_7.13		169.1212_4.39
	169.1212_4.39	151.1105_3.67	169.1212_4.39		252.1061_0.59
	252.1061_0.59	169.1211_4.86	369.1508_1.49		369.1508_1.49
	369.1508_1.49	348.1994_3.66	203.082_4.75		611.157_4.14
	203.082_4.75	369.15_2.95	171.1005_3.58		203.082_4.75
KSH	155.1057_2.77	155.1057_2.77	169.1211_3.66	169.1211_3.66	
	307.1003_4.95	183.1005_3.33	307.1003_4.95	307.1003_4.95	
	317.1579_2.81	307.1003_4.95	331.173_3.66	331.173_3.66	
	331.173_3.66	317.1579_2.81	369.15_2.95	353.1548_3.66	
	364.1944_2.96	331.173_3.66	511.1749_4.94	369.15_2.95	

3. Materials and Methods

3.1. Chemical Reagents and Standards

Methanol (MeOH) and acetonitrile (ACN) of HPLC grade were supplied from were supplied from Carlo Erba (Milano, Italy) and Fisher Scientific (Pittsburgh, PA, USA), respectively. Trifluoroacetic acid (TFA) was obtained from Acros Organics (Fair Lawn, NJ, USA) and water was purified using Milli-Q (RG) filter systems from Millipore Corporation (Billerica, MA, USA).

3.2. Sample Collection

Crocus Sativus L. dried styles (saffron) were kindly supplied by the Cooperative De Safran, (Krokos Kozanis, West Macedonia, Greece). The *saffron* samples from Morocco, Italy, Iran, India, Kashmir and Afghanistan were purchased from Sahar Saffron Company (Cleveland, OH, USA). All samples were kept refrigerated at 5 °C until analysis.

3.3. Sample Preparation

50 mg of *saffron* stigmas were soaked in methanol water 1:1 (v/v) for 200 days in dark under ambient temperature. The stigmas were extracted with 10mL MeOH:water (1:1, v/v) for 24 h at 25 °C in the absence of light with continuous stirring, and then centrifuged, filtered through a 0.2-μm filter and evaporated to dryness employing a Speed Vac system (Labconco Corp., Kansas City, MO, USA). Samples were reconstituted in MeOH:water (1:1, v/v), transferred to 1.5 mL autosampler vials and an appropriate volume was injected to the LC–MS system.

3.4. UPLC—HR MS Metabolomics Analysis

A quality control sample (QC) taken from all samples was prepared in order to periodically assess the reproducibility of the measurements. The separation of the analytes contained in the saffron samples was achieved with a Fortis UPLC C_{18} column (2.1 mm × 100 mm, 1.7 μm, Fortis Technologies Ltd., Cheshire, UK). The hyphenated LC-HRMS system comprised of an Accela UHPLC equipped with an autosampler, a vacuum degasser, a binary pump and a temperature-controlled column (Thermo Scientific, Germany) coupled to an Orbitrap Discovery XL, which was equipped with an IonMAX ion source (Thermo Scientific, Bremen, Germany). The mobile phase consisted of 0.1% aq. formic acid (v/v) (solvent A) and 0.1% formic acid in LC–MS grade ACN (v/v) (solvent B). The gradient program was for solvent B: 5% at 0 min, 5% at 3 min, 95% at 24 min, 95% at 26 min, 5% at 28 min, 5% at 30 min. The overall analysis time spanned for 30 min, whereas the injection volume was 5 μl keeping a flow rate of 400 μl min^{-1}. The positive ionization ESI mode was used using a mass range of 100–1000 amu. The "big three" approach, employing parallel scans, was used. The samples were centrifuged using a Mikro 200R centrifuge (Hettich Lab Technology, Tuttlingen, Germany), and for the solvent evaporation was performed on a GeneVac HT-4X EZ-2 series evaporator Lyospeed ENABLED (Genevac Ltd., Ipswich, UK).

3.5. Statistical Analysis

The raw data were imported to the Mzmine 2.51 [39] and the Automated Data Analysis Pipeline (ADAP) pipeline was employed, using the wavelets methodology for the chromatogram deconvolution as implemented to ADAP [40]. The feature list was analyzed by SIMCA 14.1 (Umetrics, Umea, Sweden) for the construction of the multivariate models, whereas all univariate analyses were performed by Jamovi. The multiple correction for t-testing, which used the false discovery rate approach, was performed by the qvalue R package [41]. All multivariate models were validated by n-fold as well as by permutation testing, employing 100 random permutations. The CV-ANOVA was used with $p < 0.05$ to verify the validity of the produced models [42].

3.6. Feature Identification

The peak list MS features were annotated using the KEGG, CheBI, MetaCyc, LIPIDMAPS, FOR-IDENT, and HMDB libraries. The Met-Frag online version was employed [43] for the annotation and an additional home-assembled MS library was also used.

4. Conclusions

The metabolomic profiling of saffron (*Crocus sativus* L. stigma) from different geographical regions, employing UPLC-HR MS analysis combined with multivariate statistical analysis, provided evidence that the phytochemical content in the samples of *C. sativus* L. was diverse in the different countries of origin. This diversity apparently arises from the different geoclimatic characteristics of the area of cultivation in combination with the distinct preparation procedures in the respective countries. Our results indicated that there are characteristic ions that could differentiate a certain group from its counterparts such as the Indian-Afghan and the Greek-Morocco saffron samples that could be considered to belong to the same group. The metabolomics approach was deemed to be the most suitable choice in order to evaluate the enormous array of putative metabolites of saffron, and thus provide a comparative phytochemical screening among the saffron samples studied. In addition, this UPLC-HR MS-based metabolomics approach could be also employed for probing possible adulteration of saffron samples. In view of saffron's health-promoting effects through the modulation of various biological and physiological processes, the selection of the appropriate saffron sample guided by the respective metabolomic profiling could be an important step. That, in turn, may aid the emerging popularity and interest in alternative medicine-based treatments within health practices.

Author Contributions: E.G. and A.T.; Conceptualization; E.G., N.S.K. and A.T.; methodology development, E.G. and N.S.K. formal analysis, E.G.; statistical analysis, E.G. and A.T.; coordinated and supervised the study, E.G., N.S.K. and A.T.; writing—original draft preparation. All authors have read and agreed to the published version of the manuscript.

Funding: This work was supported by the "Large Scale Cooperative Project" (TreatAD, 09SYN-21-1003) co-financed by the European Social Fund (ESF) and the General Secretariat for Research and Technology in Greece.

Institutional Review Board Statement: Not available.

Informed Consent Statement: Not available.

Data Availability Statement: The data presented in this study are available in this article.

Acknowledgments: We would like to thank Günter Allmaier and Ernst Pittenauer from the Institute of Chemical Technologies and Analytics, Vienna University of Technologies and Analytics, Vienna, Austria for their helpful discussions on the crocus project.

Conflicts of Interest: The authors declare no conflict of interest.

Sample Availability: The samples are not available from the authors.

References

1. Serrano-Díaz, J.; Sánchez, A.M.; Martínez-Tomé, M.; Winterhalter, P.; Alonso, G.L. A contribution to nutritional studies on *Crocus sativus* flowers and their value as food. *J. Food Compos. Anal.* **2013**, *31*, 101–108. [CrossRef]
2. Alavizadeh, S.H.; Hosseinzadeh, H. Bioactivity assessment and toxicity of crocin: A comprehensive review. *Food Chem. Toxicol.* **2014**, *64*, 65–80. [CrossRef] [PubMed]
3. Day, J. Crocuses in Context: A Diachronic Survey of the Crocus Motif in the Aegean Bronze Age. *Hesperia* **2011**, *80*, 337–379. [CrossRef]
4. Ferrence, S.C.; Bendersky, G. Therapy with saffron and the goddess at Thera. *Perspect. Biol. Med.* **2004**, *47*, 199–226. [CrossRef]
5. Mathew, B. *The Crocus: A revision of the genus Crocus (Iridaceae)*; BT Batsford Ltd.: London, UK, 1982; Volume 127, p. 96.
6. Zubor, A.; Suranyi, G.; Györi, Z.; Borbely, G.; Prokisch, J. Molecular biological approach of the systematics of *Crocus sativus* L. and its allies. *Acta Hortic.* **2004**, *650*, 85–93. [CrossRef]
7. Brandizzi, F.; Caiola, M.G. Flow cytometric analysis of nuclear DNA inCrocus sativus and allies (Iridaceae). *Plant Syst. Evol.* **1998**, *211*, 149–154. [CrossRef]
8. Agayev, Y.; Zarifi, E.; Fernandez, J. Study of karyotypes in the *Crocus sativus* L. aggregate and origin of cultivated saffron. *Acta Hortic.* **2010**, *850*, 47–54. [CrossRef]
9. Caiola, M.G.; Caputo, P.; Zanier, R. RAPD Analysis in *Crocus sativus* L. Accessions and Related Crocus Species. *Biol. Plant.* **2004**, *48*, 375–380. [CrossRef]
10. Winterhalter, P.; Straubinger, M. Saffron—Renewed Interest in an Ancient Spice. *Food Rev. Int.* **2000**, *16*, 39–59. [CrossRef]
11. Moradzadeh, M.; Kalani, M.R.; Avan, A. The antileukemic effects of saffron (*Crocus sativus* L.) and its related molecular targets: A mini review. *J. Cell Biochem.* **2019**, *120*, 4732–4738. [CrossRef]
12. Tarantilis, P.A.; Polissiou, M.G. Isolation and identification of the aroma components from saffron (*Crocus sativus*). *J. Agric. Food Chem.* **1997**, *45*, 459–462. [CrossRef]
13. Carmona, M.; Zalacain, A.; Salinas, M.R.; Alonso, G.L.; Delgado, M.C. A New Approach to Saffron Aroma. *Crit. Rev. Food Sci. Nutr.* **2007**, *47*, 145–159. [CrossRef] [PubMed]
14. Anastasaki, E.; Kanakis, C.; Pappas, C.; Maggi, L.; del Campo, C.P.; Carmona, M.; Alonso, G.L.; Polissiou, M.G. Geographical differentiation of saffron by GC–MS/FID and chemometrics. *Eur. Food. Res. Technol.* **2009**, *229*, 899–905. [CrossRef]
15. Xu, S.; Ge, X.; Li, S.; Guo, X.; Dai, D.; Yang, T. Discrimination of Different Parts of Saffron by Metabolomic-Based Ultra-Performance Liquid Chromatography Coupled with High-Definition Mass Spectrometry. *Chem. Biodivers.* **2019**, *16*, e1900363. [CrossRef]

16. Sunanda, B.P.V.; Rammohan, B.; Kumar, A. The effective study of aqueous extract of *Crocus sativus* Linn. (Saffron) in depressed mice. *Int. J. PharmTech Res.* **2014**, *6*, 1143–1152.
17. Poma, A.; Fontecchio, G.; Carlucci, G.; Chichiriccò, G. Anti-inflammatory properties of drugs from saffron crocus. *Antiinflamm. Antiallergy. Agents Med. Chem.* **2012**, *11*, 37–51. [CrossRef]
18. Samarghandian, S.; Borji, A. Anticarcinogenic effect of saffron (*Crocus sativus* L.) and its ingredients. *Pharmacogn. Res.* **2014**, *6*, 99–107. [CrossRef]
19. Papandreou, M.A.; Kanakis, C.D.; Polissiou, M.G.; Efthimiopoulos, S.; Cordopatis, P.; Margarity, M.; Lamari, F.N. Inhibitory Activity on Amyloid-β Aggregation and Antioxidant Properties of *Crocus sativus* Stigmas Extract and Its Crocin Constituents. *J. Agric. Food Chem.* **2006**, *54*, 8762–8768. [CrossRef]
20. Sheng, L.; Qian, Z.; Zheng, S.; Xi, L. Mechanism of hypolipidemic effect of crocin in rats: Crocin inhibits pancreatic lipase. *Eur. J. Pharmacol.* **2006**, *543*, 116–122. [CrossRef]
21. Lopresti, A.L.; Drummond, P.D. Saffron (*Crocus sativus*) for depression: A systematic review of clinical studies and examination of underlying antidepressant mechanisms of action. *Human Psychopharmacol. Clin. Exp.* **2014**, *29*, 517–527. [CrossRef]
22. Hosseinzadeh, H.; Karimi, G.; Niapoor, M. Antidepressant effect of *Crocus sativus* L. stigma extracts and their constituents, crocin and saffranal, in mice. *Acta Hortic.* **2004**, *650*, 435–445. [CrossRef]
23. Pitsikas, N.; Zisopoulou, S.; Tarantilis, P.A.; Kanakis, C.D.; Polissiou, M.G.; Sakellaridis, N. Effects of the active constituents of *Crocus sativus* L., crocins on recognition and spatial rats' memory. *Behav. Brain Res.* **2007**, *183*, 141–146. [CrossRef]
24. Finley, J.W.; Gao, S. A Perspective on *Crocus sativus* L. (Saffron) Constituent Crocin: A Potent Water-Soluble Antioxidant and Potential Therapy for Alzheimer's Disease. *J. Agric. Food Chem.* **2017**, *65*, 1005–1020. [CrossRef]
25. Koulakiotis, N.S.; Pittenauer, E.; Halabalaki, M.; Tsarbopoulos, A.; Allmaier, G. Comparison of different tandem mass spectrometric techniques (ESI-IT, ESI- and IP-MALDI-QRTOF and vMALDI-TOF/RTOF) for the analysis of crocins and picrocrocin from the stigmas of *Crocus sativus* L. *Rapid Commun. Mass Spectrom.* **2012**, *26*, 670–678. [CrossRef]
26. Srivastava, R.; Ahmed, H.; Dixit, R.; Dharamveer; Saraf, S. *Crocus sativus* L.: A comprehensive review. *Pharmacogn. Rev.* **2010**, *4*, 200–208. [CrossRef]
27. Pitsikas, N.; Boultadakis, A.; Georgiadou, G.; Tarantilis, P.; Sakellaridis, N. Effects of the active constituents of *Crocus sativus* L., crocins, in an animal model of anxiety. *Phytomedicine* **2008**, *15*, 1135–1139. [CrossRef]
28. Maggi, M.A.; Bisti, S.; Picco, C. Saffron: Chemical Composition and Neuroprotective Activity. *Molecules* **2020**, *25*, 5618. [CrossRef]
29. Koulakiotis, N.S.; Purhonen, P.; Gikas, E.; Hebert, H.; Tsarbopoulos, A. Crocus-derived compounds alter the aggregation pathway of Alzheimer's Disease—Associated beta amyloid protein. *Sci. Rep.* **2020**, *10*, 1–10. [CrossRef]
30. Selkoe, D.J.; Hardy, J. The amyloid hypothesis of Alzheimer's disease at 25 years. *EMBO Mol. Med.* **2016**, *8*, 595–608. [CrossRef]
31. Pavarini, D.P.; Pavarini, S.P.; Niehues, M.; Lopes, N.P. Exogenous influences on plant secondary metabolite levels. *Anim. Feed. Sci. Technol.* **2012**, *176*, 5–16. [CrossRef]
32. Sampaio, B.L.; Edrada-Ebel, R.; Da Costa, F.B. Effect of the environment on the secondary metabolic profile of Tithonia diversifolia: A model for environmental metabolomics of plants. *Sci. Rep.* **2016**, *6*, 29265. [CrossRef]
33. Cirak, C.; Radusiene, J.; Ivanauskas, L.; Jakstas, V.; Camas, N. Changes in the content of bioactive substances among Hypericum montbretii populations from Turkey. *Rev. Bras. Farm.* **2014**, *24*, 20–24. [CrossRef]
34. Schymanski, E.L.; Jeon, J.; Gulde, R.; Fenner, K.; Ruff, M.; Singer, H.P.; Hollender, J. Identifying Small Molecules via High Resolution Mass Spectrometry: Communicating Confidence. *Environ. Sci. Technol.* **2014**, *48*, 2097–2098. [CrossRef]
35. Tarantilis, P.A.; Tsoupras, G.; Polissiou, M. Determination of Saffron (*Crocus-Sativus* L) Components in Crude Plant-Extract Using High-Performance Liquid-Chromatography Uv-Visible Photodiode-Array Detection-Mass Spectrometry. *J. Chromatogr. A* **1995**, *699*, 107–118. [CrossRef]
36. Carmona, M.; Sanchez, A.M.; Ferreres, F.; Zalacain, A.; Tomas-Barberan, F.; Alonso, G.L. Identification of the flavonoid fraction in saffron spice by LC/DAD/MS/MS: Comparative study of samples from different geographical origins. *Food Chem.* **2007**, *100*, 445–450. [CrossRef]
37. Koulakiotis, N.S.; Gikas, E.; Iatrou, G.; Lamari, F.N.; Tsarbopoulos, A. Quantitation of Crocins and Picrocrocin in Saffron by HPLC: Application to Quality Control and Phytochemical Differentiation from Other Crocus Taxa. *Planta Medica* **2015**, *81*, 606–612. [CrossRef]
38. Pittenauer, E.; Koulakiotis, N.S.; Tsarbopoulos, A.; Allmaier, G. In-Chain neutral hydrocarbon loss from crocin apocarotenoid ester glycosides and the crocetin aglycon (*Crocus sativus* L.) by ESI-MS^n. *J. Mass Spectrom.* **2013**, *48*, 1299–1307.
39. Pluskal, T.; Castillo, S.; Villar-Briones, A.; Orešič, M. MZmine 2: Modular framework for processing, visualizing, and analyzing mass spectrometry-based molecular profile data. *BMC Bioinform.* **2010**, *11*, 395. [CrossRef]
40. Myers, O.D.; Sumner, S.J.; Li, S.; Barnes, S.; Du, X. One Step Forward for Reducing False Positive and False Negative Compound Identifications from Mass Spectrometry Metabolomics Data: New Algorithms for Constructing Extracted Ion Chromatograms and Detecting Chromatographic Peaks. *Anal. Chem.* **2017**, *89*, 8696–8703. [CrossRef]
41. Storey, J.D.; Bass, A.J.; Dabney, A.; Robinson, D. Qvalue: Q-value Estimation for False Discovery Rate Control. R Package Version 2.22.0. Available online: http://github.com/jdstorey/qvalue (accessed on 7 April 2021).

42. Eriksson, L.; Trygg, J.; Wold, S. CV-ANOVA for significance testing of PLS and OPLS® models. *J. Chemom.* **2008**, *22*, 594–600. [CrossRef]
43. Ruttkies, C.; Schymanski, E.L.; Wolf, S.; Hollender, J.; Neumann, S. MetFrag relaunched: Incorporating strategies beyond in silico fragmentation. *J. Cheminform.* **2016**, *8*, 1–16. [CrossRef] [PubMed]

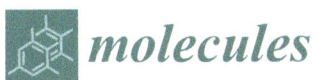

Article

Bioanalytical Method Development and Validation Study of Neuroprotective Extract of Kashmiri Saffron Using Ultra-Fast Liquid Chromatography-Tandem Mass Spectrometry (UFLC-MS/MS): In Vivo Pharmacokinetics of Apocarotenoids and Carotenoids

Aboli Girme *, Sandeep Pawar, Chetana Ghule, Sushant Shengule, Ganesh Saste, Arun Kumar Balasubramaniam, Amol Deshmukh and Lal Hingorani

Pharmanza Herbal Pvt. Ltd., Anand, Gujarat 388435, India; lcms@pharmanzaherbals.com (S.P.); adic@pharmanza.com (C.G.); rdbiotech@pharmanza.com (S.S.); ard@pharmanzaherbals.com (G.S.); process@pharmanza.com (A.K.B.); rd@pharmanza.com (A.D.); lal@pharmanzaherbals.com (L.H.)
* Correspondence: ardm@pharmanzaherbals.com; Tel.: +91-704-353-4016 or +91-982-506-3959

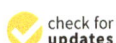

Citation: Girme, A.; Pawar, S.; Ghule, C.; Shengule, S.; Saste, G.; Balasubramaniam, A.K.; Deshmukh, A.; Hingorani, L. Bioanalytical Method Development and Validation Study of Neuroprotective Extract of Kashmiri Saffron Using Ultra-Fast Liquid Chromatography-Tandem Mass Spectrometry (UFLC-MS/MS): In Vivo Pharmacokinetics of Apocarotenoids and Carotenoids. *Molecules* **2021**, *26*, 1815. https://doi.org/10.3390/molecules26061815

Academic Editors: Nikolaos Pitsikas, Konstantinos Dimas and Karel Šmejkal

Received: 12 February 2021
Accepted: 19 March 2021
Published: 23 March 2021

Publisher's Note: MDPI stays neutral with regard to jurisdictional claims in published maps and institutional affiliations.

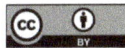

Copyright: © 2021 by the authors. Licensee MDPI, Basel, Switzerland. This article is an open access article distributed under the terms and conditions of the Creative Commons Attribution (CC BY) license (https://creativecommons.org/licenses/by/4.0/).

Abstract: Kashmir saffron (*Crocus sativus* L.), also known as Indian saffron, is an important Asian medicinal plant with protective therapeutic applications in brain health. The main bioactive in Kashmir or Indian Saffron (KCS) and its extract (CSE) are apocarotenoids picrocrocin (PIC) and safranal (SAF) with carotenoids, crocetin esters (crocins), and crocetins. The ultra-fast liquid chromatography(UFLC)- photodiode array standardization confirmed the presence of biomarkers PIC, *trans*-4-GG-crocin (T4C), *trans*-3-Gg-crocin (T3C), *cis*-4-GG-crocin (C4C), *trans*-2-gg-crocin (T2C), *trans*-crocetin (TCT), and SAF in CSE. This study's objectives were to develop and validate a sensitive and rapid UFLC-tandem mass spectrometry method for PIC and SAF along T4C and TCT in rat plasma with internal standards (IS). The calibration curves were linear ($R^2 > 0.990$), with the lower limit of quantification (LLOQ) as 10 ng/mL. The UFLC-MS/MS assay-based precision (RSD, <15%) and accuracy (RE, −11.03–9.96) on analytical quality control (QC) levels were well within the acceptance criteria with excellent recoveries (91.18–106.86%) in plasma samples. The method was applied to investigate the in vivo pharmacokinetic parameters after oral administration of 40 mg/kg CSE in the rats (*n* = 6). The active metabolite TCT and T4C, PIC, SAF were quantified for the first time with T3C, C4C, T2C by this validated bioanalytical method, which will be useful for preclinical/clinical trials of CSE as a potential neuroprotective dietary supplement.

Keywords: crocetin; crocin; picrocrocin; safranal; dietary supplement; nutraceutical

1. Introduction

Crocus sativus L. (CS), also known as saffron, is a popular food condiment. Cultivation of CS occurs in many countries, including Iran, India, Italy, Spain, and Greece. The flower stigmas of saffron have usage worldwide for traditional and medicinal use. This saffron mainly grows in India's Kashmir region, known as Kashmir or Indian Saffron (KCS).

This KCS is rich in bioactive constituents, carotenoids (crocetin esters, i.e., crocins, crocetin), and apocarotenoids such as picrocrocin (PIC) with safranal (SAF) (Figure 1) [1–4]. The Srinagar, Pulwama, Kishwar, and Badgam districts have been geographically and climatically suitable for the growth and enrichment of bioactive compounds in saffron [3–5]. Geographical indicators (GIs) for the production of Kashmir saffron have been validated [5]. It shows the growth and scope of production and the consistent supply of KCS with agricultural benefit.

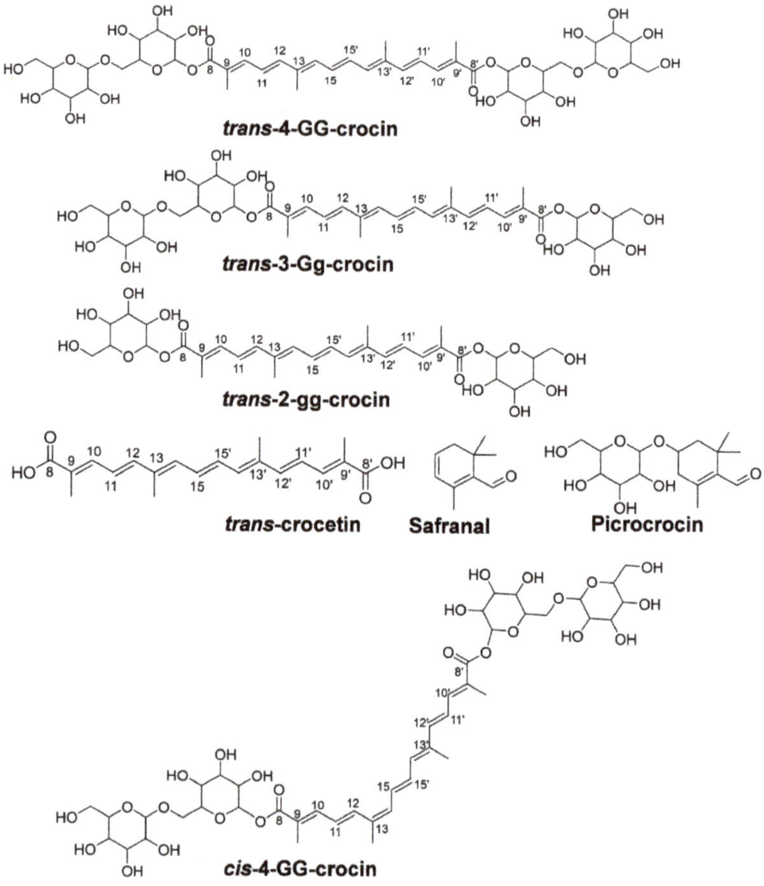

Figure 1. Compounds of Kashmir saffron extract (CSE)-*trans*-4-gg-crocin (T4C); *trans*-3-Gg-crocin (T3C); *trans*-2gg-crocin (T2C); *trans*-crocetin (TCT); safranal (SAF); picrocrocin (PIC), and *cis*-4GG-crocin (C4C).

Saffron's stigma mainly contains the water-soluble carotenoids crocetins, and its esters, known as crocins responsible for this spice's coloring properties. The esterification of crocetins with sugars like neapolitanose, gentiobiose (G), and glucose (g) gives the geometric isomers of crocins, where *trans* isomers dominate *cis* form [3,4]. The general crocins content ranges between 16–28% in the CS, and in some harvest years, it can represent up to 30% [4,6,7]. The apocarotenoid PIC is mainly responsible for the taste of CS, which is 7–16% in the dried stigmas of CS and can reach up to 20% [6,8–10]. Safranal is the bioactive precursor form of PIC which contributes to its aroma and is usually found as 0.1–0.6% in concentration in the CS on a dried weight basis (w/w) [6,11–17].

Saffron and their associated carotenoid–apocarotenoids were extensively studied over the last decade for their biomedical properties, especially for their brain health and chemopreventive potential. The compounds have found a highly antioxidant effect in neurodegenerative diseases with its relevance to Alzheimer's (AD) and Parkinson's Disease [3,18–21].

Kashmir or Indian Saffron holds importance in culinary and remedial values in India's regional and traditional medicines. It has curative properties in nervous system functions and insomnia, depression, cataracts, night blindness, low vision while normalizing heart functions. Kashmir or Indian Saffron is traditionally used in India as antispasmodic and aphrodisiac, treating dermal diseases, kidney–urinary disorders, and rheumatoid arthritis with widespread cosmetics usage as per folklore, Ayurveda, Siddha, Sowa Rigpa, and Unani medicinal systems [1,22–27]. The recent scientific studies on KCS have shown its potential in AD, cardiac functions, immunomodulatory activity, and anti-tumor agents [3,28–34]. This increased valuation and consistent growth in the KCS consumption in health benefits have prompted the demand and interest in research as a dietary supplement and nutraceutical.

The data for bioanalytical studies showed that HPLC-based quantification had been reported for the presence of *trans*-4-GG-crocin (T4C) or crocin-1 and *trans*-crocetin (TCT) in CS [4,35–37]. But there is no report of the methodology for bioactive apocarotenoids PIC and SAF along with other carotenoids *trans*-3-Gg-crocin (T3C), *trans*-2-gg-crocin (T2C), *cis*-4-GG-crocin (C4C) from CS [35–37]. This research also lacks confirmation and detection of these compounds in biological samples after CS or its extract or product consumption. There is a need to develop a short and adaptable LC-based method with MS/MS to identify and quantify these compounds in a validated way. Current bioanalytical studies lack validation data and sensitivity for the bioactive compounds T2C, T3C, C4C, SAF, and PIC from CS as per the literature [4,38–41].

In the previous studies, the neuroprotective effect of KCS extract has been evaluated. An integral approach to prevent or delay AD is the blood-brain barrier (BBB) integrity and amyloid β-protein (Aβ) clearance. In an in vitro study, KCS extract enhanced the tightness of bEnd-3 cells-based BBB in the concentration of 0.2–0.22 mg/mL, thereby increasing Aβ clearance which helps in AD condition. This KCS extract has upregulated synaptic proteins and reduced neuroinflammation associated with Aβ pathology in 5XFAD (AD model) mice brains. The treatment of active metabolite crocetin resulted in improved memory function by inducing autophagy mediated by AMPK pathway activation in mice in a separate study, which states the study requirement for in vivo therapeutics data [3,4,42].

The UFLC-PDA standardization showed bioactive compounds PIC, T4C, T3C, C4C, T2C, TCT, and SAF in the KCS extract (CSE). Therefore, the present study aimed to develop and validate a sensitive and short UFLC-MS/MS bioanalytical method for the simultaneous determination of apocarotenoids (PIC, SAF) and carotenoids (T4C, TCT) in the rat plasma. This methodology was further validated with internal standards reserpine and chloramphenicol as per the USFDA (United States Food and Drug Administration)and EMA(European Medicines Agency guidance for linearity, precision, accuracy, recovery, extraction efficiency, stability, dilution integrity, and matrix effect. [40,41] This novel method was utilized for in vivo oral pharmacokinetics investigations of CSE in rats. The PIC, SAF, T4C, TCT, T3C, C4C, T2C, were detected in rat plasma using this validated bioanalytical method. This method and results will be beneficial in the further investigation of KCS and CSE. According to the phytopharmaceutical guidelines of the Drugs Controller General (DCG) (India) and other regulations, this bioanalytical method will be useful for preclinical or phase 1 clinical trials.

2. Results

The quantitation results of CSE (n = 3) with the concentrations of PIC, SAF, T4C, T3C, C4C, T2C with TCT was found as shown in Table 1.

Table 1. Quantitation of Kashmir saffron extract (CSE) (n = 3) (%, w/w) for compounds PIC, SAF, T4C, T3C, C4C, T2C and TCT.

Analytes	T4C	T3C	T2C	C4C	TCT	SAF	PIC
CSE	13.76 ± 0.280	5.50 ± 0.418	0.875 ± 0.0255	0.624 ± 0.011	0.0378 ± 0.0015	0.033 ± 0.00050	18.09 ± 0.586

2.1. Optimization of Chromatographic Conditions

The ultra-fast liquid chromatography-tandem mass spectrometry (UFLC-MS/MS) methodology was optimized by selecting the mobile phase system and promoting the retention of targeted analytes in pre-column and cleaning interferences. The water and acetonitrile (ACN) (80% to 10%) containing formic acid (0.01% to 0.1%) were compared, and water (0.1% formic acid) with ACN was selected as a mobile phase. Different mobile phase additives were tested systematically in the mobile phase optimization, including ammonium formate, ammonium acetate, and formic acid in ascending concentrations from 0 to 10 mmol/L and 0.01% to 0.1% to enhance the sensitivity and resolution of target compounds.

The mobile phase flow rate was optimized to increase the method's separation and reproducibility as 0.8 mL/min after various trials of 0.4, 0.5, 0.6, and 0.7 mL/min flow rates (system pressure of UFLC < 4000 psi). The analyte transfer's ideal time entirely from precolumn to the analytical column was optimized by switching at times 0, 0.5, 1 min, and 0.0 min. It was found that the response was proportional to the injection volume; hence optimization of injection volume was done with 5, 10, 20, and 50 µL. An increase in system pressure observed at 50 µL injection volume when compared to the rest. The lower limit of quantification (LLOQ) decreased ten-fold by changing the injection volume of 20 µL to 5 µL. Theoretically, the sample's sensitivity is directly proportional to the injection volume loaded into the analytical column. Therefore, the column conditions with optimized injection volume influence the retention process, efficiency, peak shape, which found 20 µL. Under the optimized conditions, the retention times (tR) of T4C, T3C, T2C, C4C, TCT, PIC, SAF, reserpine (IS1), and chloramphenicol (IS2) were found as 3.90, 4.12, 4.74, 4.53, 5.96, 1.93, 6.19, 4.82 and 4.42 min, respectively. (Table 2).

Table 2. Precursor/product ion pairs and parameters for multiple reaction monitoring (MRM) of compounds used in this study.

Analyte	Formula	MW (g/mol)	Ionization Mode	Precursor Ion (m/z)	Product ion (m/z)	Dwell Time (msec)	Q1 Pre-Bias (eV)	CE (eV)	Q3 Pre-Bias (eV)	Retention Time, tR (min)
T4C	$C_{44}H_{64}O_{24}$	976.38	-ve	975.70	651.25 / 327.20	53.00 / 53.00	22.00 / 28.00	23.00 / 37.00	34.00 / 22.00	3.90
T3C	$C_{38}H_{54}O_{19}$	814.33	-ve	813.30	327.20 / 651.20	53.00 / 53.00	18.00 / 18.00	28.00 / 14.00	16.00 / 18.00	4.12
T2C	$C_{32}H_{44}O_{14}$	652.27	-ve	651.25	327.15 / 283.20	53.00 / 53.00	14.00 / 22.00	20.00 / 26.00	16.00 / 32.00	4.74
C4C	$C_{44}H_{64}O_{24}$	976.38	-ve	975.70	651.25 / 327.20	53.00 / 53.00	22.00 / 22.00	23.00 / 38.00	34.00 / 15.00	4.53
TCT	$C_{20}H_{24}O_4$	328.17	-ve	327.10	283.10 / 239.35	53.00 / 53.00	12.00 / 12.00	9.00 / 12.00	13.00 / 26.00	5.96
PIC	$C_{16}H_{26}O_7$	330.17	+ve	151.25	81.05 / 123.15	62.00 / 62.00	−16.00 / −10.00	−22.00 / −17.00	−14.00 / −24.00	1.93
SAF	$C_{10}H_{14}O$	150.10	+ve	151.25	81.05 / 123.15	53.00 / 53.00	−16.00 / −10.00	−22.00 / −17.00	−14.00 / −24.00	6.19
IS1	$C_{33}H_{40}N_2O_9$	608.27	+ve	609.70	195.10 / 448.05	53.00 / 53.00	−22.00 / −22.00	−40.00 / −31.00	−20.00 / −22.00	4.82
IS2	$C_{11}H_{12}Cl_2N_2O_5$	322.01	-ve	321.00	152.00 / 257.00	53.00 / 53.00	16.00 / 11.00	11.00 / 16.00	18.00 / 15.00	4.42

T4C—*trans*-4-gg-crocin; T3C—*trans*-3Gg-crocin; T2C—*trans*-2gg-crocin; C4C—*cis*-4GG-crocin; TCT—*trans* crocetin; PIC—picrocrocin; SAF—safranal; IS1—internal standard 1; IS2—internal standard 2.

2.2. Optimization of Mass Spectrometric Conditions

The optimization of MS conditions was performed on precursors and product ions of the analytes and IS. The electrospray ionization (ESI) interface was selected as T4C, T3C, T2C, C4C, and TCT with IS2 in a negative mode and SAF, PIC, with IS1 in a positive mode for a maximum and stable response. The mass parameters such as Q1 pre-bias and (DP), Q3 pre-bias, and collision energy values for all the analytes and IS1 and IS2 were optimized and shown in Table 2.

Carotenoids are fragile and naturally occurring isomerized compounds in CSE. The T4C and C4C are isomers with four sugar moieties at a molecular weight of 976.38 g/mol. Similarly, T3C is a carotenoid with three sugar moieties (814.33 g/mol) and T2C with two sugar moieties (652.27 g/mol). The basic chemical skeleton of these molecules is TCT with 328.17 g/mol. Similarly, the main apocarotenoid, PIC, has a molecular weight of 330.17 g/mol with a similar SAF structure, with a molecular weight of 150.10 g/mol with the sugar moiety.

The Q3 MS spectra stabilized for all these compounds T4C, T3C, C4C, T2C, TCT, PIC, and SAF in this method. The spectra of product ions (qualifier and quantifier) showed transitions for T4C, T3C, C4C at 651.25/327.20, for T2C 327.15/283.20. The TCT showed a major transition at 283.10/239.35. In comparison, apocarotenoids PIC and SAF showed transition at 123.15/81.05 and 123.15/81.05, whereas 448.05/195.10 and 257.00/152.00 were used for IS1 and IS2 in multiple reaction monitoring (MRM) scan mode. (Figures 2 and 3)

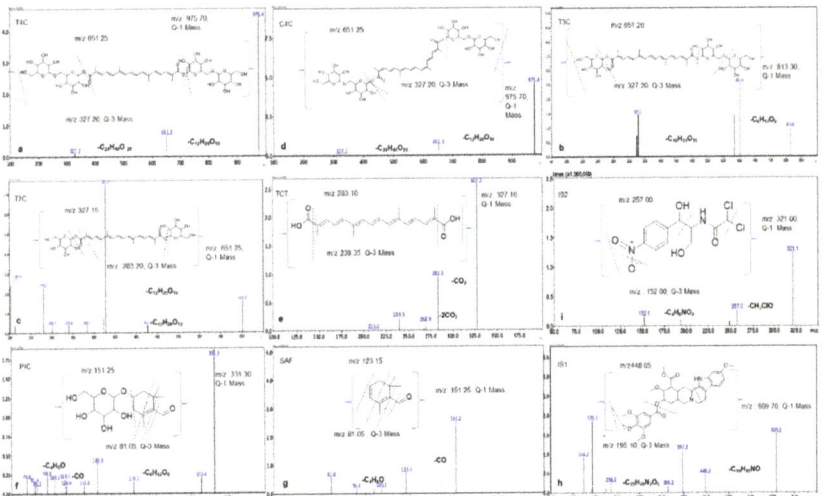

Figure 2. Possible mass fragmentation pattern and (m/z) values of precursor (Q1) and product (Q3) ions for T4C, T3C, T2C, C4C, TCT, IS2 (negative mode) and PIC, SAF, IS1 (positive mode) in the optimized ultra-fast liquid chromatography-tandem mass spectrometry (UFLC-MS/MS) based MRM conditions.

2.2.1. Carotenoids–Apocarotenoids: Mass Fragmentation Analysis by UFLC-MS/MS

The precursor and fragmented ions from UFLC-MS/MS methodology were further studied for all carotenoids and apocarotenoid's possible mass fragmentation pattern, as shown in Figure 2.

The ESI-MS (negative) spectrum of T4C (tR = 3.90 min) displayed a molecular ion at m/z 975.70 [M–H]$^-$ and other two diagnostic peaks were observed at m/z 651.25 [M–H–$C_{12}H_{20}O_{10}$]$^-$ and m/z 327.20 [M–H–$C_{24}H_{40}O_{20}$]$^-$, confirming the presence of four glucose moieties [43]. The deprotonated molecular ion peak of the ESI-MS (negative) spectrum of T3C (tR = 4.12 min) displayed an ion at m/z 813.30 [M–H]$^-$. The other two additional diagnostic peaks were observed at m/z 651.20 [M–H–$C_6H_{10}O_5$]$^-$ and m/z 327.20 [M–H–$C_{18}H_{31}O_{15}$]$^-$ confirm the presence of three glucose moieties. The deprotonated molecular ion peak of ESI-MS (negative) spectrum of T2C (tR = 4.74 min) displayed an ion at m/z 651.25 [M–H]$^-$ and another two additional diagnostic peaks were observed at m/z 327.15 [M–H–$C_{12}H_{20}O_{10}$]$^-$ and m/z 283.20 [M–H–$C_{13}H_{20}O_{12}$]$^-$ which confirm the presence of two glucose moieties.

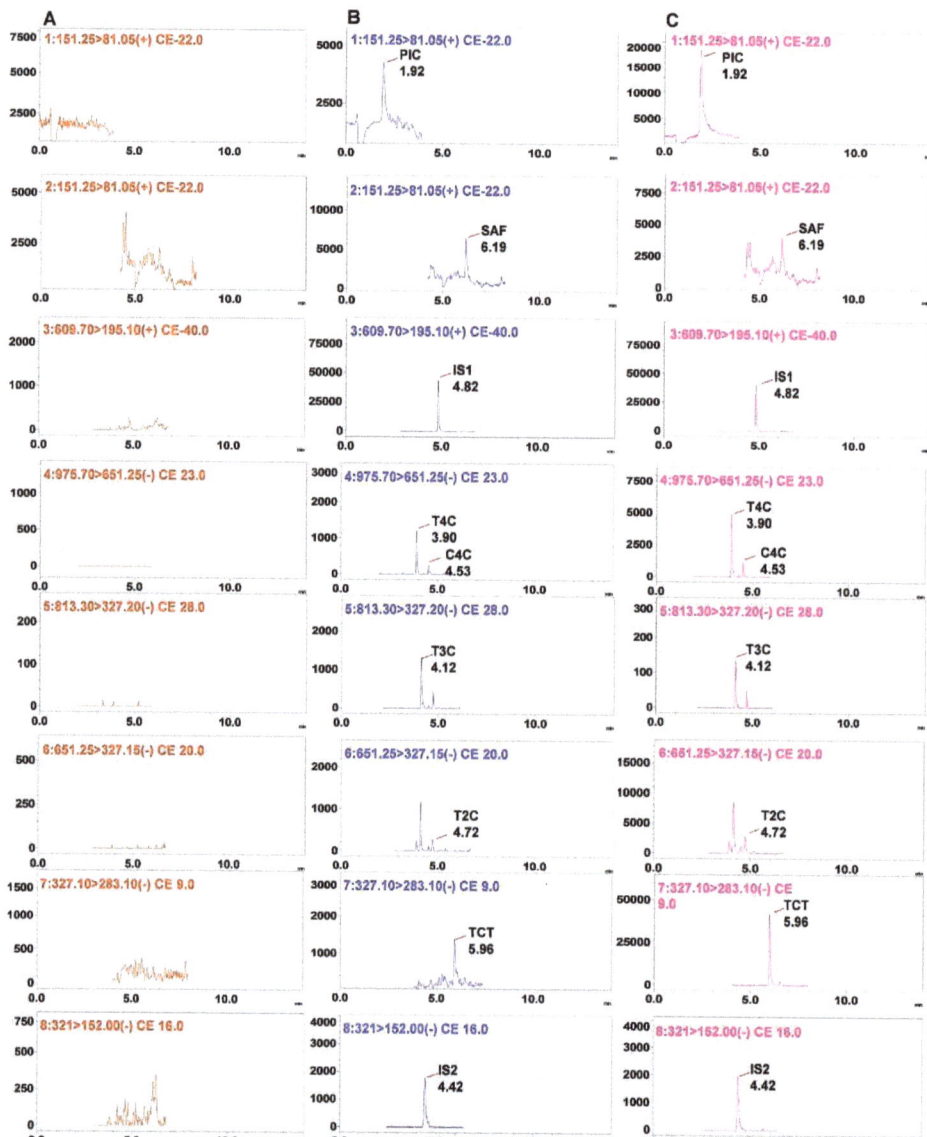

Figure 3. Typical MRM chromatograms of the seven components in rats: (**A**) blank plasma; (**B**) blank plasma sample spiked with standard mixtures and internal standard; (**C**) rat plasma samples collected after oral administration of the CSE. PIC, T4C, T3C, C4C, T2C, reserpine (IS1), TCT, SAF, chloramphenicol (IS2).

The ESI-MS (negative) spectrum of C4C (tR= 4.53 min) displayed a molecular ion at m/z 975.70 $[M-H]^-$ and two additional diagnostic peaks were observed at m/z 651.25 $[M-H-C_{12}H_{20}O_{10}]^-$ and m/z 327.20 $[M-H-C_{24}H_{40}O_{20}]^-$, which confirmed the presence of four glucose moieties. The deprotonated molecular ion peak of ESI-MS (negative) spectrum of TCT (tR= 5.96 min) displayed a molecular ion at m/z 327.10 $[M-H]^-$ [44], and other two additional diagnostic peaks were observed at m/z 283.10 $[M-H-CO_2]^-$ and m/z 239.35 $[M-H-2CO_2]^-$.

The apocarotenoids are carotenoids derived compounds with isoprenoids units present in CS [45]. In MS/MS analysis, protonated molecular ion peak observed for PIC as m/z

151.25 [M+H]$^+$ at tR=1.93 min, with additional signals as m/z 123.15 [M+H–CO]$^+$ and m/z 81.05 [M+H–C$_4$H$_6$O]$^+$. While for SAF, the molecular ion at m/z 151.25 [M+H]$^+$, with additional signals at m/z 123.15 [M-H-CO]$^+$ and m/z 81.05 [M+H–C$_4$H$_6$O]$^+$, was observed at tR=6.19 min. Both compounds could be separately identified by analyzing reference standards and retention time.

The [M+H]$^+$ spectrum of reserpine (IS1) (tR 4.82 min) displayed a molecular ion at m/z 609.70 [M+H]$^+$, and two additional signals were observed at m/z 448.05 [M+H–C$_{10}$H$_{10}$NO]$^+$, and m/z 195.10 [M+H–C$_{23}$H$_{29}$N$_2$O$_5$]$^+$. The spectrum of chloramphenicol (IS2) (tR=4.42 min) displayed a molecular ion at m/z 321.00 [M–H]$^-$ and two additional signals were observed at m/z 152.00 [M–H–C$_4$H$_6$NO$_2$]$^-$ and m/z 257.00 [M–H–CH$_3$OCl] (Figure 2). This data gives us possible ion fragmentation and application of this methodology in the proposed MS-based fragmentation pattern of these analytes from CSE.

2.2.2. Linearity and Lower Limit of Quantification (LLOQ)

The calibration curves, correlation coefficients (R^2), linear ranges, and LLOQ of the analytes are shown in Table 3. The linearity of the calibration curves was determined by plotting the peak area ratio (analytes/IS) against the nominal concentration of the calibration standards in rat plasma covering the expected range (10–3200 ng/mL) by linear regression analysis with the use of a 1/X^2 (x is the concentration) weighing factor. The calibration curves of the analytes exhibited linearity at a specific concentration range in rat plasma.

Table 3. The linear equation, linear range, and LLOQ of the T4C, T3C, T2C, C4C, TCT, PIC, and SAF in rat plasma samples.

Analyte	Linear Equation	Range (ng/mL)	R^2	LOD (ng/mL)	LLOQ (ng/mL)
T4C	10.00 to 3200.00	y = 0.001106907x + 0.0007873082	0.9968	2.00	10.00
T3C	10.00 to 3200.00	y = 0.002373485x − 0.000003492705	0.9954	2.00	10.00
T2C	10.00 to 3200.00	y = 0.002490268x − 0.0001086531	0.9990	5.00	10.00
C4C	10.00 to 3200.00	y = 0.0002475676x + 0.0003535316	0.9960	5.00	10.00
TCT	10.00 to 3200.00	y = 0.002001102x + 0.002474666	0.9952	2.00	10.00
PIC	10.00 to 3200.00	y = 0.002674921x + 0.004357420	0.9975	5.00	10.00
SAF	10.00 to 3200.00	y = 0.007429112x + 0.02994744	0.9985	2.00	10.00

The LOD was determined on the analyte concentration, which showed a peak response with a signal-to-noise ratio (S/N) of >3.3. Further, the LLOQ was determined with a signal-to-noise ratio > 10 at 10 ng/mL level (n = 5) for each analyte [40,41], which indicated that the method was sufficiently sensitive for pharmacokinetic studies. It is the lowest concentration of the standard curve that can be accurately and precisely measured.

2.3. Bioanalytical Method Validation

The following validation results were recorded and analyzed for four bioactive compounds (i.e., TCT, T4C, PIC) and SAF by UFLC-MS/MS in rat plasma.2.3.1. Optimization of Analytes Extraction from the Plasma

2.3.1. Optimization of Analytes Extraction from the Plasma

While processing the rat plasma samples, analytes extraction is a critical step for accurate and consistent MS/MS analysis. Protein precipitation extraction (PPE) and liquid-liquid extraction (LLE) methods were compared for sample preparation. The carotenoids and apocarotenoids classes are the least stable in natural products. In CSE, the polar solvents are the solvent of choice for better solubility and consistent extraction. After different trials, acetonitrile and methanol were found as efficient solvents. Methanol was found to have better precipitation and stability of the analytes and IS experiments for CSE and was chosen as the optimized solvent for experimentation.

The simple and stable protein precipitation (PPE) method was optimized for the CSE analyte and internal standard extraction. The accuracy and matrix effect achieved in the PPE method using acidified methanol with formic acid also enhanced recovery and efficiency. This extraction method was suitable for stabilizing SAF content in the rat plasma compared to other trials. The quantification was done by using a response factor of IS. This concentration-dependent strategy was found helpful for CSE carotenoids–apocarotenoids for encountering variable responses.

2.3.2. System Suitability Test

The system suitability test was applied to each batch at the LQC level ($n = 5$), during and after the batch analysis. The relative standard deviation of peak area response and retention time for each analyte was $\leq$10% and 5%, respectively.

2.3.3. Specificity and Sensitivity

Validation was carried out as per USFDA and EMA guidelines [40,41]. The specificity and selectivity were investigated by comparing the retention times in chromatograms of blank plasma added with analytes and blank plasma, and plasma sample after oral administration of CSE; no interference peak was observed at a retention time of analytes of endogenous substances in the plasma samples. (Figure 3) The mean signal-to-noise ratios for T4C, TCT, PIC, SAF, IS1, and IS2 were 18.90 $\pm$ 4.28, 24.97 $\pm$ 4.82, 17.02 $\pm$ 3.39, 34.70 $\pm$ 7.08, 77.72 $\pm$ 8.28, 88.69 $\pm$ 10.77, respectively.

2.3.4. Quality Control Samples

The accuracy and precision parameters determined on the four QC levels and other parameters and assay were calculated with three QC levels based on linearity and LLOQ [41] (Table 3). The QC samples were prepared at four levels by spiking the analyte in plasma to get the LLQC (10 ng/mL), LQC (three times of LLOQ, 30 ng/mL), MQC (50% of the upper CC range, 1600 ng/mL), and HQC (75% of the upper CC range, 2400 ng/mL).

2.3.5. Accuracy and Precision

Precision and accuracy were determined by analyzing QC samples at four level concentrations ($n = 6$) on the same days (01–04) and a different day ($n = 6 \times 3$). The accuracy was evaluated by relative error (RE). In contrast, precision was expressed in relative standard deviation (RSD), as given in Table 4. The range of precision from 1.29 to 10.18% for intra-day ranged from 1.16 to 10.51% for inter-day, respectively. The accuracy expressed was within $\pm$15% in all QC levels. All the results met the acceptance criteria. This data indicated that this developed UFLC-MS/MS method was accurate and reliable for determining compounds.

Table 4. Intra- and inter-day precision and accuracies of the analytes in rat plasma, (ng/mL).

Analyte	Nominal Concentration (ng/mL)	Intra-Day 01 ($n = 6$)		Intra-Day 02 ($n = 6$)		Intra-Day 03 ($n = 6$)		Intra-Day 04 ($n = 6$)		Inter-Day ($n = 6 \times 3$)	
		Precision (RSD, %)	Accuracy (RE, %)	Precision (RSD, %)	Accuracy (RE, %)	Precision (RSD, %)	Accuracy (RE, %)	Precision (RSD, %)	Accuracy (RE, %)	Precision (RSD, %)	Accuracy (RE, %)
T4C	10.00	6.76	−2.78	6.76	−2.78	7.96	−1.09	5.72	−6.03	6.93	5.53
	30.00	6.65	−2.33	6.65	−2.33	6.65	−3.97	2.98	−1.95	5.53	−7.62
	1600.00	1.23	−2.73	1.23	−2.73	3.43	−6.39	2.92	−7.50	1.16	−8.92
	2400.00	5.15	−0.19	5.15	−0.19	5.48	−1.94	2.25	−7.77	1.69	2.15
TCT	10.00	7.40	0.92	7.40	0.92	7.18	−1.16	6.97	−5.52	6.07	1.12
	30.00	4.95	−0.63	4.95	−0.63	5.67	−3.12	6.31	−3.91	5.74	−4.83
	1600.00	1.98	2.29	1.98	2.29	5.63	−4.44	1.29	−7.14	3.49	−8.48
	2400.00	5.81	1.68	5.82	1.68	4.38	−1.21	1.94	−3.99	2.48	−1.32
PIC	10.00	7.04	−11.03	7.04	−11.03	9.96	−3.71	6.70	0.25	5.24	4.63
	30.00	5.95	−6.23	5.95	−6.23	8.00	−3.20	4.83	−0.77	10.51	−5.14
	1600.00	2.50	−1.50	2.50	−1.50	3.99	−5.72	2.90	−3.97	2.08	−8.32
	2400.00	1.57	0.24	1.57	0.24	3.35	−1.83	4.09	−4.98	3.34	−0.61
SAF	10.00	5.11	4.90	5.11	4.90	6.61	3.83	10.18	−4.73	7.41	6.35
	30.00	5.15	−1.26	5.15	−1.26	5.45	−1.18	5.21	1.77	7.14	−1.49
	1600.00	2.24	−2.95	2.24	−2.95	3.21	−4.85	2.59	−7.35	2.33	−7.63
	2400.00	2.91	−0.20	2.91	−0.20	3.88	−1.51	1.96	−5.11	1.95	0.66

2.3.6. Extraction Recovery, Dilution Integrity, and Carryover

The results of the extraction recoveries and dilution integrity of the four compounds are listed in Tables 5 and 6. The mean extraction recoveries of the analytes in plasma at three quality control (QC) concentration levels were found from $91.18 \pm 0.73\%$ to $106.86 \pm 1.73\%$.

Table 5. Extraction recovery(ng/mL) of the compounds in rat plasma samples, ($n = 6$).

Analyte	Nominal Concentration (ng/mL)	Extraction Recovery (%, mean ± SD)	Precision (RSD, %)	Accuracy (RE, %)
T4C	30.00	91.18 ± 0.73	0.80	−9.29
	1600.00	99.09 ± 1.55	1.56	−1.15
	2400.00	101.60 ± 0.46	0.45	1.56
TCT	30.00	106.23 ± 3.62	3.41	5.99
	1600.00	105.22 ± 3.48	3.30	4.45
	2400.00	101.45 ± 1.01	1.00	−2.18
PIC	30.00	96.74 ± 1.04	1.07	−4.30
	1600.00	102.89 ± 1.76	1.71	2.04
	2400.00	106.86 ± 1.73	1.61	4.67
SAF	30.00	100.72 ± 0.58	0.57	0.91
	1600.00	103.05 ± 2.95	2.86	2.38
	2400.00	105.29 ± 1.83	1.74	4.98

Table 6. Dilution Integrity of analytes in two-fold and four-fold dilution (ng/mL) ($n = 6$).

Analyte	Nominal Concentration (ng/mL)	Two-Fold Dilution (ng/mL)	Precision (RSD, %)	Accuracy (RE, %)	Four-Fold Dilution (ng/mL)	Precision (RSD, %)	Accuracy (RE, %)
T4C	5000.00	4663.09 ± 92.81	1.99	−6.74	4642.16 ± 118.87	2.56	−7.16
TCT		4634.89 ± 137.40	2.96	−7.30	4689.90 ± 182.80	3.90	−6.20
PIC		4740.06 ± 164.85	3.48	−5.20	4744.10 ± 118.81	2.50	−5.12
SAF		4706.07 ± 57.69	1.23	−5.88	4722.58 ± 62.50	1.32	−5.55

Dilution integrity determined by analyte spiking above the upper limit of quantification (ULOQ) and diluted with blank plasma brought into the calibration curve was analyzed to obtain acceptable concentration after proper dilution with blank plasma. The results showed that the precision and accuracy of the diluted QCs were within the 15% limit (Table 6).

2.3.7. Matrix Effect and Stability Studies

The four compounds' matrix effects were found to be in the range of $95.88 \pm 8.44\%$ to $100.78 \pm 2.59\%$, suggesting no significant ion suppression or enhancement in this LC-MS method as the guidelines in Table 7.

Table 7. Matrix effect (ng/mL) for the determination of compounds in rat plasma ($n = 6$).

Analyte	Nominal Concentration (ng/mL)	Matrix Effect (%, mean ± SD)	Precision (RSD, %)	Accuracy (RE, %)
T4C	30.00	100.03 ± 5.21	5.21	−7.63
	2400.00	98.98 ± 4.17	4.21	3.33
TCT	30.00	97.68 ± 8.35	8.55	−2.25
	2400.00	100.78 ± 2.59	2.57	−2.08
PIC	30.00	95.88 ± 8.44	8.81	2.14
	2400.00	98.91 ± 6.91	6.99	0.71
SAF	30.00	96.43 ± 6.51	6.75	2.18
	2400.00	99.19 ± 2.53	2.55	1.51

The analyte stability in plasma was demonstrated by analyzing LQC and HQC samples (n = 6) at storage conditions as per Table 8 for processed plasma samples of CSE. It showed that T4C, TCT, PIC, and SAF were stable but under restricted storage conditions due to their sensitive nature. The precision was found for autosampler stability conditions from approximately 3.08% to 4.76% with accuracy (RE, −0.19–3.40), for room temperature from 2.38% to 5.35% with accuracy (RE, −0.26–1.33), and freeze-thaw stability 2.43% to 8.25% with accuracy (RE, −0.06–4.13).

Table 8. Stability assays for the determination of compounds in rat plasma (n = 6).

Analyte	Nominal Concentration (ng/mL)	Autosampler Stability (%, mean ± SD)	Precision (RSD, %)	Accuracy (RE, %)	Room Temperature Stability (%, mean ± SD)	Precision (RSD, %)	Accuracy (RE, %)	Freeze-Thaw Stability (%, mean ± SD)	Precision (RSD, %)	Accuracy (RE, %)
T4C	30.00	29.01 ± 1.38	4.76	−3.29	27.80 ± 1.29	4.64	−7.34	28.45 ± 1.06	3.74	−5.18
	2400.00	2481.58 ± 86.48	3.49	3.40	2413.86 ± 73.67	3.05	0.58	2369.47 ± 195.39	8.25	−1.27
TCT	30.00	29.94 ± 1.29	4.30	−0.19	28.59 ± 1.18	4.12	−4.69	29.79 ± 1.58	5.30	−0.69
	2400.00	2467.92 ± 101.06	4.09	2.83	2425.78 ± 112.27	4.63	1.07	2383.90 ± 133.23	5.59	−0.67
PIC	30.00	29.52 ± 1.26	4.26	−1.61	30.40 ± 0.92	3.01	1.33	29.98 ± 1.66	5.55	−0.06
	2400.00	2463.69 ± 113.42	4.60	2.65	2406.19 ± 94.01	3.91	−0.26	2498.53 ± 111.53	4.46	4.11
SAF	30.00	29.97 ± 0.90	3.08	−2.44	28.07 ± 0.67	2.38	−6.43	29.66 ± 1.42	4.78	−1.13
	2400.00	2472.88 ± 0.90	4.08	3.04	2370.67 ± 126.71	5.35	−1.22	2499.17 ± 60.75	2.43	4.13

2.3.8. Application of Bioanalytical Method to Oral Pharmacokinetics Study

The method parameters were confirmed and validated for TCT, T4C, PIC, and SAF based on bioanalytical guidelines in the rat plasma. This method was applied to the study of carotenoids and apocarotenoids in plasma after oral administration of CSE in rats. The compounds PIC, SAF T4C, TCT with T3C, C4C, and T2C were determined using the validated UFLC-MS/MS method. The response of compounds T3C, T2C, and C4C were confirmed based on the retention time, relative retention factor from IS1, and optimized MS/MS profile. (Table 2) These compounds were quantified against individual linearity and area response in rat plasma in each analysis [4] (Figure 4)

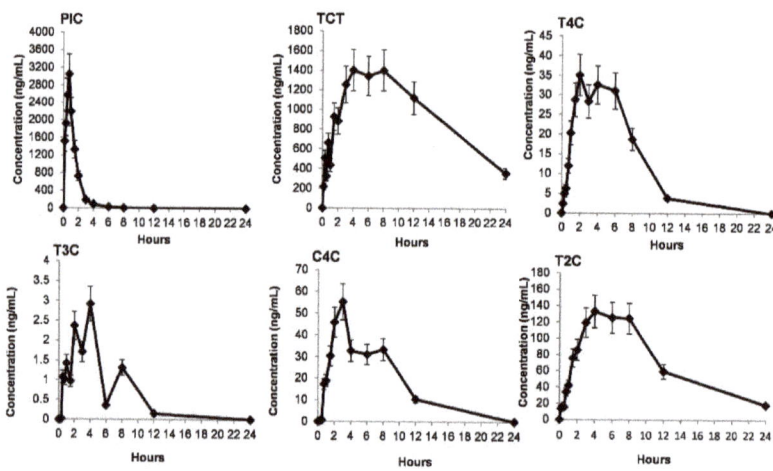

Figure 4. Mean plasma concentration-time curves of six constituents identified and quantified after oral administration of Kashmir saffron extract (CSE) at the dose of 40 mg/kg in rats (mean ± SEM, n = 6). PIC, T4C, TCT, T3C, C4C, and T2C.

2.4. Pharmacokinetic Results

As is known, natural products may work through the combined effects of constituents with similar structures [44]. Satisfactory therapeutic effects are obtained even though some of the constituents may be at low blood concentrations. The quantification showed a significant amount of T4C, T3C, and PIC with C4C, T2C, TCT, and SAF in CSE by UFLC-PDA. The validated bioanalytical UFLC-MS/MS method was applied to the simultaneous determination of these seven compounds after single oral administration of CSE (40 mg/kg) in rats ($n = 6$). The quantification was done for apocarotenoids PIC and SAF and carotenoids T4C, T3C, C4C, T2C, TCT.

The PK parameters were calculated by non-compartmental analysis. The PK parameters, such as maximum plasma concentration (C_{max}) and the time to reach the maximum plasma concentration (T_{max}), were derived directly from the experimental data. The trapezoidal equation calculated the areas under the plasma concentration-time curves from 0 to the time of the last quantifiable concentration (AUC_{0-t}). The AUC was extrapolated to infinity $AUC_{0-\infty}$ using C_t/K_{el}, where C_t is the last measured MET concentration. K_{el} is the elimination rate constant determined from the terminal slope of the log concentration-time plot. The K_{el} was obtained from the linear regression curve slope by fitting the terminal concentrations' natural logarithms versus time. The terminal elimination half-life ($t_{1/2}$) was calculated by $0.693/K_{el}$. The clearance (CL) was calculated as the quotient of the dose (D) and $AUC_{0-\infty}$. All values were expressed as mean ± SEM.

As a result, in this study, the crocins detected in plasma were all acquired. This is the first report on the PK profiles of seven compounds of CSE in rats. The PK parameters were calculated and are listed in Table 9. The mean plasma concentration-time curves of six compounds are shown in Figure 4, except SAF due to the low concentration in vivo. The PK parameters of SAF could not be calculated because of the lack of sufficient data points, as its original amount in the CSE was comparatively low.

Table 9. Pharmacokinetics (PK) parameters of six compounds after an oral administration of Kashmir saffron extract (CSE) ($n = 6$).

PK Parameters	T4C	T3C	T2C	C4C	TCT	PIC
C_{max} (ng/mL)	49.27 ± 11.15	7.59 ± 4.71	160.44 ± 15.17	86.14 ± 15.65	2076.21 ± 373.61	2722.95 ± 231.41
T_{max} (h)	3.5 ± 0.57	3.5 ± 1.09	4.34 ± 0.51	3.25 ± 1.05	6.84 ± 1.69	0.792 ± 0.10
AUC_{0-t} (h.ng/mL)	277.04 ± 67.69	20.36 ± 9.64	1529.1 ± 197.40	395.64 ± 113.41	23,590 ± 3119.25	3691.19 ± 274.38
$AUC_{0-\infty}$ (h.ng/mL)	370.45 ± 75.64	55.46 ± 31.21	1676.12 ± 238.38	407.21 ± 187.28	30,679.13 ± 3706.46	3818.76 ± 256.67
$t_{1/2}$ (h)	3.36 ± 1.00	4.6 ± 2.74	5.75 ± 0.73	1.57 ± 1.57	8.98 ± 2.00	0.793 ± 0.078
CL (mL/h/kg)	19,568.35 ± 4835.41	114,958.33 ± 71,000.46	234.77 ± 31.12	326.37 ± 445.89	0.547 ± 0.094	1935.88 ± 123.45
V_d (L/kg)	69.250 ± 16.150	325.573 ± 13.099	2.006 ± 0.457	4.29 ± 1.94	0.00617 ± 0.00104	2.258 ± 0.3168

C_{max}- maximal observed concentration; T_{max}- maximum observed time; AUC_{0-t}- area under the curve from time zero to the last measurable concentration; $AUC_{0-\infty}$- area under the curve from time zero extrapolated to infinite time; $t_{1/2}$ - half-life; CL- clearance; V_d-volume of distribution; h-hour; ng-nanogram; mL-milliliter; L-liter; kg-kilogram.

All six compounds were detected at a first-time point (i.e., 10 min). The TCT reached C_{max} at 6.83 ± 1.68 h in the plasma, which is higher than the previously reported maximum plasma concentration (C_{max}), i.e., 66.3 ± 9.2 min in rat plasma [42]. The five CS analytes T4C, T3C, C4C, T2C, and TCT, achieved C_{max} at between 3 and 7 h, i.e., time to reach the maximum plasma concentration (T_{max}) except PIC, which attained C_{max} at 0.67 h in the plasma. The concentration-dependent responses of PIC, T4C, C4C, T2C, T3C, and TCT are shown in Figure 4 except for SAF due to its low abundance and AUC in samples.

This is the first study that reports the PK parameters of the PIC in the rats. As shown in Table 9, the $t_{1/2}$ of TCT was more than 11 h, suggesting that the compounds' absorption and elimination rates were slower than most carotenoid ingredients after oral administration of CSE in rats. The slow elimination of components might help to maintain effects. The absorption rate of TCT, which had the highest concentration among all components, was relatively slow, maybe because of transformation from T4C, T3C, C4C, and T2C by intestinal bacteria [46,47], and this validated method was found to be efficient to confirm and quantify these analytes responses in rat plasma samples. This concludes that PIC is also a significant biomarker in vivo and TCT after oral KCS and CSE consumption.

3. Discussion

While the latest methodologies and reports are [17,22,29] targeting only T4C study in PK or bioanalysis, this research gives a novel method of quantification and study for five more bioactive compounds from CS (i.e., T3C, T2C, C4C, PIC, and SAF) for further application in any preclinical or clinical studies. Most of the saffron bioanalytical studies lack the validation data needed for the reproducibility and robustness of these carotenoids and apocarotenoids quantification methods. The current study gives a stable matrix-based extraction and validation of UFLC-MS/MS-based methodology, consistent and sensitive for all these compounds.

Some pharmacokinetic studies on CS reported that the intestinal deglycosylation of various crocins is primarily due to the enzymatic processes in the epithelial cells. In these reports, minor crocins may be deglycosylated by the fecal microbiome, facilitating transformation into TCT finally [36,37]. The values of C_{max} and AUC_{0-t} of TCT in the present study were much higher than other crocins. This phenomenon might be the biotransformation of crocins to TCT by intestinal bacteria and enzymes in vivo, leading to a higher concentration of TCT in plasma. The comparative results indicated that coexisting compounds in CS might enhance the absorption of TCT by increasing absorption or bioavailability. However, the exact absorption mechanism of these components is still unclear.

4. Materials and Methods

4.1. Chemicals and Reagents

Compounds used in this study are *trans*-4-GG-crocin (T4C) (Pubchem CID-24721245), *trans*-3-Gg-crocin (T3C) (Pubchem CID-9940690), *trans*-2-gg-crocin (T2C) (Pubchem ID-25244294), *cis*-4-GG-crocin (C4C) (Pubchem CID-101662426), *trans* crocetin (TCT) (Pubchem CID-124350893), picrocrocin (PIC) (Pubchem CID-130796), safranal (SAF) (Pubchem CID-61041), reserpine (Pubchem CID-5770), and chloramphenicol (Pubchem CID-5959). The reference compounds were procured from the following suppliers: T4C and T3C procured from Chromadex (Los Angeles, CA, USA) and PhytoLab, (Vestenbergsgreuth, Germany), respectively. SAF, reserpine, and chloramphenicol were procured from Sigma–Aldrich (St. Louis, MO, USA). Both PIC and TCT were isolated in-house using previously reported extraction and column chromatography methods [4], further characterized by nuclear magnetic resonance (NMR), MS/MS, and UHPLC-PDA analysis. Both C4C and T2C were received as a gift sample from CSIR-IIIM (Jammu, India) [3,4,48]. The purity of reference compounds was checked by analyzing high-concentration (1 mg/mL) solution by UHPLC-PDA and found (>90.0%). Acetonitrile, methanol, water (JT Baker, India), and formic acid, MS grade (Fluka, Honeywell, India), were used in the UFLC-MS/MS study.

4.2. Preparation and Standardization of Kashmir Saffron Extract (CSE)

The Kashmir saffron sample was procured from Jammu and Kashmir, India, (KCS) and authenticated by the Botanical Survey of India, Jodhpur. The dried stigmas of saffron were ground to a coarse powder (200 g) and extracted with ethanol-water at 40 °C for 3 h. Extraction was repeated twice, followed by distillation of solvent below 50 °C with yield (20%). The powder obtained after distillation was stored in an amber-colored bottle below 2 °C (CSE). The CSE (110g), suspended in water and then partitioned with hexane-ethyl acetate (5:95). Further from this, hexane-ethyl acetate layer fraction (12 g), PIC (28 mg), and TCT (34 mg) were isolated and further characterized by nuclear magnetic resonance (NMR) and MS/MS analysis [4].

The contents of PIC, SAF, T4C, T3C, C4C, T2C, and TCT, the CSE was standardized and quantified by an external standard method by similar chromatographic conditions as the experimental section by the UFLC-PDA method [49–51]. The PIC and SAF's identification and quantification were recorded at 254 nm and 320 nm against the reference standards.

All the isomers of crocins and TCT were identified and quantified at 440 nm against T4C and TCT, respectively. (Figure S1).

4.3. Animals

Male Sprague–Dawley rats (250–300 g) were purchased from Crystal Biological Solution, Pune, Maharashtra, India. The animal studies were sanctioned by the Animal Ethics Committee of Crystal Biological Solution, Pune. It was carried out following the Animal Ethics Procedures and Guidelines of Control and Supervision of Experiments on Animals (CPCSEA) committee requirements. Animals were housed 3–4 per cage in rooms with constant temperature (25 ± 2 °C), humidity (50 ± 20%), and 12 h dark-light cycle. All animals in the oral group fasted overnight before the dosing, and food was provided 8 h post-dose, and water was ad libitum. The investigational CSE was fed orally to an individual rat as per its body weight.

4.4. Ultrafast Liquid Chromatography-Mass Spectrometry (UFLC-MS/MS)

The UFLC-MS/MS analysis was performed on a Shimadzu UFLC system (Kyoto, Japan) consisting of a DGU-20A5R degasser, LC-30AD pump, SIL-30AC autosampler, CTO-20AC column oven. The chromatographic separation was carried out in a single analytical run divided into loading and eluting phases by alternating the electronic valve. At the loading phase (−1–0 min), the auto-sampler was responsible for injecting 50 µL of the sample. The LC-30AD pump was responsible for delivering water containing 0.1% formic acid to the pre-column (Phenomenex Security Guard ULTRA with C8 Cartridge) at 0.8 mL/min to remove protein and retain analytes. At the eluting phase (0–12 min), the retained components were flushed from the pre-column into the analytical column (Dr. Maisch GmbH Reprosil Gold XBD C8, 50 mm × 4.6 mm, i.d., 1.8 µm) eluting as per time programmed gradient. The flow rate of the mobile phase was 0.8 mL/min. The mobile phase consists of a mixture of water containing 0.1% formic acid (%v/v) (A) and 100% acetonitrile (B). The gradient elution program was carried out for chromatographic separation: 0.01–1.91 min, 20% B; 1.91–5.91 min, 2090% B; 5.91–6.91 min, 90–80% B; 6.91–8.24 min, 80–20% B; and 8.24–12 min, 20% B. The column oven temperature was set at 30 °C. The MS/MS analysis was carried out on an LCMS-8045 triple-quadrupole mass spectrometer (Shimadzu, Kyoto, Japan) equipped with positive and negative electrospray ionization (ESI) interfaces using the MRM mode. The compound and source dependent parameters were defined as follows: nitrogen was used as nebulizing and drying gas; argon was used as the collision gas. Quadruple voltage was set at Q1 RF gain: 4998 Q1 RF offset 4990 and Q1 post-rod bias: −5.0 V CID CELL exit lens: −4.0 V, interface: ESI, interface temperature: 350 °C, desolvation line (DL) temperature: 250 °C, nebulizing gas flow: 2.50 L/min, heating gas flow: 10.00 L/min heat block: 300 °C; drying gas flow: 10.00 L/min.

The ESI source was operated in the negative and positive ion mode. The MRM analysis was done by monitoring transitions of the precursor to product ions transition of compounds, i.e., m/z 975.7/651.3 for T4C, m/z 813.3/327.2 for T3C, m/z 651.3/327.2 for T2C, m/z 975.5/651.4 for C4C, m/z 327.1/283.1 for TCT, m/z 609.7/195.1 for reserpine, and 321.00/152.00 for chloramphenicol. The IS1 (reserpine) was used to analyze PIC and SAF in positive mode, whereas IS2 (chloramphenicol) was used to analyze T4C, T3C, T2C, C4C, and TCT in a negative mode. The apocarotenoids PIC showed m/z 151.3/81.1, similar to the SAF m/z 151.3/81.1 but separated by LC based on retention time 1.925 and 6.190 min, respectively (Figure 3). The other instrument parameters, viz. dwell time (msec), Q1 Pre-Bias (eV), CE (eV), Q3 Pre-Bias (eV), tR (min), were optimized as per Table 2. All data were controlled and analyzed by Lab Solution and Lab Solution Insight Software (Versions 3.2) of Shimadzu Tech. (Kyoto, Japan).

4.5. Preparation of Standard Solution, Calibration Standards, and Quality Control Samples

Each standard stock solution of T4C, T3C, T2C, C4C, TCT, PIC, and SAF (1.0 mg/mL) with IS1and IS2 (1.0 mg/mL) was prepared separately in the methanol to prepare calibration standards and quality control samples. The primary stock solutions were made up of methanol to prepare mixed working solutions (WSa). All the standard stock solutions were stored at 4 °C. The calibration curve (CC) stock solutions (WSa) were diluted with methanol to prepared working solutions with a range of 100 to 32,000 ng/mL (WSb). The stock solutions of IS1 and IS2 were diluted to prepare 0.1 mg/mL (WSc).

The blank plasma samples of volume 45 µL were spiked with each of 5 µL standards (WSa) and IS (WSc) solutions, respectively. With further 200 µL, methanol was added and vortex for 2 min, followed by centrifugation for 10 min at 2000 RPM. The supernatant was collected in HPLC vials for analysis. A nine-point CC (10, 30, 100, 200, 400, 800, 1600, 2400, and 3200 ng/mL) was prepared for analysis. Quality control samples were prepared separately by spiking respective working standard solutions to achieved LLOQ (10 ng/mL), LOQ (30 ng/mL), MOQ (1600 ng/mL), and HOQ (2400 ng/mL).

4.5.1. Preparation of Plasma Samples

An aliquot of 45 µL of rat plasma was spiked with each 5 µL of IS1 and IS2, and 200 µL of methanol was added, vortexed for 1–2 min, then centrifuged for 10 min at 2000 RPM. Collect the supernatant into HPLC vials and injected it into the UFLC-MS/MS system for analysis.

4.5.2. Linearity and Calibration Curve (CC)

The linearity of T4C, T3C, T2C, C4C TCT, PIC, and SAF over nine points (10, 30, 100, 200, 400, 800, 1600, 2400, and 3200 ng/mL) were prepared by spiking of 45 µL drug-free rat plasma with the appropriate amount of analyte and IS1 and IS2. The linearity was assessed with three different calibration curves with maintaining the standard internal concentration at 10 ng/mL. A nine-point CC was set up by plotting T4C, T3C, T2C, C4C, TCT, PIC, and SAF peak area ratio against the control matrix's nominal concentration of calibration standards. Calculation of linear regression data with $1/X^2$ weighting factor.

4.6. Bioanalytical Validation: UFLC-MS/MS Method

The optimized method for carotenoids T4C, T3C, C4C, T2C, TCT, and apocarotenoids PIC and SAF were further validated for four bioactive compounds, i.e., TCT, T4C, PIC, and SAF based on the reference compound's availability. The compounds T3C, T2C, and C4C were confirmed based on the retention time, relative retention factor from IS, and MS/MS profile [3].

4.6.1. System Suitability Test

A system suitability test (SST) was performed before the batch analysis. The LLQC ($n = 7$) sample was followed by a blank ($n = 8$) injected in the system to assess the reproducibility of tR and peak area response in the method. Acceptance criteria for the relative standard deviation (RSD) of the analyte peaks' area response obtained from the seven-system suitability; plasma samples were <10.00%.

4.6.2. Specificity, Selectivity, and Sensitivity (LLOQ)

The method's specificity and selectivity were determined by analyzing samples from at least six different blank rat plasma sources for significance interference at the LC peak elution zone of T4C, TCT, PIC, SAF, and IS. Further plasma samples spiked with IS1 and IS2 were analyzed as zero calibrators and spiked with mixed analyte at LLOQ level for any co-eluting peak interference at the LC peak elution zone. Sensitivity was evaluated at the LLOQ with acceptable precision, accuracy, and signal-to-noise (S/N) ratio was >10.

4.6.3. Quality Control Samples

After determining the linearity of T4C, TCT, PIC, and SAF nine points calibration curve (in Section 4.5.2), four QC levels were calculated [41]. The QC samples were prepared at four levels by spiking the analytes in plasma to get the LLOQ (lower limit of specification),

LQC (three times of LLOQ), MQC (50% of the upper CC range), and HQC (75% of the upper CC range).

4.6.4. Accuracy and Precision

The intraday accuracy and precision were ascertained by analyzing QC samples spiked at four levels within the calibration curve (10 ng/mL, 30 ng/mL, 1600 ng/mL, 2400 ng/mL) in blank rat plasma. Intraday precision and accuracy of the method were estimated in multiple analyses of batches ($n = 6$) of quality control samples for repeatability. And for the inter-day analysis, the same sample set was analyzed on three consecutive days. The acceptance criterion for each back-calculated standard concentration was 85–115% accuracy from the nominal value, except for the LLOQ (<80–120%). The precision criterion was <15% RSD (Tables 3 and 4) except for the LLOQ (<20%).

4.6.5. Extraction Recovery, Matrix Effect, and Carryover

Analyte recovery was calculated at three quality control levels in blank plasma. QC samples were prepared ($n = 6$) at the low, medium, and higher QC (30, 1600, 2400 ng/mL), by spiking freshly prepared mix analyte and IS (1.0 µg/mL) into the blank matrix. Following extraction, recovery (%) was determined by comparing QC samples' mean response at pre-extraction spiking with corresponding post-extraction spiking. The matrix effect was demonstrated as a matrix factor at two quality control levels in blank plasma. The QC samples (LQC and HQC) were prepared ($n = 6$), containing the analyte and IS spiked into a blank plasma matrix (post-extraction samples). The other containing Analyte and IS spiked into the mobile phase (diluent). The matrix factor was evaluated as the ratio of peak response of analyte and IS in the presence of matrix divided by IS and analyte's peak response in the absence of matrix. The carryover was studied by comparing the response in a blank after calibration standard at the ULOQ ($n = 3$). The total response was noted and monitored for not exceeding 20% of LLOQ.

4.6.6. Stability Studies of Carotenoids and Apocarotenoids

The stability was performed at different sets of working and storage conditions. As carotenoids and apocarotenoids are sensitive compounds, their presence in CSE was studied carefully. The degradation of T4C, TCT, PIC, and SAF was observed in plasma at LQC and HQC levels. The stability conditions of the method studied were at ambient temperature for 4 h (room-temperature stability), in the autosampler at 8 °C conditions for 24 h (autosampler stability), and with three freeze-thaw cycles at -20 ± 4 °C condition (freeze-thaw stability). The samples were prudent to be stable if the measured concentration was within ±15% of the nominal concentration [40,41].

4.7. Application of Validated Methodology in Investigation of Pharmacokinetic Parameters of CSE

This sensitive and validated UFLC-MS/MS method was applied for the simultaneous determination of CSE apocarotenoids and carotenoids in rat plasma. The PK parameters were investigated after oral administration of CSE in the rats ($n = 6$). The in vivo pharmacokinetic study of KCS was studied for active metabolite TCT and T4C with PIC, SAF with T3C, C4C, and T2C.

4.8. Pharmacokinetic Study

Twelve male animals were free to access the water and food until 12 h before the experiment. In the study, the animals were administered 40 mg/kg CSE by oral gavage. The dose was selected based on previous research [3,4,52]. After drug administration, twelve animals were further subdivided into two groups with six animals (for alternate time-point blood samples). Blood samples (0.2 mL) were collected from the ophthalmic venous plexus into heparinized tubes at pre-dose, 0.16, 0.33, 0.5, 0.75, 1, 1.5, 2, 3, 4, 6, 8, 12, and 24 h post-dosing, respectively. Heparin sodium (1 g/100 mL) with 10 µL was added to a tube and dried into the heparinized tube. In the experiment, the saline and sugar solutions were provided every two h to promote the recovery of the rat's blood volume. The blood samples were collected from six rats at each time point. Each blood sample was centrifuged at 5000 rpm for 10 min, and then the plasma layer was transferred into clean tubes and stored at −80 °C until analysis.

5. Conclusions

India's Kashmir region has been found suitable for the growth and quality supply of KCS with regional agricultural benefit. The KCS and its extract (CSE) has become a popular dietary supplement with bioactive as apocarotenoids (PIC, SAF) and carotenoids (crocins, crocetin) [3,28–34]. These dietary supplements have been regulated widely and require a validated methodology and data. [53,54]. The studies showed the potential of KCS and CSE in brain health. Therefore, the quantitative relationship of apocarotenoids, carotenoids, and active metabolites like crocetin in the CSE and it's in vivo therapeutics data hold importance showed an improved memory function.

Thus, in this research, a sensitive and reproducible UFLC-MS/MS method was developed for the simultaneous determination of seven CSE compounds in rat plasma. The method showed excellent linearity ($R^2 > 0.990$) with the lower limit of quantification (LLOQ) (10 ng/mL) for apocarotenoids PIC and SAF and carotenoids T4C, T3C, C4C, T2C, TCT.

This UFLC-MS/MS method was validated to determine PIC, SAF TCT, and T4C with internal standards reserpine and chloramphenicol in the rat plasma. The precision (RSD, <15%) and accuracy (RE, −11.03–9.96) studies on UFLC-MS/MS assay based on the three analytical quality control (QC) levels were well within the acceptance criteria from FDA guidance for bioanalytical method validation with recoveries (91.18–106.86%) [40]. The method was applied to investigate the PK parameters after oral administration of 40 mg/kg CSE in the rats ($n = 6$).

This is the first report on the in vivo oral pharmacokinetics investigations that disclosed active metabolite PIC with TCT, T4C quantitatively related to CSE. The T3C, C4C, T2C, and SAF were also detected by this validated bioanalytical method after oral CSE consumption. This will help preclinical/clinical trials of KCS dietary supplements focusing on apocarotenoids and carotenoids in various therapeutic applications and their neuroprotective role.

6. Patents

Sustained-release formulations of Crocus sativus. IN201711036084, WO2019077621A1, EP18796784.9, US16753969.

Supplementary Materials: The following are available online. Figure S1: HPLC Standardization of *Crocus sativus* extract A- Chromatograms of standards PIC, T4C, TCT, SAF; B- Chromatograms of KCS extract at 254 nm/440 nm/320 nm.

Author Contributions: Conceptualization, A.G., S.S., A.D. and L.H.; Data curation, S.P., G.S. and A.K.B.; Formal analysis, S.P., S.S., A.K.B. and A.D.; Funding acquisition, L.H.; Investigation, A.G., S.P., C.G. and L.H.; Methodology, A.G., S.P., C.G., S.S., G.S. and A.D.; Project administration, A.G. and L.H.; Resources, L.H.; Software, S.P., C.G. and A.K.B.; Supervision, A.G., S.S. and L.H.; Validation, S.P., C.G., S.S., G.S., A.K.B. and A.D.; Visualization, A.G., C.G. and G.S.; Writing—original draft, A.G., S.P., C.G., S.S., G.S., A.K.B. and A.D.; Writing—review & editing, A.G., and L.H. All authors have read and agreed to the published version of the manuscript.

Funding: This research received no external funding.

Institutional Review Board Statement: The Institutional Animal Ethics Committee (Animal House Registration no. 2030/PO/RcBiBt/S/18/CPCSEA) had reviewed and approved the experimental protocol (No. CRY/1920/008). All animals used in the study were handled with humane care and as per CPESEA guidelines.

Acknowledgments: The authors would like to acknowledge CSIR-IIIM (Jammu, India) for the technology's initial development and its transfer to Pharmanza Herbal Pvt. Ltd. The authors acknowledge Ram Vishwakarma (Director CSIR-IIIIM, India) and Sandip Bharate for providing reference compounds in this study. Also, the authors acknowledge Utpal Nandi (PK-PD, Toxicology and Formulation Division, CSIR-IIIIM, India) and Vijay Thawani (Director, Centre for Scientific Research and Development (CSRD), India) for expert assistance in reviewing the manuscript. Amit Mirgal and Pradeep Solanki (Pharmanza Herbal Pvt. Ltd.) for authentication of plant material and sample preparation.

Conflicts of Interest: The authors declare no conflict of interest.

Sample Availability: Samples of the compounds are available from the authors.

References

1. Hosseinzadeh, H.; Nassiri-Asl, M. Avicenna's (Ibn Sina) the Canon of Medicine and Saffron (Crocus sativus): A review. *Phytother. Res.* **2013**, *27*, 475–483. [CrossRef] [PubMed]
2. Srivastava, R.; Ahmed, H.; Dixit, R.K. *Crocus sativus* L.: A comprehensive review. *Pharmacogn. Rev.* **2010**, *4*, 200. [CrossRef]
3. Batarseh, Y.S.; Bharate, S.S.; Kumar, V.; Kumar, A.; Vishwakarma, R.A.; Bharate, S.B.; Kaddoumi, A. *Crocus sativus* extract tightens the blood-brain barrier, reduces amyloid β load and related toxicity in 5XFAD mice. *ACS Chem. Neurosci.* **2017**, *8*, 1756–1766. [CrossRef]
4. Bharate, S.S.; Kumar, V.; Singh, G.; Singh, A.; Gupta, M.; Singh, D.; Kumar, A.; Vishwakarma, R.A.; Bharate, S.B. Preclinical development of *Crocus sativus*-based botanical lead IIIM-141 for Alzheimer's disease: Chemical standardization, efficacy, formulation development, pharmacokinetics, and safety pharmacology. *ACS Omega* **2018**, *3*, 9572–9585. [CrossRef] [PubMed]
5. GI-Geographical Indications Kashmir Saffron. Available online: http://ipindiaservices.gov.in/GIRPublic/Application/Details/635 (accessed on 17 October 2020).
6. Carmona, M.; Zalacain, A.; Sánchez, A.M.; Novella, J.L.; Alonso, G.L. Crocetin esters, picrocrocin, and its related compounds present in *Crocus sativus* stigmas and Gardenia jasminoides fruits. Tentative identification of seven new compounds by LC-ESI-MS. *J. Agric. Food Chem.* **2006**, *54*, 973–979. [CrossRef] [PubMed]
7. Moratalla-López, N.; Bagur, M.J.; Lorenzo, C.; Martínez-Navarro, M.E.; Salinas, M.R.; Alonso, G.L. Bioactivity and bioavailability of the major metabolites of *Crocus sativus* L. Flower. *Molecules* **2019**, *24*, 2827. [CrossRef]
8. Maggi, L.; Carmona, M.; Sánchez, A.M.; Alonso, G.L. Saffron flavor: Compounds involved, biogenesis, and human perception. *Funct. Plant. Biol.* **2010**, *4*, 45–55.
9. Chrysanthou, A.; Pouliou, E.; Kyriakoudi, A.; Tsimidou, M.Z. Sensory threshold studies of picrocrocin, the major bitter compound of saffron. *J. Food Sci.* **2016**, *81*, S189–S198. [CrossRef]
10. Del Campo, C.P.; Carmona, M.; Maggi, L.; Kanakis, C.D.; Anastasaki, E.G.; Tarantilis, P.A.; Polissiou, M.G.; Alonso, G.L. Picrocrocin content and quality categories in different (345) worldwide samples of Saffron (*Crocus sativus* L.). *J. Agric. Food Chem.* **2010**, *58*, 1305–1312. [CrossRef] [PubMed]
11. Alonson, G.L.; Salinas, M.R.; Sánchez-Fernández, M.A.; Garijo, J. Note. Safranal content in spanish Saffron. *Food Sci. Technol. Int.* **2001**, *7*, 225–229. [CrossRef]
12. Condurso, C.; Cincotta, F.; Tripodi, G.; Verzera, A. Bioactive volatiles in Sicilian (South Italy) saffron: Safranal and its related compounds. *J. Essent. Oil Res.* **2017**, *29*, 221–227. [CrossRef]
13. Alonso, G.L.; Salinas, M.R.; Garijo, J. Method to determine the authenticity of the aroma of Saffron (*Crocus sativus* L.). *J. Food Prot.* **1998**, *61*, 1525–1528. [CrossRef] [PubMed]
14. Carmona, M.; Zalacain, A.; Salinas, M.R.; Alonso, G.L. A new approach to saffron aroma. *Crit. Rev. Food Sci. Nutr.* **2007**, *47*, 145–159. [CrossRef] [PubMed]
15. Sánchez, A.M.; Winterhalter, P. Carotenoid cleavage products in saffron (*Crocus sativus* L.). In *Carotenoid Cleavage Products*; Winterhalter, P., Ebeler, S.E., Eds.; American Chemical Society: Washington, DC, USA, 2013; Volume 1134, pp. 45–63. [CrossRef]
16. Kanakis, C.D.; Daferera, D.J.; Tarantilis, P.A.; Polissiou, M.G. Qualitative determination of volatile compounds and quantitative evaluation of safranal and 4-hydroxy-2, 6, 6-trimethyl-1-cyclohexene-1-carboxaldehyde (HTCC) in Greek Saffron. *J. Agric. Food Chem.* **2004**, *52*, 4515–4521. [CrossRef] [PubMed]
17. García-Rodríguez, M.V.; López-Córcoles, H.; Alonso, G.L.; Pappas, C.S.; Polissiou, M.G.; Tarantilis, P.A. Comparative evaluation of an ISO 3632 method and an HPLC-DAD method for safranal quantity determination in Saffron. *Food Chem.* **2017**, *221*, 838–843. [CrossRef]

18. Hatziagapiou, K.; Kakouri, E.; Lambrou, G.I.; Bethanis, K.; Tarantilis, P.A. Antioxidant properties of *Crocus sativus* L. and its constituents and relevance to neurodegenerative diseases; focus on Alzheimer's and Parkinson's disease. *Curr. Neuropharmacol.* **2019**, *17*, 377–402. [CrossRef]
19. Singh, D. Neuropharmacological aspects of *Crocus sativus* L.: A review of preclinical studies and ongoing clinical research. *CNS Neurol. Disord. Drug Targets* **2015**, *14*, 880–902. [CrossRef]
20. Tsolaki, M.; Karathanasi, E.; Lazarou, I.; Dovas, K.; Verykouki, E.; Karakostas, A.; Georgiadis, K.; Tsolaki, A.; Adam, K.; Kompatsiaris, I.; et al. Efficacy and safety of *Crocus sativus* L. in patients with mild cognitive impairment: One year single-blind randomized, with parallel groups, clinical trial. *J. Alzheimers Dis.* **2016**, *54*, 129–133. [CrossRef]
21. Akhondzadeh, S.; Sabet, M.S.; Harirchian, M.H.; Togha, M.; Cheraghmakani, H.; Razeghi, S.; Hejazi, S.S.; Yousefi, M.H.; Alimardani, R.; Jamshidi, A.; et al. A 22-week, multicenter, randomized, double-blind controlled trial of *Crocus sativus* in the treatment of mild-to-moderate Alzheimer's disease. *Psychopharmacology* **2010**, *207*, 637–643. [CrossRef] [PubMed]
22. Srivastava, T.N.; Rajasekharan, S.; Badola, D.P.; Shah, D.C. Important medicinal plants of Jammu and Kashmir, I. Kesar (Saffron). *Anc. Sci. Life.* **1985**, *5*, 68–73.
23. Kafi, A.; Koocheki, A.; Rashed, M.H.; Nassiri, M. *Saffron (Crocus sativus): Production and Processing*; Science Publisher; CRC Press: Boca Raton, FL, USA, 2006; pp. 7–8.
24. Ballabh, B.; Chaurasia, O.P.; Ahmed, Z.; Singh, S.B. Traditional medicinal plants of cold desert Ladakh-used against kidney and urinary disorders. *J. Ethanopharmacol.* **2008**, *118*, 331–339. [CrossRef]
25. Dash, B. Saffron in Ayurveda and Tibetan medicine. *Tibet J.* **1976**, *1*, 59–66. Available online: https://jstor.org/stable/43299808 (accessed on 25 November 2020).
26. Sahni, M. Parenting in Saffron. *J. Intellect. Prop. Rights* **2002**, *7*, 530–535. Available online: http://nopr.niscair.res.in/bitstream/123456789/4937/1/JIPR%207%286%29%20530-535.pdf (accessed on 25 November 2020).
27. National Medicinal Plants Board, Ministry of AYUSH (Ayurveda, Yoga & Naturopathy, Unani, Siddha & Homoeopathy), Government of India, Indian Medicinal plants List. Available online: http://www.medicinalplants.in/ (accessed on 25 November 2020).
28. Mazumder, A.G.; Sharma, P.; Patial, V.; Singh, D. Crocin attenuates kindling development and associated cognitive impairments in mice via inhibiting reactive oxygen species-mediated NF-κB activation. *Basic Clin. Pharmacol.Toxicol.* **2017**, *120*, 426–433. [CrossRef] [PubMed]
29. Bani, S.; Pandey, A.; Agnihotri, V.K.; Pathania, V.; Singh, B. Selective Th2 upregulation by Crocus sativus: A neutraceutical spice. *Evid. Based Complement Alternat. Med.* 2011. [CrossRef]
30. Sachdeva, J.; Tanwar, V.; Golechha, M.; Siddiqui, K.M.; Nag, T.C.; Ray, R.; Kumari, S.; Arya, D.S. *Crocus sativus* L.(Saffron) attenuates isoproterenol-induced myocardial injury via preserving cardiac functions and strengthening antioxidant defense system. *Exp. Toxicol.Pathol.* **2012**, *64*, 557–564. [CrossRef] [PubMed]
31. Patel, S.; Sarwat, M.; Khan, T.H. Mechanism behind the anti-tumour potential of Saffron (*Crocus sativus* L.): The molecular perspective. *Crit. Rev. Oncol. Hematol.* **2017**, *115*, 27–35. [CrossRef]
32. Bukhari, S.I.; Pattnaik, B.; Rayees, S.; Kaul, S.; Dhar, M.K. Safranal of *Crocus sativus* L. inhibits inducible nitric oxide synthase and attenuates asthma in a mouse model of asthma. *Phytother. Res.* **2015**, *29*, 617–627. [CrossRef]
33. Premkumar, K.; Thirunavukkarasu, C.; Abraham, S.K.; Santhiya, S.T.; Ramesh, A. Protective effect of Saffron (*Crocus sativus* L.) aqueous extract against genetic damage induced by anti-tumor agents in mice. *Hum. Exp. Toxicol.* **2006**, *25*, 79–84. [CrossRef]
34. Mir, M.A.; Ganai, S.A.; Mansoor, S.; Jan, S.; Mani, P.; Masoodi, K.Z.; Amin, H.; Rehman, M.U.; Ahmad, P. Isolation, purification and characterization of naturally derived crocetin beta-d-glucosyl ester from *Crocus sativus* L. against breast cancer and its binding chemistry with ER-alpha/HDAC2. *Saudi J. Biol. Sci.* **2020**, *27*, 975–984. [CrossRef]
35. Xi, L.; Qian, Z.; Du, P.; Fu, J. Pharmacokinetic properties of crocin (crocetin digentiobiose ester) following oral administration in rats. *Phytomedicine* **2007**, *14*, 633–636. [CrossRef]
36. Christodoulou, E.; Grafakou, M.E.; Skaltsa, E.; Kadoglou, N.; Kostomitsopoulos, N.; Valsami, G. Preparation, chemical characterization, and determination of crocetin's pharmacokinetics after oral and intravenous administration of Saffron (*Crocus sativus* L.) aqueous extract to C57/BL 6J mice. *J. Pharm. Pharmacol.* **2019**, *71*, 753–764. [CrossRef] [PubMed]
37. Umigai, N.; Murakami, K.; Ulit, M.V.; Antonio, L.S.; Shirotori, M.; Morikawa, H.; Nakano, T. Thepharmacokinetic profile of crocetin in healthy adult human volunteers after a single oral administration. *Phytomedicine* **2011**, *18*, 575–578. [CrossRef]
38. Almodóvar, P.; Briskey, D.; Rao, A.; Prodanov, M.; Inarejos-García, A.M. Bioaccessibility and Pharmacokinetics of a Commercial Saffron (*Crocus sativus* L.) Extract. *Evid. Based Complementary Altern. Med.* **2020**, *2020*. [CrossRef] [PubMed]
39. Karkoula, E.; Dagla, I.V.; Baira, E.; Kokras, N.; Dalla, C.; Skaltsounis, A.L.; Gikas, E.; Tsarbopoulos, A. A novel UHPLC-HRMS based metabolomics strategy enables the discovery of potential neuroactive metabolites in mice plasma, following i.p. administration of the main *Crocus sativus* L. bioactive component. *J. Pharmaceut. Biomed.* **2020**, *177*, 112878. [CrossRef]
40. United States Food and Drug Administration (USFDA)—Department of Health and Human Services.Bioanalytical Method Validation, Guidance for Industry. 2018. Available online: https://www.fda.gov/files/drugs/published/Bioanalytical-Method-Validation-Guidance-for-Industry.pdf/ (accessed on 17 December 2019).
41. European Medicines Agency. Guideline on Bioanalytical Method Validation. 2011. Available online: www.ema.europa.eu/docs/en_GB/document_library/Scientifc_guideline/2011/08/WC500109686.pdf/ (accessed on 17 December 2019).

42. Wani, A.; Al Rihani, S.B.; Sharma, A.; Weadick, B.; Govindarajan, R.; Khan, S.U.; Sharma, S.U.; Sharma, P.R.; Dogra, A.; Nandi, U.; et al. Crocetin promotes clearance of amyloid-β by inducing autophagy via the STK11/LKB1-mediated AMPK pathway. *Autophagy* **2021**, 1–20. [CrossRef]
43. Van Calsteren, M.R.; Bissonnette, M.C.; Cormier, F.; Dufresne, C.; Ichi, T.; LeBlanc, J.Y.; Perreault, D.; Roewer, I. Spectroscopic characterization of crocetin derivatives from *Crocus sativus* and Gardenia jasminoides. *J. Agric. Food Chem.* **1997**, *45*, 1055–1061. [CrossRef]
44. Ekor, M. The growing use of herbal medicines: Issues relating to adverse reactions and challenges in monitoring safety. *Front Phamacol.* **2014**, *4*, 177. [CrossRef] [PubMed]
45. Liu, T.Z.; Qian, Z.Y. Pharmacokinetics of crocetin in rats. *Yao XueXue Bao* **2002**, *37*, 367–369.
46. Jafarisani, M.; Bathaie, S.Z.; Mousavi, M.F. Saffron carotenoids (crocin and crocetin) binding to human serum albumin as investigated by different spectroscopic methods and molecular docking. *J. Biomol. Struct. Dyn.* **2018**, *36*, 1681–1690. [CrossRef]
47. Lautenschlager, M.; Sendker, J.; Huwel, S.; Galla, H.; Brandt, S.; Dufer, M. Intestinal formation of *trans*-crocetin from saffron extract (*Crocus sativus* L.) and in vitro permeation through intestinal and blood-brain barrier. *Phytomedicine* **2015**, *22*, 36–44. [CrossRef] [PubMed]
48. Reddy, C.N.; Bharate, S.B.; Vishwakarma, R.A.; Bharate, S.S. Chemical analysis of Saffron by HPLC based crocetin estimation. *J. Pharm. Biomed. Anal.* **2020**, *181*, 113094. [CrossRef] [PubMed]
49. Chen, Y.; Zhang, H.; Tian, X.; Zhao, C.; Cai, L.; Liu, Y.; Jia, L.; Yin, H.X.; Chen, C. Antioxidant potential of crocins and ethanol extracts of Gardenia jasminoides ELLIS and *Crocus sativus* L. A relationship investigation between antioxidant activity and crocin contents. *Food Chem.* **2008**, *109*, 484–492. [CrossRef]
50. Tong, Y.; Yan, Y.; Zhu, X.; Liu, R.; Gong, F.; Zhang, L.; Wang, P. Simultaneous quantification of crocetin esters and picrocrocin changes in Chinese Saffron by high-performance liquid chromatography-diode array detector during 15 years of storage. *Pharmacogn. Mag.* **2015**, *11*, 540–545. [CrossRef]
51. D'Archivio, A.A.; Di Donato, F.; Foschi, M.; Maggi, M.A.; Ruggieri, F. UHPLC analysis of Saffron (*Crocus sativus* L.): Optimization of separation using chemometrics and detection of minor crocetin esters. *Molecules* **2018**, *23*, 1851. [CrossRef] [PubMed]
52. Samarghandian, S.; Azimi-Nezhad, M.; Farkhondeh, T. Immunomodulatory and antioxidant effects of saffron aqueous extract (*Crocus sativus* L.) on streptozotocin-induced diabetes in rats. *Indian Heart J.* **2017**, *69*, 151–159. [CrossRef]
53. Brown, P.N.; Chan, M.; Betz, J.M.; Shahid, M.; Cannon, S.; Palissery, J.; Puglisi, M.P. Regulation of nutraceuticals in Canada and the United States. In *Nutraceuticals and Human Health: The Food-to-Supplement Paradigm*; Spagnuolo, P.A., Ed.; Royal Society of Chemistry: Piccadilly, London, UK, 2020; pp. 7–26.
54. Tripathi, C.; Girme, A.; Champaneri, S.; Patel, R.J.; Hingorani, L. Nutraceutical regulations: An opportunity in ASEAN countries. *Nutrition* **2020**, *74*, 110729. [CrossRef] [PubMed]

MDPI
St. Alban-Anlage 66
4052 Basel
Switzerland
Tel. +41 61 683 77 34
Fax +41 61 302 89 18
www.mdpi.com

Molecules Editorial Office
E-mail: molecules@mdpi.com
www.mdpi.com/journal/molecules

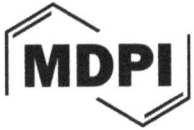

www.ingramcontent.com/pod-product-compliance
Lightning Source LLC
LaVergne TN
LVHW070707100526
838202LV00013B/1045